Acute Medicine in the Frail Elderly

HENRY WOODFORD

BSc, FRCP
Consultant in Elderly Medicine
North Tyneside Hospital, North Shields

and

JAMES GEORGE

MBChB, MMEd, FRCP
Consultant in Medicine for the Elderly
Cumberland Infirmary, Carlisle

Foreword by

PROFESSOR DAVID OLIVER

National Clinical Director for Older Peoples Services (England)
Consultant Geriatrician, Royal Berkshire NHS Foundation Trust

Radcliffe Publishing
London • New York

Radcliffe Publishing Ltd
33–41 Dallington Street
London
EC1V 0BB
United Kingdom

www.radcliffehealth.com

British Library Cataloguing in Publication Data

A catalogue record for this book is available from the British Library.

ISBN-13: 978 190891 158 2

The paper used for the text pages of this book
is FSC® certified. FSC (The Forest Stewardship
Council®) is an international network to promote
responsible management of the world's forests.

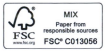

MIX
Paper from
responsible sources
FSC® C013056

Typeset by Darkriver Design, Auckland, New Zealand
Printed and bound by TJI Digital, Padstow, Cornwall

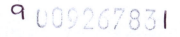

Contents

Foreword

When the NHS was founded in 1948, nearly half the population died before they reached 65 – many from infectious diseases, cancers, heart disease or stroke, and life expectancy was only 65 for men and 70 for women. Now, in 2013, only 18% of the population in England die before they reach 65 and this figure has been constant for the past two decades, so that the fastest growing demographic is the 'oldest old' – those over 85.

There are already over 8 million over-65s in England and life expectancy at 70 is now 17 years for men and 19 years for women. In many ways, this is a cause for celebration. Population ageing is a victory for increasing societal wealth, better housing, nutrition, workplace and environmental safety and preventative public health. It also represents an opportunity for most of us to live a long and flourishing life. And of course it is also partly the consequence of modern medicine. Death rates from those common killers have all fallen dramatically since the Second World War – partly due to lifestyle factors, partly better management of chronic conditions in primary care and partly due to more effective interventions when people do present in crisis. Although most older people report high levels of happiness and satisfaction with their own health, the inevitable downside is that after 75 most people live with three or more long-term conditions. These include common and often neglected conditions of ageing such as dementia, poor mobility, bone fragility, incontinence or frailty, and although most older people are not disabled, most people with disabilities such as impaired vision, hearing, mobility or cognition are older. It is these patients who are most likely to be dependent on formal or informal care and to rely on a range of health and social care services. And these who are most likely to benefit from comprehensive geriatric assessment, from multidisciplinary care, from targeted rehabilitation and discharge planning and from the skills of geriatric medicine – in particular acknowledging that misleadingly called 'functional' or 'social' problems are often fully or partially reversible if a diagnosis is sought and a treatment plan formulated.

Sadly, we know from a series of recent reports on the care of older people in hospital in the NHS and on age discrimination in health services that older people do not always receive the standard of assessment and treatment that they and their families should expect, or that younger patients are more likely to receive. There is constant talk of keeping older people away from hospitals which are labelled as 'the wrong environment for them'. In reality, patients over 65 already account for around 60% of admissions and 70% of bed days in NHS hospitals. Many of these have multiple long-term conditions, frailty, disability or social vulnerability and acute illness precipitating a crisis and with hospital admission rates and emergency readmission rates still rising, we need to catch up with the reality that older people in acute hospitals are here to stay and are where the biggest activity, the biggest spend and biggest care gaps and variation lie. Twenty-first century hospitals are still too often designed as if they were still caring for younger patients with 'single organ' disease and are still not adequately geared around the needs of the patients who actually use them. Medical under-graduate and post-graduate training is still skewed excessively to 'single disease' thinking and needs to be rebalanced to reflect the reality of modern medical practice.

Geriatricians and the multidisciplinary teams who work with such older patients would pride themselves on having the right skills and knowledge to deliver good care to older inpatients. However, we can never look after every older person as they are to be found throughout all adult ward areas and in the emergency department. And it is vital that all clinicians have some good basic skills and knowledge in assessment of older patients, in rehabilitation and discharge planning, in dealing with common geriatric problems such as falls, dementia, delirium, poor mobility and incontinence as well as presentations common in older age such as stroke and cardiac failure. These skills are also required in surgery and anaesthetics. We need only look at the typical hip frac-ture patient to see this – median age of 84, high mortality and morbidity and high incidence of dementia, delirium, falls and bone fragility.

What this excellent new book adds to the field is a very clear focus on the emergency care of older patients. It can be an excellent resource for specialists in other fields wanting to improve their own skills and knowledge when caring for older patients with complex needs. I also believe it will be of great use to nurses and allied health professionals, to trainees in geriatric medicine and to consultants. Despite being an experienced geriatrician, I certainly learned a lot from reading the chapters and will be calling on the book for my own teaching, writing and clinical practice, and will be pointing my trainees to it.

This book covers everything from key facts about population ageing and health, to assessment and investigation of older patients, to the common 'geri-atric giants' of falls, immobility, confusion and incontinence and on to more specialised chapters around, for instance, stroke medicine or assessment of older surgical patients.

This will be an excellent resource for clinical practice – it has really added to the field and is highly readable and informative. I for one will be recommending it to colleagues.

Professor David Oliver
National Clinical Director for Older Peoples Services (England)
Consultant Geriatrician, Royal Berkshire NHS Foundation Trust
Visiting Professor of Medicine for Older People, City University, London
Clinical Expert Advisor, NHS Emergency Care Intensive Support Team
Visiting Senior Fellow, The King's Fund
January 2013

Preface

Frail older people now contribute the majority of the acute emergency take both medical and surgical. Despite this, there is often a lack of confidence and knowledge among doctors and nurses in treating older people in the emergency department and on emergency assessment units. Emergency care of frail older people is often seen as less glamorous and less rewarding than other branches of medicine. The philosophy of this book is precisely the opposite – emergency care of frail older people is seen as both challenging and very rewarding. The authors have many years' combined experience of working at the front door of the hospital, assessing and treating older patients. This book encapsulates their experience and also their enthusiasm. Older people tend to be more complex and therefore their assessment needs to be more extensive and to include comprehensive geriatric assessment. It is the 'extras' in their assessment that are not usually needed in younger patients, such as cognitive, functional and social evaluations that make the difference in achieving a better outcome. As regards treatment, older people are at a disadvantage in that the evidence base for successful intervention is sometimes harder to find – this book is extensively referenced for this reason, so that the reader can check for him- or herself. The aim of the book is to provide doctors, nurses and therapists with both the background and essential information to provide the excellent acute care that older people now deserve. In order to keep the text accessible, we have focused on the more common and serious acute presentations and diagnoses.

Henry Woodford
James George
January 2013

About the authors

Henry Woodford was born in York and went to school in Yorkshire. He then went to medical school at King's College London. During this time he undertook an intercalated degree incorporating physiology. His elective period was spent in British Columbia, Canada. He did his house jobs in the south-east of England but then moved to the north-east for further training. He did his specialist registrar rotation based around Newcastle upon Tyne. One year was taken out of the programme to work at Westmead Hospital in Sydney, Australia. He worked as a consultant geriatrician in Carlisle from 2006 until 2012, when he moved to take up a post in North Tyneside, UK. He is married and has two daughters.

James George was born in Derbyshire and qualified in Liverpool. After early training in Liverpool, Leeds and Bradford he was appointed as a Consultant in 1986 in Carlisle. He is the Clinical Lead for Research for North Cumbria University Hospitals NHS Trust. He was a member of the National Institute for Health and Clinical Excellence (NICE) Clinical Guideline Group for the 2010 NICE guidelines on delirium. He is married and has one daughter, who is an occupational therapist.

List of abbreviations

AAA	abdominal aortic aneurysm
ACE	angiotensin-converting enzyme
ACS	acute coronary syndrome
ADH	antidiuretic hormone
ADL	activities of daily living
ADR	adverse drug reaction
AF	atrial fibrillation
AKI	acute kidney injury
AMT	Abbreviated Mental Test
AMT4	four-question Abbreviated Mental Test
anti-CCP	anti-cyclic citrullinated peptide
ASB	asymptomatic bacteriuria
BMI	body mass index
BP	blood pressure
BPPV	benign paroxysmal position vertigo
CAM	Confusion Assessment Method
CAP	community-acquired pneumonia
CDI	*Clostridium difficile* infection
CDT	Clock Drawing Test
CGA	comprehensive geriatric assessment
CI	confidence interval
COMT	catechol-O-methyltransferase
COPD	chronic obstructive pulmonary disease
CPR	cardiopulmonary resuscitation
CRP	C-reactive protein
CSF	cerebrospinal fluid
CT	computed tomography
DI	diabetes insipidus
DKA	diabetic ketoacidosis
ECG	electrocardiogram
ED	emergency department

EEG	electroencephalography
ESR	erythrocyte sedimentation rate
FI	faecal incontinence
GCS	Glasgow Coma Scale
GDS	Geriatric Depression Scale
GDS-15	15-question Geriatric Depression Scale
GFR	glomerular filtration rate
GI	gastrointestinal
GP	general practitioner
HHS	hyperosmolar hyperglycaemic state
HSV	herpes simplex virus
ICH	intracerebral haemorrhage
IE	infective endocarditis
IF	iliac fossa
ITU	intensive therapy unit
iv	intravenous
LFT	liver function test
LP	lumbar puncture
MAOIs	monoamine oxidase inhibitors
MI	myocardial infarction
MMSE	Mini-Mental State Examination
MNA	Mini Nutritional Assessment
MNA-SF	Mini Nutritional Assessment Short Form
MoCA	Montreal Cognitive Assessment
MRI	magnetic resonance imaging
MRSA	methicillin-resistant *Staphylococcus aureus*
MUST	Malnutrition Universal Screening Tool
NH	nursing home
NHAP	nursing home-acquired pneumonia
NMDA	N-methyl-D-aspartate
NMLS	neuroleptic malignant-like syndrome
NSAID	non-steroidal anti-inflammatory drug
OH	orthostatic hypotension
OT	occupational therapist
PCR	polymerase chain reaction
PD	Parkinson's disease
PPI	proton pump inhibitor
PTH	parathyroid hormone
PU	pressure ulcer

QCS	Quick Confusion Scale
RH	residential care home
SAH	subarachnoid haemorrhage
SDH	subdural haematoma
SIADH	syndrome of inappropriate antidiuretic hormone
SIS	Six-Item Screener
SSRI	selective serotonin reuptake inhibitor
TB	tuberculosis
TIA	transient ischaemic attack
TTH	tension-type headache
UI	urinary incontinence
UK	United Kingdom
UQ	upper quadrant
UTI	urinary tract infection
VDRL	venereal disease research laboratory test
VF	ventricular fibrillation
VSV	varicella zoster virus
VT	ventricular tachycardia
WCC	white cell count
ZN	Ziehl–Neelsen

CHAPTER 1

Introduction

Ageing is the process by which we accumulate cellular damage over time, and this leads to a generalised decline in function, an increased susceptibility to disease and a higher probability of death. It is a complex, multifactorial process and there is much inter-individual variation in the manner and timing of its presentation (seen as differences in 'biological' and 'chronological' age). It is determined by both internal (i.e. genetics) and external factors (e.g. smoking, diet and sunlight exposure). Ageing is related to reactive oxygen species (or 'free radical') production mainly in the mitochondria, which causes damage to cellular structures, such as DNA and proteins (including enzymes).[1] We have an imperfect ability to repair our somatic cells' DNA, resulting in the accumulation of defects. The 'disposable soma' theory of ageing explains this as a balance between energy used in repair against that used for reproduction. Wild animals die of predation, starvation and accidents before they have time to age. Therefore, historically, it made more sense to invest resources in producing offspring rather than in maintaining the perfect repair of a doomed body. The ability to live to old age should be celebrated as one of humanity's achievements, but in the field of healthcare it has created new challenges.

WHAT IS OLD AGE?

Traditionally, the age of 60 or 65 years has been used to define an older person, which coincided with the typical age of retirement from work. However, over recent years, life expectancy in the developed world has been steadily increasing (*see* Figure 1.1), and current life expectancy at birth in the UK is around 78 years for men and 82 years for women. The proportion of the population made up of older people is also increasing (*see* Figure 1.2). Coupled with this has been a reduction in age-related disability levels – that is, our disease-free lifespan has also increased. At the present time, the majority of people aged in their 60s are physiologically very similar to younger adults. The distinction that doctors wish to make is to describe those patients who are physiologically different and require a different approach to that of younger adults. If we were to adopt an age cut-off to achieve this, most of the time it would probably be somewhere over 75 years. The elderly are sometimes classified as the 'young old' (60/65–74 years), 'old old' (75–84 years) and the 'oldest old' (85+ years).

Given the wide variation in the ageing process seen between individuals, age alone is usually insufficient to identify those who need a specialised 'elderly care' approach. Other criteria that have been adopted in hospital settings include residing in a care home or presenting with either an acute or chronic geriatric syndrome (confusion, falls, immobility or incontinence).[2] Some diagnoses are seen much more frequently in older adults (e.g. dementia) and are usually best cared for by someone experienced in looking after the old. In reality, we use a combination of age, functional status, method of presentation and co-morbidities to define those patients who are best managed under the banner of elderly medicine. The unifying factor is that these patients are considered frail (hence the title for this book). We will discuss frailty later in this chapter. First, let's outline the physiological changes that accompany ageing.

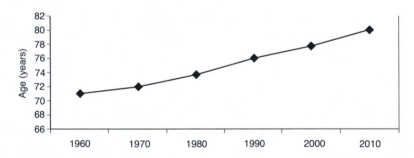

FIGURE 1.1 Life expectancy at birth in the UK (men and women combined average)

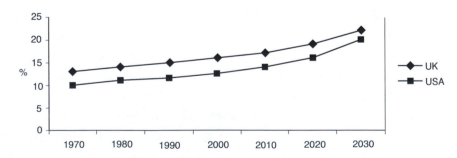

FIGURE 1.2 The changing proportion of population aged 65 and over in the UK and USA with estimates for future change

CHANGES IN PHYSIOLOGY

Ageing is associated with impairments in physiological systems within the body. These are usually compensated for in non-stressful situations, but increased bodily demands imposed by acute illness are more likely to precipitate organ system failure. A summary of the key changes is given in Table 1.1.

TABLE 1.1 A summary of key physiological changes seen in the frail elderly

Bodily system	Change
General composition	↑ Fat
	↓ Muscle, bone mass and intracellular water
Cardiovascular	↑ Systolic blood pressure and risk of arrhythmia
	↓ Cardiac diastolic relaxation, peak heart rate and maximal cardiac output
Respiratory	↑ Residual volume
	↓ Chest wall mobility, respiratory muscle strength and diffusion capacity
Renal	↑ Risk of dehydration and nephrotoxicity from drugs
	↓ Glomerular filtration rate and number of glomeruli
Neurological	↑ White matter lesions, prevalence of hearing and visual impairment
	↓ Brain volume
Gastrointestinal	↑ Colonic transit time, gall stones and bowel diverticula
	↓ Dentition, saliva, sense of taste/smell and liver mass
Immunological	↑ Autoantibodies
	↓ Specific antibody production and number of T-cells

Bodily composition

As we age, our bodily composition changes, with an increased proportion of fat and less water. Comparing young adults with those in their 80s, body fat increases between 18%–36% for men and 33%–44% for women.[3] Fat also tends to be more centrally distributed. This raises the risk of type 2 diabetes and hypertension. Bodily water content falls by around 14% in the elderly compared with young adults, and the reduction mainly affects intracellular fluid.[4] There is a gradual reduction in bone mass after the third decade. Older people are at risk of developing osteoporosis. In addition, vitamin D is predominantly formed by the action of sunlight on our skin, and so those who do not go outdoors as often (e.g. the immobile elderly) are at an increased risk of osteomalacia.

Sarcopenia is a term for the reduction in muscle mass, with evidence of reduced muscle strength or reduced physical functioning, that occurs in older age.[5] It is likely to be multifactorial in its aetiology, including motor neuron loss, endocrine changes (e.g. sex and growth hormones), nutritional changes, and atrophy secondary to immobility. It is distinct from cachexia (a catabolic state induced by disease). Unfortunately, there is currently no universally accepted method of defining sarcopenia. On average, muscle strength in those aged 60–80 years is 20%–40% lower than that seen in young adults, and it is 50% lower in those aged over 80.[6] The observed loss of muscle strength is greater than can be explained by loss of muscle mass alone, suggesting a concomitant reduction in muscle quality.[7] However, it is not an irreversible process and high-resistance weight training can lead to significant increases in muscle strength and size even in those aged in their 90s.[8]

Basal metabolic rate declines because of the reduction in muscle mass. Total energy needs typically fall further because of lower activity levels (e.g. secondary to osteoarthritis). The combined result is a drop in overall energy requirements by approximately 30% from age 30 to age 90. This means less food is necessary to meet energy demands, but protein and micronutrient needs remain similar, which requires a diet relatively high in protein and micronutrients to maintain optimal health. Body weight tends to peak around the age of 60 and gradually decline afterwards. The recommended daily intake for water is around 30 mL/kg/day, and for fibre it is around 30 g/day. Failure to achieve these targets increases the risk of constipation.

Cardiovascular

Ageing is associated with a reduction in elastin content and an increase in collagen and calcium deposition within the arterial walls and myocardium.[9] The resulting increased stiffness of the blood vessels raises vascular resistance and leads to systolic hypertension and an increased pulse wave velocity.[10] The vascular endothelium typically becomes less responsive to vasoactive substances such as nitric oxide and endothelin-1. There is also reduced baroreflex sensitivity, which may lead to a labile blood pressure.[11] Protein glycation may further increase vessel stiffness, especially in people with diabetes. Amyloid deposition in the walls of cerebral vessels increases the risk of intracerebral haemorrhage.

Stiffness of the heart leads to reduced diastolic relaxation and an increased risk of diastolic heart failure.[12] The ejection fraction is preserved in normal ageing. Vascular resistance causes the left ventricular wall to become thickened and the left atrium enlarged.[9] Dilatation of the left atrium increases the likelihood of developing atrial fibrillation. There is a reduction in the number of myocytes (by around 35%) but with hypertrophy of the remainder.[10] Fibrosis of the conducting system results in higher rates of arrhythmias and bundle branch block.[13] Common ECG changes in the old include prolongation of the PR interval, QRS and QT durations, left axis deviation, and an increased incidence of ectopic beats. Heart valves acquire degenerative changes and become calcified. The prevalences of coronary artery disease and valvular heart disease increase with age.

There is little change in resting cardiovascular status, but a reduction in maximal capacity (i.e. heart rate and cardiac output) results in compromise in situations of stress.[10] The ageing heart appears less responsive to beta-adrenergic stimulation, possibly secondary to reduced receptor function. Peak heart rate can be quickly, but inaccurately, estimated by the formula 220 – age. The lower maximal heart rate makes the old more reliant on increasing stroke volume, which is dependent on preload, to raise cardiac output.

Respiratory

As we age the thoracic cage becomes less mobile and the lungs less elastic. The reduced chest wall compliance may be made worse by osteoporotic fractures and the resultant kyphosis. Respiratory muscle strength is diminished in the frail. The decline in lung elasticity leads to uneven alveolar ventilation, causing air trapping and ventilation–perfusion mismatch. Total lung capacity remains the same, but there is an increase in residual volume resulting in a decline in vital capacity. Forced expiratory volume in 1 second and forced vital capacity are both reduced. A fall in diffusion capacity and ventilation–perfusion mismatch lead to a reduced partial pressure of oxygen, but partial pressure of carbon dioxide is unchanged. Ventilatory responses to hypoxia and hypercapnia are diminished because of reduced chemoreceptor function. The net effect is an increased risk of hypoxia in stress situations. There may also be a reduction in cough ability to clear secretions.

Renal

Ageing is associated with a progressive decline in renal function, although the severity of this varies between individuals, with some having only minimal decline over time. On average, glomerular filtration rate (GFR) declines by around 10% per decade from the fourth decade onwards, or around $0.8 \, mL/min/1.73 \, m^2$ per year.[14] Some of this change may be partly due to the higher prevalence of co-morbidities in older age (e.g. hypertension). Those with diabetes or chronic renal impairment (GFR $<30 \, mL/min/1.73 \, m^2$) decline at a faster rate.[15] Renal mass peaks in the fourth decade of life and then progressively declines and is reduced by about 25% by age 90.[14] Most of the loss is from the cortex, not the medulla. There is a reduction in renal blood flow at a rate of around 10% per decade from the fourth decade onwards (from 600 mL/min down to around 300 mL/min); this is associated with an increase in renal arterial resistance. The basement membrane becomes thickened, there is focal cortical glomerulosclerosis, tubular atrophy and interstitial fibrosis. The number of glomeruli reduces by around 40% by age 70.[14] A decline in muscle mass (sarcopenia) means that serum creatinine concentration may change little despite the decline in function, which makes it harder to estimate GFR.

The decreased renal reserve and concentrating ability lead to a reduced ability to conserve sodium and excrete hydrogen ions, which makes it harder to compensate for fluid or electrolyte imbalances. There is an increased risk of nephrotoxicity from drugs or radiocontrast agents. There is reduced activity of the renin–angiotensin system and organ responsiveness to antidiuretic hormone. This coupled with reduced thirst perception increases the risk of dehydration in the elderly. Proteinuria is not a feature of normal ageing. Bladder collagen levels become increased resulting in reduced distensibility and impaired emptying.

Neurological

With advancing age there is a tendency to develop a degree of cerebral atrophy. MRI studies have demonstrated enlargement of the lateral ventricles and widening of the sulci of those without disease.[16] This is mainly because of the loss of supporting architecture rather than loss of neurons. However, these changes are more pronounced in those with dementia, hypertension or high alcohol intake. Post-mortem examinations of the brains of older adults who did not have dementia have detected neurofibrillary tangles and beta-amyloid plaques in around 40%–50% of cases.[17] Cerebral white matter lesions (or leukoaraiosis) are commonly seen on brain images. In a sample of 822 randomly selected people over the age of 65 (mean age, 73 years), 66% had either focal (17%) or diffuse (49%) white matter lesions on MRI.[18] They should not be considered a benign change, as they occur more commonly in those with vascular disease and are associated with an increased risk of falls, functional decline and cognitive impairment.[18–20]

Hearing loss is common. A study of patients aged 75 and over found that 42% reported some hearing impairment, with 8% reporting severe impairment.[21] Twenty-six per cent failed a hearing test. Following removal of earwax, when present, the number failing the test fell to 23%. Over half of the patients who failed the test did not own a hearing aid, and of those who did only 60% used it regularly. Presbycusis is a term for age-related hearing loss. This is typically a bilateral deficit most affecting ability to hear high frequency sounds. Visual impairments are also common. Presbyopia is a term for age-related reduction in ability to focus on near objects; it is caused by reduced lens flexibility. In addition, there are higher prevalences for many ocular conditions, including cataracts and age-related macular degeneration.

Cognitive changes with normal ageing are likely to be minor. Studies have found that 30% of people over the age of 70 showed no decline in cognition over an 8-year period, and that the average decline in those in good health is likely to be <0.1 points on the Mini-Mental State Examination (out of 30 points) per year.[22,23]

Gastrointestinal

Through our adult lives we have progressive tooth decay and subsequent poor dentition. There may be a reduction in saliva due to an age-related decline in production, higher prevalence of co-morbidities associated with the sicca syndrome (e.g. rheumatoid arthritis), or medication effects (e.g. anticholinergics). This can impair normal swallowing. Sense of taste and smell typically decline, which can reduce the pleasurable sensation of eating.

Oesophageal motility declines. Upper and lower oesophageal sphincter pressures are reduced. Gastric acid secretion may be reduced secondary to medications or atrophic gastritis. Atrophic gastritis can develop because of either autoimmune disease or chronic *Helicobacter pylori* infection. This can impair the absorption of vitamin B_{12}. There is less secretion of prostaglandins that protect the gastric wall. Hepatic mass and blood flow decrease by 30%–40% by age 80 compared with young adults.[24,25] Liver enzymes are unchanged in healthy elders. Gallstones are more prevalent in older age. Colonic transit time is increased, which may predispose to constipation. Diverticuli become more prevalent because of reduced colonic wall tensile strength and increased evacuation pressure (e.g. secondary to constipation). Bacterial overgrowth becomes more prevalent and can increase the risk of malnutrition.

Immune system

Although B cell numbers are relatively preserved in older age, there is reduced specific antibody production and a higher prevalence of monoclonal gammopathies and autoantibodies. For example, older adults are more likely to have a positive rheumatoid factor without clinical evidence of disease than younger adults. T-cell numbers are reduced, resulting in reduced reactivity to antigens and impaired immunological memory. This increases susceptibility to infection and reduces the efficacy of vaccines. Other factors that increase the risk of infection in older adults include a higher prevalence of co-morbidities (e.g. chronic obstructive pulmonary disease (COPD) and diabetes), frailty, malnutrition, and poor-quality housing. The febrile response to sepsis is absent or diminished in 20%–30% of elderly patients with underlying serious infection.[26] This is most likely to be due to a reduced immunological reaction to pathogens.

- Both life expectancy and the proportion of population classified as old have been steadily increasing over recent decades.
- Through ageing we accumulate cellular damage that causes a decline in function; this leads to some impairment in every bodily system.
- The accumulated impairments may not be obvious in most situations but do become apparent at times of physiological stress, such as acute illness.
- There is also a change in bodily composition with a lower proportion of water, muscle and bone, and an increased proportion of fat.
- However, ageing is not a uniform process – it has differing effects on individual people. Age alone is a poor determinant of physical function.

FRAILTY

What is frailty?

Frailty is an expression for the observed loss of physiological reserve seen in association with the ageing process. It results in a reduction in homeostatic mechanisms leaving the individual more susceptible to the effects of disease. As diseases themselves can lead to further functional decline, the effect can be a progressive cycle of deterioration (*see* Figure 1.3).

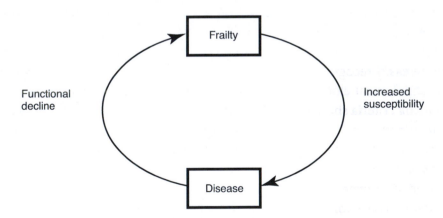

FIGURE 1.3 The relationship between frailty and disease

Frailty is seen as a combination of sarcopenia, functional impairment, neuroendocrine dysregulation and reduced immunity. It is typically associated with weight loss but can occur in overweight patients. Unfortunately, no standardised definition exists.[27] Some argue that it is purely a physical function disorder, but others feel it should also relate to cognitive and social factors. It has been described as a 'phenotype' including five measurable items, with frailty said to be present if three or more of the criteria are met.[28]

1. Exhaustion or low energy level (self-reported)
2. Weight loss
3. Weak grip strength (measured by a dynamometer)
4. Slow walking
5. Reduced activity levels.

Gait speed may be the most reliable of these items, with speeds below 1 m/s suggestive of frailty.[29] The Study of Osteoporotic Fractures index is a three-item system for rapidly identifying frailty: weight loss of 5% or more, inability to rise five times from a chair without using arms, and answering 'no' to the question 'do you feel full of energy?' It may be as accurate as longer scales in detecting frailty.[30] Others have suggested a 'frailty index' calculated by summing the number of physical disorders of an individual.[31] The Edmonton Frail Scale is another assessment tool based on a series of questions and brief assessments that takes less than 5 minutes to administer.[32] However, the various definitions proposed identify different patients.[33] This makes it hard to accurately quantify the prevalence of frailty until consensus on the best detection method is reached.

While precise definitions are useful in clinical research, it is impractical to systematically test them on all of our patients. In addition, assessing weight loss requires a prior measurement to compare to that is likely to not be available at the time of acute illness, and illness itself may result in feelings of exhaustion or reduced activity. In clinical practice, frailty (sometimes likened to beauty) may be easily recognised even if hard to accurately define. As a simple guide we recommend that elderly patients requiring hospitalisation who fulfil any of the following criteria should be considered frail:

➤ requirement of mobility aids or immobile
➤ needing assistance with activities of daily living
➤ residing in a care home
➤ aged 85 or over
➤ diagnosis of dementia
➤ presentation with falls, confusion or 'off legs'.

Why is it important?

It is important to recognise the frail in clinical medicine, as these patients require a different approach to assessment and treatment, as we will outline throughout this book. They typically have multiple medical and social problems, and are prone to the effects of common stressors. They are likely to present in atypical or non-specific ways (e.g. falls, confusion and 'off legs'). They usually take multiple medications and are at a higher risk of side effects and adverse reactions. It is especially important that we balance the potential benefits of any treatment against the risk of causing harm. They often require the support of others to exist in the community, which makes discharges harder to arrange. They are more likely to develop complications in hospital and are less likely to survive acute illnesses.

OLDER PEOPLE IN ACUTE HOSPITALS

As the population ages, older people are making up a larger proportion of emergency department (ED) patients, with the largest percentage rises seen in those aged over 70 years.[34] These patients often present with poorly classified complaints.[35] They are likely to have multiple concurrent problems, making them not fit into traditional disease-oriented models of care, and they may fall between hyper-specialist services. This is a problem with the healthcare system, not the patient. Given longer average lengths of stay, older patients occupy a large proportion of emergency beds. In the UK it is estimated that 60%–70% of acute hospital beds are used by people aged over 65, and 25% of bed days used by those aged over 85.[34,36,37]

Emergency physicians have reported finding the management of older patients more difficult and time-consuming than of the same presentations in younger individuals.[38] They tend to be less confident in dealing with older adults than with younger adults and they overestimate the proportion of older patients that they treat in the ED, suggesting a perception of burden.[39] It is widely recognised that improved ED staff training in geriatric emergency medicine would be beneficial.[38-42] Key competencies for older patients that should be achieved by those training in emergency medicine have been defined.[43]

Why do geriatrics?

The nature of geriatrics does not appeal to all physicians. It can seem less 'heroic'. We more often deal with non-curable conditions and rely on other healthcare professions in a multidisciplinary team (e.g. nursing, physiotherapy and occupational therapy). However, just because we cannot cure a condition it does not mean we cannot lessen the effects of disease. After all, medicine does not cure many serious conditions and we all ultimately die, so is it all futile? We think not.

Unfortunately, geriatrics is currently an unpopular career choice with many medical students and junior doctors. Some will not see past the lack of private practice income. Currently only small amounts of time for junior doctors are dedicated to education in geriatric medicine.[44-46] However, everyone who works in adult hospital specialties can expect to spend an increasing amount of time caring for elderly patients in the future. We hope to be able to show you that caring for older people is every bit as worthwhile and rewarding as caring for younger adults when you know what to look for and how to react when problems are found. But perhaps you already know that – you did pick up this book.

Providing high-quality care

The quality of care for older people should be just as high as that of younger people. Yet there is evidence from primary care that the quality of assessment and treatment of geriatric conditions (falls, dementia and urinary incontinence) is less than that observed for other general medical conditions.[47] A recent Health Service Ombudsman report of care for elderly patients in English hospitals highlights examples of suboptimal care.[48] Recurrent themes are poor communication, lack of basic care (e.g. nutrition and hygiene) and lack of compassion. Unfortunately, there is some evidence of a decline in doctors' empathy during clinical training.[49] Lack of empathy and compassion coupled with the common atypical presentations of older people can lead to under-recognition of acute illness and this can have grave consequences.[50]

Qualitative studies of the care of older people in hospital have suggested that high-quality care includes good communication with patients and their families, maintenance of the individual's personal identity and involvement in decision-making.[51] Older people are typically appreciative of the care they receive. Areas that often could be improved include giving patients the opportunity to explain their condition (which may include several problems), giving appropriate information about diagnosis and treatment rationale, acknowledgement of long waiting times, addressing sensory deficits (e.g. using glasses or hearing aids), avoiding depersonalising or stigmatising comments, ensuring comfort, privacy and dignity are maintained, and respecting patients' opinions.[52] A positive approach toward the care of older people should be present throughout the hospital, from boardroom to ward, with appropriate training provided where needed.[53]

Multidisciplinary input is essential (*see* p. 22). The overall aims are to promote self-care, mobility, continence and optimal nutrition. Non-pharmacological approaches to challenging behaviour should be adopted wherever possible (*see* p. 118). Urinary catheterisation should only be performed when necessary and removed as soon as feasible (*see* p. 90). Physical restraints should not be used. It can seem daunting to be faced with patients with multiple problems. Sometimes it is better not to try to tackle everything at once, but to prioritise the key problems for initial intervention.

The medical handover has been identified as a 'high risk' step in patient care pathways.[54,55] Arrangements for frail older patients are important because of their multiple co-morbidities and increased vulnerability. This is particularly so in acute hospitals where older patients are often transferred from ED to medical assessments units and then to specialist wards. Information may become lost, reducing the safety and quality of care. Handovers can be verbal, written or, preferably, in both formats. A useful approach to handovers is the SBAR tool (**S**ituation, **B**ackground, **A**ssessment and **R**ecommendation) – *see* Table 1.2.[56] This can be used for transfers between hospital wards, escalations of care or for discharge into the community.

TABLE 1.2 An example of the use of the SBAR tool for a medical handover in hospital

Situation	'AB' is an 80-year-old man admitted with a fall, but no apparent injury. He is unsteady on his feet, unsafe mobilising and has lost his confidence.
Background	He lives alone, does not remember the details of his fall and may have lost consciousness. He is receiving treatment for hypertension.
Assessment	The fall is likely to be due to postural hypotension, as a 30 mmHg drop in his systolic blood pressure has been recorded, which was associated with feeling light-headed.
Recommendation	We need to monitor his blood pressure, both lying and standing. His medication needs to be clarified with his general practitioner, and we will probably need to reduce any antihypertensive drugs. He will need to be reviewed by the physiotherapy and occupational therapy teams. It is recommended that he be referred to the falls service following discharge.

Ward environment

The typical ED environment is not optimised for the specific needs of older people. The layout is primarily designed to aid rapid diagnosis and throughput. EDs are usually noisy and full of people rushing about. The beds are narrow trolleys with only limited cushioning, making them unsuitable to minimise the risk of pressure ulcers. Overhead fluorescent lights and lack of windows can be disorienting to time of day. These factors have led some to suggest that an ED specifically designed to treat elderly patients would be a better future model of care.[57] Another problem for the frail elderly is multiple ward moves.[37] These reduce continuity of care, increase the risk of delirium and increase lengths of stay.

An ideal environment for an acutely ill older person includes access to specialist medical treatment and investigations but also should be 'older-friendly'. Older-friendly includes consideration for privacy and dignity, encouragement of independence and mobility in a homely rehabilitative setting. A ward environment suitable for caring for older people would have appropriate flooring, orientation cues (large clocks and calendars), handrails and equipment such as raised toilet seats. While carpeted floors may be less slippery, more like home and lessen the impact of falls, they are difficult to clean effectively and are therefore an infection hazard. There is evidence that older patients cared for on specific geriatrics wards have shorter lengths of stay, less functional decline and lower rates of institutionalisation than those on standard medical wards.[58,59]

By definition, frail older people have 'unstable disability' and there is also a need for regular medical review and reassessment during a hospital stay.[60] The right environment and a rehabilitative approach can help prevent common hospital complications, such as depression, falls, delirium and deconditioning (muscle weakness and wasting due to inactivity), which all extend length of stay. In simple terms, older people do better in hospital if the care is directed at help- ing you see what you are doing, hear what is happening, and in an environment where you are encouraged to self-care, get enough to eat and drink and where people talk to you and tell you what is going on.[61] Simply providing a liaison serv- ice that makes recommendations to the treating team seems to be less effective.[62]

KEY POINTS

- Frailty is an expression for the observed loss of physiological reserve seen in association with the ageing process.
- Frail patients can be challenging to care for, as they tend to present atypically, have multiple problems, and take multiple drugs, and they are prone to adverse effects when exposed to only minor stressors.
- Over time, the proportion of older, frailer patients in acute hospitals will increase; this will be true for most medical and surgical specialities.
- The worst way to address this is to blame these patients and provide them with lower quality care or label them as 'bed-blockers' or 'social admissions'.
- The best way to address the problem is to learn how to provide optimal care to this important part of our society.
- Older patients should receive high-quality care that involves their input and aims to optimise physical function and dignity.
- Poor medical and nursing handovers reduce the quality of care and increase clinical risk – use the SBAR tool.

REASONS FOR ATTENDING HOSPITAL

Old age is not an illness and does not make people unwell. Elderly people do not come to hospital because they are old; they come to hospital because they have an illness. Some clinicians do not appreciate this. Admissions to hospital can be seen as inappropriate, risking negative labels such as 'bed-blocker'. Such attitudes increase the risk of inadequate assessment.

People aged over 65 years account for around 15%–18% of ED visits, with attendance rates being highest for those aged over 80 years.[63-65] Compared with those aged below 65 years, they are less likely to present with an injury (33% vs 60%), more likely to arrive by ambulance and more likely to be admitted (32%–46% vs 8%–14%).[63,65-70]

Older people often present 'atypically' (i.e. unlike the classic textbook descriptions of illnesses). Such presentations are common (and so typical) in the frail elderly (*see* p. 67). They include the 'geriatric giants' (falls, immobility, confusion and incontinence), alone or in combination, which are caused by the breakdown of complex systems. Such acute declines in cognitive and functional status may be due to a new illness or decompensation of a pre-existing chronic one. Also older people frequently have multiple problems, often including functional dependence, poor social support or living alone, co-morbidities, polypharmacy, cognitive impairment and depression. As might be expected, functional decline commonly accompanies subacute presentations of illnesses and may be the deciding factor that prompts acute hospital attendance.[71] This may prompt the inexperienced to label the presentation as purely 'social'. Patients may even be discharged from hospital without a specific diagnosis. There is evidence that the number of episodes of inpatient emergency care for older adults in England who have ill-defined conditions is rising.[72] This may lead to inappropriate treatment being given, higher readmission rates and have financial consequences related to inaccurate coding.

A study of 1298 patients aged over 75 years presenting to a rural ED found the commonest reasons for attendance were 'general status deterioration' (21.5%), dyspnoea (15%), falls or trauma (15%), abdominal problems (13%), chest pain (9%), syncope or dizziness (7%) and stroke (5.5%).[73] Only 0.2% presented with a social problem. Overall 69% of the patients were admitted, 85% to medical and 15% to surgical wards. Another study looked at patients aged 65 and over presenting to ED (n = 5,038).[74] The commonest initial diagnoses or presenting symptoms were as follows:

Chest pain (including ischaemic heart disease)	8.1%
Congestive cardiac failure	3.6%
Pneumonia	3.1%
Stroke or transient ischaemic attack	2.8%
Abdominal pain	2.5%

Syncope	2.4%
Urinary tract infection	2.3%*
COPD	2.0%

*Note, value may be artificially high (*see* p. 184).

Other studies have found higher rates of falls (7%–44%) and abdominal pain (6%) in patients aged over 65 presenting to ED.[75-78] Differences may reflect different populations studied or different coding of non-specific presentations.

Acute admissions from care homes

Compared with community-dwelling adults aged over 65 years, those residing in care homes who attend ED are more likely to be older (mean age 85 vs 76 years), female (71% vs 53%), be admitted (65% vs 55%) and die in hospital (7.8% vs 3.5%).[79] They are also more likely to be diagnosed with pneumonia, urinary tract infection or hip fracture. The commonest chief complaints of nursing home (NH) residents who attend an ED are respiratory symptoms (14%), altered mental status (10%), gastrointestinal symptoms (10%) and falls (8%).[80] Some people have questioned whether this resource use by NH residents is worthwhile; however, when evaluated, 77%– 90% of such attendances seem to be appropriate.[81-83]

A recent review of admissions from NHs to hospitals in the United States suggested that 67% were potentially avoidable; however, mechanisms to avoid admission included on-site physicians and nurse practitioners, rapid access to laboratory investigations and the ability to give intravenous fluids.[84] This highlights the difference in definition of a NH between the United States and the UK, where many US facilities are more like UK community hospitals (sometimes termed 'skilled nursing facilities' or 'long-term care facilities').

OUTCOMES

Older age is associated with worse outcomes following hospital admission. Patients aged over 75 admitted to an acute medical unit have been found to have a 30-day mortality rate of 20.7%, compared with 4.5% in those aged below 75.[85] A degree of functional decline can also be expected following presentation to hospital with an acute illness. A study found that around 60% of patients over the age of 80 years presenting to an ED were dependent on a person or device for performing one or more activities of daily living (ADL) (*see* p. 48).[86] Two months after admission, around 40% of those originally independent had developed some degree of dependency. Patients over the age of 70 with new deficits in functional ability following hospital discharge have a higher risk of death (41% vs 18%) and a smaller chance of attaining baseline functional level (30% vs 67%) at 1 year than those without new deficits.[87] The oldest patients seem to be the least likely to return to baseline function and the most likely to develop new problems during admission.[88]

The elderly, especially those with baseline impairments, are more likely to report worse health than the non-elderly at 3 weeks following discharge from the ED (20% vs 4%).[89] Baseline frailty also suggests a worse prognosis. Patients with functional or cognitive impairment or those with depression are more likely to die within 2 years of hospital admission.[90] Another factor is the condition prompting admission. Of 1851 patients aged over 65 (mean age, 77 years) discharged from an ED, 31% had a diagnosis of injury or musculoskeletal disorder, and this group of patients had a lower risk of subsequent adverse health outcomes (hazard ratio, 0.69; 95% confidence interval (CI), 0.50–0.96).[91] Those seen for exacerbations of chronic conditions (e.g. COPD and heart failure) were at greatest risk of death or hospital admission within 30 days (hazard ratio, 1.86; 95% CI, 1.37–2.52).

A study found that 90 days after emergency admission to hospital of patients aged over 65, 85% had returned to their previous residence, 9% were dead, and 6% were still in hospital or were now in residential care.[92] In the over-85s the figures were 77% in prior residence, 11% dead and 12% in residential care. Physical function was the best predictor of outcome. Length of stay had a mean and median duration of 17.7 and 12 days, respectively.

Given the risk of adverse events in all acutely ill adults, a number of criteria have been proposed to allow the earlier identification and appropriate intervention to improve outcomes. Triage tools reliably used in younger populations may be less sensitive to predict adverse outcomes in the elderly.[93]

Modified Early Warning Score

The Modified Early Warning Score is a value (range, 0–15) based on physiological parameters (blood pressure, heart rate, respiratory rate, temperature and conscious level) that can be used to predict those patients who need hospital admission and those at risk of death.[94] Despite theoretical limitations in elderly patients (e.g. absent pyrexial response to severe sepsis (see p. 176)), it still appears to be a valid tool to detect those at risk of a poor outcome during admission. In a study of older patients (mean age, 79 years), the in-hospital mortality rate rose from 3% for those with an admission score of 0 to 40% for those with a score of 5 or more.[95] A number of other similar assessment scales are also available.

Serum lactate and albumin

Serum lactate is a marker of tissue hypoperfusion and may have a prognostic role. In patients aged over 65 (mean age, 80 years) presenting with blunt trauma, but with a systolic blood pressure of 90 mmHg or more, serum lactate levels of 0–2.4, 2.5–4.0 and >4.0 were associated with mortality rates of 15%, 23% and 40%, respectively.[96] A study of patients aged 65 and over (mean age, 77 years) in an ED found that a serum lactate level above 2.0 mmol/L was associated with an increased risk of death at 30 days in those with and without infections.[97] A low serum albumin level is another marker of worse prognosis.[98]

INTENSIVE THERAPY UNIT AND HIGH DEPENDENCY UNIT CARE

Intensive therapy unit (ITU) care provides temporary physiological support for patients with potentially reversible conditions. It is not, by itself, a treatment. This should be taken into account when selecting patients who may benefit.

Patients aged 80 years and over account for around 5%–10% of ITU admissions at the present time.[99,100] Length of stay appears to be similar to that for younger individuals. Age per se does not seem to be predictive of mortality, whereas emergency admission, non-operative status, more severe illness and functional impairment are predictive.[100-102] However, older patients selected for ITU care are presumably those who are physiologically fitter prior to admission. In another study of patients aged 80 years and over (n = 233; mean age, 86 years), the mortality rate on the ITU and the 2 days after discharge was 20%.[103] After 3 years 29% of patients were still alive. Having an underlying fatal disease or severe functional limitation were both predictive of death. These data suggest that selected patients aged over 80 can do well after ITU care.

A frequent factor in deciding which patients to admit to ITU is the physician's perception of the patient's background functional and cognitive abilities, but these subjective assessments can be inaccurate.[104] Baseline functional status and patient preferences should be properly evaluated. ITU care itself can be hazardous. Elderly people have higher risks of barotrauma and nosocomial pneumonia, and may be more difficult to wean off ventilation.[105]

An alternative, but typically less invasive, option to ITU care is that provided on a high dependency unit. The results from a high dependency unit designed for older patients seem to suggest that outcomes can be achieved that are comparable with those of ITU care.[106] This may be a cost-effective alternative model for selected patients.

RESUSCITATION

Older patients are more likely to have a cardiac arrest. A recent review in the UK found the median age of patients to be 77 years.[107] Overall survival to hospital discharge following an out-of-hospital cardiac arrest is estimated to be around 8%; it is around 18% for those occurring in hospitals.[108] In older people, survival following any cardiac arrest is estimated to be around 10%–29%, including rates of around 14%–24% for out-of-hospital ventricular fibrillation arrests.[105] Which suggests that age alone should not be a limitation to receiving cardiopulmonary resuscitation (CPR). However, it would be expected that the best outcomes would be seen in the least frail, and the data for efficacy in NH populations is less clear. One study found that none of 14 NH residents requiring CPR in an ED survived to hospital discharge.[80]

Factors accounting for variability in outcome results include the location of the arrest (e.g. coronary care unit vs geriatric ward), background co-morbidities and the initial presenting rhythm. Better outcomes occur in those with a 'shock-able' rhythm (ventricular tachycardia or fibrillation) (37% of in-hospital arrests survive to discharge) compared with those with either pulseless electrical activity or asystole (11% survive to discharge).[108] The efficacy of CPR may be limited by cardiac valvular disease.[105] In the frail elderly, CPR may lead to chest injuries, including rib or sternal fractures related to osteoporosis. Even when circulation is restored there is a risk of persisting hypoxic brain injury.

Prior to the event of an in-hospital cardiac arrest, there is likely to be a window of opportunity to decide what the patient would want and what is in their best interests in such a situation. This is something that is currently happening in only around 22% of patients who go on to have a cardiac arrest in the UK during their admission, which leads to many futile attempts at CPR.[104] The explanation for this may be partly because of perceived difficulties in communication with patients and/or their relatives and carers. Perhaps it would be more appropriate to move away from the term 'do not attempt CPR' to a concept of 'allow natural/dignified death'.[107]

An in-hospital study of the preferences of patients aged over 80 (median age, 85 years) found that 55% would want to receive CPR, but just 36% of their physicians would choose to receive CPR themselves if in a similar condition.[109] This suggests that patients lack the awareness of the process and likely outcomes of resuscitation following a cardiac arrest. Wherever possible, it is appropriate to make advance decisions regarding resuscitation for all frail elderly patients. This decision to withhold a treatment is a medical one, but this is best informed by the beliefs and wishes of patients or their carers if capacity is lacking. Patient education regarding the process and likely outcomes is required. It is important to emphasise that deciding not to perform CPR in the event of a cardiac arrest is very different to not providing full, high-quality care up to the time of such an event. Decisions should be communicated sensitively and recorded clearly within the patient's records.

KEY POINTS

- People aged over 65 years account for around a sixth of ED attendances but are less likely to present following an injury, more likely to arrive by ambulance and more likely to be admitted than younger people.
- Older people come to hospital because they have an illness but this may present in a non-specific way, such as 'off legs'.
- Rarely is the primary reason for hospital attendance a 'social' one and clinicians should be very careful not to wrongly label their patients.
- Older patients are more likely to have adverse outcomes following a hospital admission – this includes a higher risk of death or functional decline.
- ITU care can be appropriate for selected frail elderly patients.
- Cardiac resuscitation can also be effective in selected frail patients but in many cases there will be no realistic chance of a successful outcome. Resuscitation decisions should be made in advance whenever possible.

HAZARDS OF HOSPITALISATION

Hospitals are dangerous places for old people and have many possible hazards.[110] Even those admitted with potentially fully reversible conditions (e.g. pneumonia) that are appropriately treated are at risk of long-term functional decline. A period of immobility is associated with loss of muscle strength and bone mass, which starts after just a few days.[111] Reversal of such changes may take weeks of rehabilitation. Pressure ulcers can develop after just a few hours of immobility. Reduced mobility increases the risk of falls and incontinence (because of reduced access to the toilet). It also promotes constipation, aspiration pneumonia, orthostatic hypotension, development of contractures, deep vein thrombosis, pulmonary embolus and depression. However, a study found that a cohort of non-demented hospitalised older adults (mean age, 74 years) who were mobile 2 weeks prior to admission spent on average 83% of their time in hospital lying in bed, 13% sitting in a chair and just 4% standing or walking (*see* Figure 1.4).[112] Patients who are less mobile during their period in hospital have worse functional outcomes.[113] This is potentially modifiable. Patients require active rehabilitation, not passive 'bed rest' or convalescence.

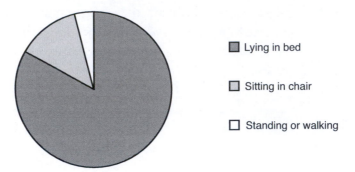

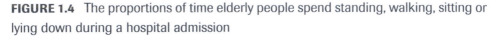

FIGURE 1.4 The proportions of time elderly people spend standing, walking, sitting or lying down during a hospital admission

The lack of orientating stimuli in hospitals increases the risk of delirium. Malnutrition and dehydration may develop because of lack of assistance feeding, unappealing meals, reduced appetite or thirst, and inadequate access to fluids. These factors all increase the risk of subsequent admission into a care home. Adverse events rates occurring in hospitals are higher in those aged over 65 years than younger patients, with many events being related to medications and potentially preventable.[114,115]

Falls in hospital

Falls represent 60% of reported incidents in UK hospitals, with 3%–5% resulting in fracture. There is evidence from a meta-analysis that multifaceted interventions can reduce the risk of falls (rate ratio, 0.82; 95% CI, 0.68–0.997), but not the number of fractures.[116] Falls can also lead to fear of falling, increased length of stay and possible complaints or litigation. The prevention of falls is discussed on page 131.

Insomnia

Older patients are at risk of insomnia, especially when in hospital environments. Doctors are often asked to prescribe sedative medications. These are potentially hazardous, increasing the risk of delirium, falls and fractures. There is also a risk they will be continued after discharge leading to long-term dependency. Studies suggest that around 30% of patients receive a sedative drug for insomnia during hospital stays.[117,118]

There are changes seen in our sleeping patterns as we age. Older people sleep for shorter periods than younger people and complain of more fragmented and less satisfying sleep.[119] This can be mistaken for insomnia. The causes of insomnia can be described as intrinsic or extrinsic to the patient.[120] Possible intrinsic causes are listed in Table 1.3. Extrinsic causes relate to the ward environment (e.g. noise and light levels). Caffeinated drinks should be avoided in the evenings.

TABLE 1.3 Possible intrinsic causes of insomnia

Cause	Comment
Delirium	Reversal of normal day–night pattern of arousal can be seen
	Patients may be more agitated in the evening ('sun-downing')
Depression or anxiety	Disturbed sleep is common in older people with depression (*see* p. 261)
Nocturia	Awoken to pass urine or already awake and so went to the toilet?
Nocturnal leg cramps	This is common, occurring in up to one in three older people
	It is usually idiopathic but may be secondary to drugs (e.g. diuretics, beta-agonists, statins or lithium)
	It is sometimes treated with quinine when frequent and severe (*see* p. 306)
Restless legs syndrome	A strong urge to move the legs that can delay the ability to get to sleep
	Can be idiopathic or secondary to iron deficient anaemia
Periodic limb movements during sleep	Repeated rapid flexions of the leg during sleep causing the patient to wake up multiple times
Paroxysmal nocturnal dyspnoea	Waking up during the night with shortness of breath due to heart failure
Daytime sleeping	This may be a feature of lack of daytime activities, medication effects (e.g. dopamine agonists) or underlying disease (e.g. obstructive sleep apnoea)
Pain	Always consider pain, especially in patients with cognitive impairment who may use non-verbal expressions (*see* p. 44)
Medications	For example, steroids, theophylline, bronchodilators and some selective serotonin reuptake inhibitors
Withdrawal	Alcohol or drugs (e.g. long-term benzodiazepines)

Evaluation of the problem requires consideration of all potential intrinsic and extrinsic factors. It can be helpful to reduce noise on the ward at night (e.g. staff conversations or the volume of alarms), move the patient to a quieter room, or possibly use earplugs. Warm, milky, non-caffeinated drinks may be beneficial. The use of sedative medication should be considered a last resort and evidence of beneficial effects to health are lacking; they do not provide equivalent sleep quality to natural sleep. It has been calculated that 13 people need to be treated with sedatives for one person to have an improvement in sleep quality, compared to just six to cause a harmful event (i.e. falls and cognitive impairment).[121] The average increase in sleep duration with sedatives compared with placebo is only around 25 minutes. It seems unlikely that the benefits outweigh the potential hazards for most patients.

REHABILITATION

Rehabilitation is at the heart of geriatric medicine. It has many definitions but perhaps the best is that rehabilitation is the restoration of the individual to his or her fullest physical, mental and social capability.[122,123] There has been a shift in recent years for as much rehabilitation to take place outside the acute hospital as possible, with decreasing hospital lengths of stay. Nevertheless, acute hospitals have an important early role in rehabilitation, especially in assessment and setting appropriate goals and preparing for discharge. Rehabilitation for older people should start as soon as possible and concurrently with making a medical diagnosis and starting medical treatment to allow the minimisation of functional decline. It should not be seen as a process isolated from acute care. Inactive periods of 'bed rest' or 'convalescence' should always be avoided.

Rehabilitation requires teamwork and consultation with other experts. A multidisciplinary team approach is established practice. It is important that teams understand and respect each other's roles and communicate effectively and have regular multidisciplinary meetings with the patients as the focus. Doctors, including general practitioners, when working alone fail to recognise up to 75% of disabilities.[124] The key roles of the members of the rehabilitation team are described here.

Physiotherapy

Physiotherapists work with patients to reduce impairment related to mobility and motor function. In older patients this includes assessing mobility and working to improve gait and balance to reduce the risk of falls. In those who have fallen they may also advise on suitable techniques for the patient to use to independently get up off the floor. They can assess and provide the most suitable walking aid to encourage safe mobility (*see* Table 1.4). These measures can improve patient confidence and instil self-help strategies. They may also assist the care of immobile patients by advising on appropriate positioning or seating to prevent complications.

Occupational therapy

Occupational therapists (OTs) work with patients to assess and reduce mental and physical disability. In older patients OTs assess their ability to do things (i.e. ADL) and function in their environment, including performing home visits. This process may pick up mental and physical deficits that have been missed by bedside testing. It may also identify any home hazards, such as trailing wires, loose rugs or poorly lit stairways. OTs work with the patients to overcome impairments and improve their daily living skills. They may also be required to assess

TABLE 1.4 Examples of commonly used mobility aids

Type of aid	Comments
Walking stick	Can use one or two
	Single stick usually held in hand contralateral to the problem (e.g. stroke) to improve balance
	They may also reduce the weight transferred through a painful limb (e.g. arthritis)
	A specialised 'Fischer' handle can be more comfortable for those with arthritis
	Those with reduced arm swing (e.g. Parkinson's disease) may find walking sticks less useful
Tripod or tetrapod stick	Stability can be improved on the flat, but less stable on uneven surfaces
	Typically too bulky to use on stairs or in confined spaces
Elbow crutches	Usually used for short periods following injury in younger people
	Used less often in the frail elderly, as offer little help with balance
Zimmer frame	A standard Zimmer frame has four 'legs'
	The patient moves the frame forwards, then steps into space behind the frame – the walking pattern is 'stop-start'
Wheeled Zimmer frame	Many Zimmer frames have two wheels on the front 'legs'; this enables the frame to be pushed along, and this can help those with limited arm strength but it may be less stable
	It can also promote a smoother gait pattern that can assist people with Parkinson's disease
Gutter frame	This frame has armrests on the top that the patient can transfer their weight through
	It can help those with a weak grip or arthritic pain in the hands
Delta frame	This frame is triangular shaped from above, with three wheeled legs
	Often they are fitted with brakes and a shopping basket and can be folded to ease transport
	The larger wheels are most suited for use outdoors
Wheelchair	Wheelchairs can be self-propelled, pushed by others or motorised. Some patients use them for all mobility; others, just when they are going long distances
	They may have specialised pressure-relieving cushions and removable sides to aid transfers in and out of the chair

the need for and arrange provision of specialist equipment or adaptations (*see* Table 1.5), including wheelchairs. They may also advise on the type and level of care patients need after discharge.

Speech and language therapy

Speech and language therapists work with patients to improve their language and communication skills. This may include the provision of aids including picture

TABLE 1.5 Examples of commonly used equipment and home adaptations

Equipment or adaptation	Comments
Handrails	Rails can be fitted next to steps, including to both sides of stairways
	They can also be placed next to toilets and baths to enable patients to get off or out
Raised toilet seat	These allow patients to stand up more easily after using the toilet
Personal care alarm	A care alarm can be worn around the wrist like a watch or around the neck like a necklace
	They are typically used for people at risk of falls – if unable to get up or if injured, they can press the button and contact help
Key safe	These are usually fitted next to the front door in house of patients who have limited mobility – a carer can enter a code to access the key and let themselves into the property
Bedside commode	These can allow maintenance of continence in patients with limited mobility that need to get up during the night to go to the toilet
Hoists	A variety of hoist designs can be used in the homes of those with limited ability to transfer themselves from bed to chair or toilet
	Their operation requires the help of one or more carers

charts or letter boards that patients can point to in order to indicate their needs. They also play a role in the assessment and management of swallowing problems, particularly following stroke. This may result in the use of a modified diet – for example, the use of thickened fluids. A speech therapy assessment may be helpful in assessing capacity in an older patient with communication problems.

Social work

Social workers are employed by social services and are usually community based. They are valuable in assessing the social and environmental background and may know the patient and carers before they were admitted. Social workers will be able to provide advice on local support services available and provide continuing advocacy and psychological support. They often help arrange packages of care for patients. These typically vary from a few calls by one person a week up to two carers calling four times a day. Overnight care is expensive and only infrequently available for patients in their own homes. Social workers are a good source of information regarding the financial implications of various forms of care and any financial benefits that patients may be entitled to. When patients require placement within a care home, they are able to provide advice about the availability and costs to patients and their families.

Nursing

Of all the hospital staff, nurses know the patients best as they provide the around-the-clock physical care. Usually a single 'named' nurse is allocated as the key link for each patient. The nurses have an essential role in coordinating the multidisciplinary team and providing psychological support and advice to the patient, family and carers. They typically take a leading role in many aspects of care for older adults, including pressure ulcers, leg ulcers and continence. Close work with physiotherapy and OT colleagues allows rehabilitation techniques to be incorporated by all staff into the patients' daily routines.

DISCHARGE PLANNING

Discharge from hospital can be a major life event for a patient and carer. In the 'real world' it is not just a question of deciding that an older patient is medically fit for discharge, as admission to hospital may be the culmination of multiple problems and difficulties, including functional and environmental. Discharge is a multidisciplinary process that involves the patient and carer, as well as members of the multidisciplinary team. Discharge planning is a problem-solving exercise that involves tackling the consequences of the medical illness in the context of the resulting impairment and disability. Ideally, discharge planning should start as soon as a patient is admitted, with the usual aim being to get the patient back to his or her own home.

The minimum requirement for a patient to go home alone is that he or she should be safely mobile and be able to make a hot drink. If the patient's functional ability has changed during the admission, then a plan for further rehabilitation may be required, or the patient may need to have a higher level of care arranged. It is important that such potentially life-changing decisions involve the patient, carers and multidisciplinary team. Discharging a patient to a NH may seem an easy solution for the hospital, but it may be disastrous for the patient and the taxpayer. Moving frail older people to another ward as a 'sleep-out' at the point of discharge is not good practice, as it often necessitates a change in nursing and therapy team, and last-minute changes in the patient's condition may go unrecognised. The process of discharge also requires the coordination of providing correct medications and transport, information exchange to community practitioners and ensuring any previous care arrangements are restarted. Some of the common considerations are shown in Table 1.6. Frail people living alone should not be discharged in the middle of the night unless temporary support is available.

TABLE 1.6 Common considerations when planning the discharge of a frail older patient

Consideration	Comments
Does the patient have a package of care?	Does the amount or frequency of care need to change following this illness? Many care agencies require 48 hours' notice to restart existing care packages.
Does the patient have stairs at home?	If a patient can no longer do stairs (including steps to a front door), it may hinder their discharge. Possible solutions include extra handrails, downstairs living (if enough space and a downstairs bathroom) or the fitting of a stair lift.
Are they able to take their medications consistently?	Patients with visual or cognitive impairment may have a carer who could help with their medication. Aids such as dosette boxes may assist (*see* p. 308). District nurses might be required to administer insulin.
Can they do their own shopping?	Some patients rely on others to be able to access food. It may be necessary to give advance warning to a carer for them to be able to ensure the fridge and cupboards are stocked up.
How will the patient get home?	If the patient requires transport provided by an ambulance then this will need to be arranged in advance. They may have friends or relatives who could take them home. This will only be possible if they can safely and comfortably travel in a standard car seat.
Do they have ongoing medical, nursing or rehabilitation needs?	Any requirements for specific monitoring or treatment should be handed over to the relevant community team. It may be possible to have more rehabilitation within their home.

READMISSIONS

Many patients are discharged from ED each day but some will return. Readmission rates in the following month after discharge from ED in those aged over 75 are around 17%–22%,[125,126] and around 44% of patients aged over 65 will have a return visit in the 6 months after the index presentation.[127] Those with difficulties in performing ADL are at an increased risk of re-presenting.[125] A proportion of patients discharged from ED (perhaps around 30%) would benefit from further geriatric assessment.[128] This seems particularly true for those who presented with falls and who live alone. Of people aged 75 who were discharged from an ED, those receiving a comprehensive assessment and multidisciplinary team follow-up were less likely to be readmitted in the following 30 days.[126] A number of other studies have also shown functional benefits resulting from intervention programmes for older patients discharged from an ED. These findings have prompted clinicians to seek an effective tool to rapidly screen for those patients at highest risk and then offer this group further intervention to prevent recurrent illness.

The BRIGHT assessment tool involves a questionnaire to be completed by the patient, a relative or carer (those with cognitive impairment were excluded from study).[129] Scores range from 0 to 11. The questions are based around functional ability, mobility, falls, depression and cognition. Compared with a standardised form of comprehensive geriatric assessment, the sensitivity and specificity of the questionnaire to detect instrumental activities of daily living deficit were 76% and 79%, respectively; to detect cognitive impairment, the sensitivity and specificity were 70% and 74%, respectively; and to detect ADL deficit, the sensitivity and specificity were 69% and 70%, respectively.

The Identification of Seniors at Risk screening tool has a self-administered, six-item format covering topics such as functional dependence, prior hospitalisation, cognitive impairment and polypharmacy.[130] A score of 2 or more (out of 6) has been used to predict those at high risk of hospital use in the next 6 months. A selected group of patients aged 65 and over who attended an ED and were found to be at risk according to the ISAR tool were then randomised to a standardised nursing assessment, with notification to doctors and carers in the community or to usual care.[131] This led to a lower rate of functional decline or death at 4 months (21% of participants vs 31% in control group). However, other studies have not found the sensitivity and specificity to be very high (73% and 51%, respectively).[132] When tested in an Italian population, it did seem predictive of adverse outcomes over the next 6 months, but over 70% of screened patients tested positive, making it of only limited use to effectively target resources.[133]

The LACE score (calculated by values for each of **L**ength of stay, **A**dmission type, **C**o-morbidity and number of **E**D attendances – range, 0–19) was developed to try to predict those patients at risk of readmission, but unfortunately it does not appear to be sufficiently accurate.[134] A number of other tools have also been created but so far they seem to have only moderate precision.[135,136]

ALTERNATIVES TO ACUTE HOSPITALS

Given the potential harms of acute hospitals for the frail elderly, it is an attractive idea that hospital admission could be avoided for some patients. 'Intermediate care' is a term for schemes that lie somewhere between the patient's own home and a traditional acute hospital bed. This covers a range of services designed to facilitate discharge from hospital ('step down') and in some cases to prevent admission to hospital ('step up'). Such schemes include 'hospital at home' and community hospitals. Overall there is a lack of evidence that intermediate care systems tested to date in the UK are either able to reduce hospital admission rates or reduce overall costs.[137–139] However, for carefully selected patients they may improve outcomes. Patients should not be referred for intermediate care without a diagnosis and a full medical assessment. A readmission rate back from community hospitals to an acute hospital of around 8% in the first week has been reported.[140] Factors increasing the risk are reduced functional and cognitive ability and increased numbers of co-morbidities.

CARE HOMES

Care homes provide long-term 24-hour care and companionship for people who can no longer manage in their own home. The proportion of people residing in care homes increases with advancing age (*see* Figure 1.5), and in the UK around two-thirds are aged over 80, with a mean age around 85 years.[141,142]

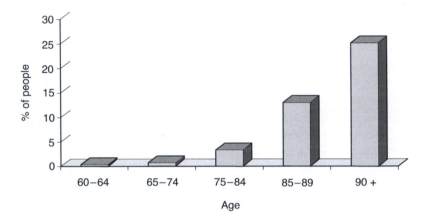
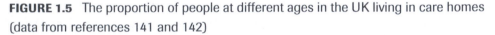

FIGURE 1.5 The proportion of people at different ages in the UK living in care homes (data from references 141 and 142)

The homes vary considerably in the level of care they are able to provide. Residential care homes (RHs) will usually provide help with personal hygiene, urinary continence management, assisting with toileting and help with mobility and dressing. They do not provide 'round-the-clock' trained nursing staff. The district nursing service can provide any short-term nursing care (e.g. dressings and pressure ulcer care) in RHs. NHs do provide 24-hour nursing care, sometimes including patients with advanced dementia or severe neurological disability. Some NHs also provide continuing physiotherapy or occupational therapy. In general terms, patients with faecal incontinence or requiring more than one person to assist with mobility usually require NH rather than RH placement. When an older patient is admitted from a care home, or discharged to a care home, it is important to check the level of service the home provides and what it is registered for.

KEY POINTS

- Hospitals are potentially hazardous places for frail elderly patients. Every effort should be made to minimise the risk of harm – especially of falls.
- Periods of inactivity promote muscle loss and functional decline – 'bed rest' or 'convalescence' should always be avoided.
- Rehabilitation is restoring the patient to their fullest physical, mental and social capability.
- Frail older patients by definition frequently have unstable disability and need frequent reassessment.
- Rehabilitation requires teamwork between doctors, nurses and therapists and a good rehabilitative environment, and it is an essential function of acute hospitals to prepare patients for discharge.
- Patients may benefit from walking aids or home adaptations to maximise their functional ability.
- Discharge is a problem-solving exercise and not just deciding when a patient appears medically stable.

REFERENCES

1. Balaban RS, Nemoto S, Finkel T. Mitochondria, oxidants, and aging. *Cell.* 2005; **120**(4): 483–95.
2. Whitaker J, Tallis R. Misplaced elderly patients in hospital: clarifying responsibilities. *Health Trends.* 1992; **24**(1): 15–17.
3. Evans WJ, Campbell WW. Sarcopenia and age-related changes in body composition and functional capacity. *J Nutr.* 1993; **123**(2 Suppl.): 465–8.
4. Fukagawa NK, Bandini LG, Dietz WH, *et al.* Effect of age on body water and resting metabolic rate. *J Gerontol.* 1996; **51**(2): M71–3.
5. Cruz-Jentoft AJ, Baeyens JP, Bauer JM, *et al.* Sarcopenia: European consensus on definition and diagnosis. *Age Ageing.* 2010; **39**(4): 412–23.
6. Doherty TJ. Aging and sarcopenia. *J Appl Physiol.* 2003; **95**(4): 1717–27.
7. Goodpaster BH, Park SW, Harris TB, *et al.* The loss of skeletal muscle strength, mass, and quality in older adults: the Health Aging and Body Composition Study. *J Gerontol.* 2006; **61**(10): 1059–64.
8. Fiatarone MA, Marks EC, Ryan ND, *et al.* High-intensity strength training in nonagenarians: effects on skeletal muscle. *JAMA.* 1990; **263**(22): 3029–34.
9. Lakatta EG. Age-associated cardiovascular changes in health: impact on cardiovascular disease in older persons. *Heart Fail Rev.* 2002; **7**(1): 29–49.
10. Oxenham H, Sharpe N. Cardiovascular aging and heart failure. *Eur J Heart Fail.* 2003; **5**(4): 427–34.
11. Ford G. Ageing and the baroreflex. *Age Ageing.* 1999; **28**(4); 337–8.
12. Salmasi A, Alimo A, Jepson E, *et al.* Age-associated changes in left ventricular diastolic function are related to increasing left ventricular mass. *Am J Hypertens.* 2003; **16**(6): 473–7.

13. Bharati S, Lev M. The pathologic changes in the conduction system beyond the age of ninety. *Am Heart J.* 1992; **124**(2): 486–96.

14. Yilmaz R, Erdem Y. Acute kidney injury in the elderly population. *Int Urol Nephrol.* 2010; **42**(1): 259–71.

15. Hemmelgarn BR, Zhang J, Manns BJ, *et al.* Progression of kidney dysfunction in the community-dwelling elderly. *Kidney Int.* 2006; **69**(12): 2155–61.

16. Drayer BP. Imaging of the aging brain: part I normal findings. *Radiology.* 1988; **166**(3): 785–96.

17. Woodford HJ, George J. Neurological and cognitive impairments detected in older people without a diagnosis of neurological or cognitive disease. *Postgrad Med J.* 2011; **87**(1025): 199–206.

18. Corti M, Baggio G, Sartori L, *et al.* White matter lesions and the risk of incident hip fracture in older persons. *Arch Intern Med.* 2007; **167**(16): 1745–51.

19. Sakakibara R, Hattori T, Uchiyama T, *et al.* Urinary function in elderly people with and without leukoaraiosis: relation to cognitive and gait function. *J Neurol Neurosurg Psychiatry.* 1999; **67**(5): 658–60.

20. Pantoni L, Poggesi A, Basile AM, *et al.* Leukoaraiosis predicts hidden global functioning impairment in nondisabled older people: The LADIS (Leukoaraiosis and Disability in the Elderly) Study. *J Am Geriatr Soc.* 2006; **54**(7): 1095–101.

21. Smeeth L, Fletcher AE, Ng ES, *et al.* Reduced hearing, ownership, and use of hearing aids in elderly people in the UK – the MRC Trial of the Assessment and Management of Older People in the Community: a cross-sectional survey. *Lancet.* 2002; **359**(9316): 1466–70.

22. Lipsitz LA, Nyquist RP Jr, Wei JY, *et al.* Postprandial reduction in blood pressure in the elderly. *N Engl J Med.* 1983; **309**(2): 81–3.

23. Starr JM, Deary IJ, Inch S, *et al.* Age-associated cognitive decline in healthy old people. *Age Ageing.* 1997; **26**(4): 295–300.

24. Wynne HA, Cope LH, James OFW, *et al.* The effect of age and frailty upon acetanilide clearance in man. *Age Ageing.* 1989; **18**(6): 415–18.

25. Vestal RE. Aging and pharmacology. *Cancer.* 1997; **80**(7): 1302–10.

26. Norman DC, Yoshikawa TT. Fever in the elderly. *Infect Dis Clin North Am.* 1996; **10**(1): 93–9.

27. Bergman H, Ferrucci L, Guralnik J, *et al.* Frailty: an emerging research and clinical paradigm – issues and controversies. *J Gerontol A Biol Sci Med Sci.* 2007; **62**(7): 731–7.

28. Fried LP, Tangen CM, Walston J, *et al.* Frailty in older adults: evidence for a phenotype. *J Gerontol A Biol Sci Med Sci.* 2001; **56**(3): M146–56.

29. Van Kan GA, Rolland Y, Houles M, *et al.* The assessment of frailty in older adults. *Clin Geriatr Med.* 2010; **26**(2): 275–86.

30. Ensrud KE, Ewing SK, Cawthon PM, *et al.* A comparison of frailty indexes for the prediction of falls, disability, fractures, and mortality in older men. *J Am Geriatr Soc.* 2009; **57**(3): 492–8.

31. Mitnitski AB, Graham JE, Mogilner AJ, *et al.* Frailty, fitness and late-life mortality in relation to chronological and biological age. *BMC Geriatr.* 2002; **2**: 1.

32. Rolfson DB, Majumdar SR, Tsuyuki RT, *et al.* Validity and reliability of the Edmonton Frail Scale. *Age Ageing.* 2006; **35**(5): 526–9.

33. Van Iersel MB, Olde Rikkert MGM. Frailty criteria give heterogeneous results when applied in clinical practice. *J Am Geriatr Soc.* 2006; **54**(4): 728–9.

34. George G, Jell C, Todd BS. Effect of population ageing on emergency department speed and

efficiency: a historical perspective from a district general hospital in the UK. *Emerg Med J*. 2006; **23**(5): 379–83.

35. Roberts DC, McKay MP, Shaffer A. Increasing rates of emergency department visits for elderly patients in the United States, 1993 to 2003. *Ann Emerg Med*. 2008; **51**(6): 769–74.

36. Department of Health. *National Service Framework for Older People*. London: Department of Health; 2001. Available at: www.dh.gov.uk/en/Publicationsandstatistics/Publications/PublicationsPolicyAndGuidance/DH_4003066 (accessed 22 January 2013).

37. Royal College of Physicians. *Hospitals on the Edge? The time for action*. London: Royal College of Physicians; 2012. Available at: www.rcplondon.ac.uk/projects/hospitals-edge-time-action (accessed 22 January 2013).

38. McNamara RM, Rousseau E, Sanders AB. Geriatric emergency medicine: a survey of practicing emergency physicians. *Ann Emerg Med*. 1992; **21**(7): 796–801.

39. Schumacher JG, Deimling GT, Meldon S, *et al*. Older adults in the emergency department: predicting physicians' burden levels. *J Emerg Med*. 2006; **30**(4): 455–60.

40. Hwang U, Morrison RS. The geriatric emergency department. *J Am Geriatr Soc*. 2007; **55**(11): 1873–6.

41. Wilber ST, Gerson LW, Terrell KM, *et al*. Geriatric emergency medicine and the 2006 Institute of Medicine reports from the Committee on the Future of Emergency Care in the US Health System. *Acad Emerg Med*. 2006; **13**(12): 1345–51.

42. Peterson LN, Fairbanks RJ, Hettinger AZ, *et al*. Emergency medical service attitudes toward geriatric prehospital care and continuing medical education in geriatrics. *J Am Geriatr Soc*. 2009; **57**(3): 530–5.

43. Hogan TM, Losman ED, Carpenter CR, *et al*. Development of geriatric competencies for emergency medicine residents using an expert consensus process. *Acad Emerg Med*. 2010; **17**(3): 316–24.

44. Warshaw GA, Thomas DC, Callahan EH, *et al*. A national survey on the current status of general internal medicine residency education in geriatric medicine. *J Gen Intern Med*. 2003; **18**(9): 679–84.

45. Warshaw GA, Bragg EJ, Thomas DC, *et al*. Are internal medicine residency programs adequately preparing physicians to care for the baby boomers? A national survey from the Association of Directors of Geriatric Academic Programs Status of Geriatrics Workforce Study. *J Am Geriatr Soc*. 2006; **54**(10): 1603–9.

46. Lally F, Crome P. Undergraduate training in geriatric medicine: getting it right. *Age Ageing*. 2007; **36**(4): 366–8.

47. Wenger NS, Solomon DH, Roth CP, *et al*. The quality of medical care provided to vulnerable community-dwelling older patients. *Ann Intern Med*. 2003; **139**(9): 740–7.

48. Parliamentary and Health Service Ombudsman. *Care and Compassion? Report of the Health Service Ombudsman on ten investigations into NHS care of older people*. London: The Stationery Office; 2011. Available at: www.official-documents.gov.uk/document/hc1011/hc07/0778/0778.pdf (accessed 22 January 2013).

49. Neumann M, Edelhauser F, Tauschel D, *et al*. Empathy decline and its reasons: a systematic review of studies with medical students and residents. *Acad Med*. 2011; **86**(8): 996–1009.

50. Oliver D. 'Acopia' and 'social admission' are not diagnoses: why older people deserve better. *J R Soc Med*. 2008; **101**(4): 168–74.

51. Bridges J, Flatley M, Meyer J. Older people's and relatives' experiences in acute care settings: systematic review and synthesis of qualitative studies. *Int J Nurs Stud*. 2010; **47**(1): 89–107.

52. Spilsbury K, Meyer J, Bridges J, *et al*. Older adults' experiences of A&E care. *Emerg Nurse*. 1999; **7**(6): 24–31.

53. Commission on Dignity in Care. *Delivering Dignity: securing dignity in care for older people in hospitals and care homes*. UK: Commission on Dignity in Care; 2012. Available at: www. nhsconfed.org/Documents/dignity.pdf (accessed 22 January 2013).

54. British Medical Association. *Safe Handover: safe patients. Guidance for clinical handover for clinicians and managers*. London: British Medical Association; 2004.

55. Royal College of Physicians. *Acute Care Toolkit 1: handover*. London: Royal College of Physicians; 2011.

56. Wacogne I, Diwakar V. Handover and note keeping: the SBAR approach. *Clin Risk*. 2010; **16**: 173–5.

57. Salvi F, Morichi V, Grilli A, *et al*. A geriatric emergency service for acutely ill elderly patients: pattern of use and comparison with a conventional emergency department in Italy. *J Am Geriatr Soc*. 2008; **56**(11): 2131–8.

58. Asplund K, Gustafson Y, Jacobsson C, *et al*. Geriatric-based versus general wards for older acute medical patients: a randomized comparison of outcomes and uses of resources. *J Am Geriatr Soc*. 2000; **48**(11): 1381–8.

59. Baztan JJ, Suarez-Garcia FM, Lopez-Arrieta J, *et al*. Effectiveness of acute geriatric units on functional decline, living at home, and case fatality among older patients admitted to hospital for acute medical disorders: meta-analysis. *BMJ*. 2009; **338**: b50.

60. Campbell AJ, Buchner DM. Unstable disability and fluctuations of frailty. *Age Ageing*. 1997; **26**(4): 315–18.

61. Vincent C. *Patient Safety*. Oxford: BMJ Books; 2010.

62. Miller DK, Lewis LM, Nork MJ, *et al*. Controlled trial of a geriatric case-finding and liaison service in an emergency department. *J Am Geriatr Soc*. 1996; **44**(5): 513–20.

63. Strange GR, Chen EH, Sanders AB. Use of emergency departments by elderly patients: projections from a multicenter data base. *Ann Emerg Med*. 1992; **21**(7): 819–24.

64. Strange GR, Chen EH. Use of emergency departments by elder patients: a five-year follow-up study. *Acad Emerg Med*. 1998; **5**(12): 1157–62.

65. Downing A, Wilson R. Older people's use of accident and emergency services. *Age Ageing*. 2005; **34**(1): 24–30.

66. Baum SA, Rubenstein LZ. Old people in the emergency room: age-related differences in emergency department use and care. *J Am Geriatr Soc*. 1987; **35**(5): 398–404.

67. Ettinger WH, Casani JA, Coon PJ, *et al*. Patterns of use of the emergency department by elderly patients. *J Gerontol*. 1987; **42**(6): 638–42.

68. Singal BM, Hedges JR, Rousseau EW, *et al*. Geriatric patient emergency visits part I: comparison of visits by geriatric and younger patients. *Ann Emerg Med*. 1992; **21**(7): 802–7.

69. Aminzadeh F, Dalziel WB. Older adults in the emergency department: a systematic review of patterns of use, adverse outcomes, and effectiveness of interventions. *Ann Emerg Med*. 2002; **39**(3): 238–47.

70. Platts-Mills TF, Leacock B, Cabanas JG, *et al*. Emergency medical services use by the elderly: analysis of a statewide database. *Prehosp Emerg Care*. 2010; **14**(3): 329–33.

71. Wilber ST, Blanda M, Gerson LW. Does functional decline prompt emergency department visits and admissions in older patients? *Acad Emerg Med*. 2006; **13**(6): 680–2.

72. Walsh B, Roberts HC, Nicholls PG, *et al*. Trends in hospital inpatient episodes for signs, symptoms and ill-defined conditions: observational study of older people's hospital episodes in England, 1995–2003. *Age Ageing*. 2008; **37**(4): 455–78.

73. Vanpee D, Swine CH, Vandenbossche P, *et al*. Epidemiological profile of geriatric patients admitted to the emergency department of a university hospital localized in a rural area. *Eur J Emerg Med*. 2001; **8**(4): 301–4.

74. Wofford JL, Schwartz E, Timerding BL, *et al.* Emergency department utilization by the elderly: analysis of the National Hospital Ambulatory Medical Care Survey. *Acad Emerg Med.* 1996; **3**(7): 694–9.

75. Davies AJ, Kenny RA. Falls presenting to the accident and emergency department: types of presentation and risk factor profile. *Age Ageing.* 1996; **25**(5): 362–6.

76. Marco CA, Schoenfeld CN, Keyl PM, *et al.* Abdominal pain in geriatric emergency patients: variables associated with adverse outcomes. *Acad Emerg Med.* 1998; **5**(12): 1163–8.

77. Close J, Ellis M, Hooper R, *et al.* Prevention of falls in the elderly trial (PROFET): a randomised controlled trial. *Lancet.* 1999; **353**(9147): 93–7.

78. Baraff LJ, Lee TJ, Kader S, *et al.* Effects of a practice guideline for emergency department care of falls in elder patients on subsequent falls and hospitalizations for injuries. *Acad Emerg Med.* 1999; **6**(12): 1224–31.

79. Ingarfield SL, Finn JC, Jacobs IG, *et al.* Use of emergency departments by older people from residential care: a population based study. *Age Ageing.* 2009; **38**(3): 314–8.

80. Ackermann RJ, Kemle KA, Vogel RL, *et al.* Emergency department use by nursing home residents. *Ann Emerg Med.* 1998; **31**(6): 749–57.

81. Bergman H, Clarfield AM. Appropriateness of patient transfer from a nursing home to an acute-care hospital: a study of emergency room visits and hospital admissions. *J Am Geriatr Soc.* 1992; **39**(12): 1164–8.

82. Jones JS, Dwyer PR, White LJ, *et al.* Patient transfer from nursing home to emergency department: outcomes and policy implications. *Acad Emerg Med.* 1997; **4**(9): 908–15.

83. Finn JC, Flicker L, Mackenzie E, *et al.* Interface between residential aged care facilities and a teaching hospital emergency department in Western Australia. *Med J Aust.* 2006; **184**(9): 432–5.

84. Ouslander JG, Lamb G, Perloe M, *et al.* Potentially avoidable hospitalizations of nursing home residents: frequency, causes, and costs. *J Am Geriatr Soc.* 2010; **58**(4): 627–35.

85. Byrne DG, Chung SL, Bennett K, *et al.* Age and outcome in acute emergency medical admissions. *Age Ageing.* 2010; **39**(6): 694–8.

86. Wu AW, Yasui Y, Alzola C, *et al.* Predicting functional status outcomes in hospitalized patients aged 80 years and older. *J Am Geriatr Soc.* 2000; **48**(5 Suppl.): S6–15.

87. Boyd CM, Landefeld CS, Counsell SR, *et al.* Recovery of activities of daily living in older adults after hospitalization for acute medical illness. *J Am Geriatr Soc.* 2008; **56**(12): 2171–9.

88. Covinsky KE, Palmer RM, Fortinsky RH, *et al.* Loss of independence in activities of daily living in older adults hospitalized with medical illnesses: increased vulnerability with age. *J Am Geriatr Soc.* 2003; **51**(4): 451–8.

89. Denman SJ, Ettinger WH, Zarkin BA, *et al.* Short-term outcomes of elderly patients discharged from an emergency department. *J Am Geriatr Soc.* 1989; **37**(10): 937–43.

90. Inouye SK, Peduzzi PN, Robison JT, *et al.* Importance of functional measures in predicting mortality among older hospitalized patients. *JAMA.* 1998; **279**(15): 1187–93.

91. Hastings SN, Whitson HE, Purser JL, *et al.* Emergency department discharge diagnosis and adverse health outcomes in older adults. *J Am Geriatr Soc.* 2009; **57**(10): 1856–61.

92. Campbell SE, Seymour DG, Primrose WR, *et al.* A multi-centre European study of factors affecting the discharge destination of older people admitted to hospital: analysis of in-hospital data from the ACME*plus* project. *Age Ageing.* 2005; **34**(5): 467–75.

93. Platts-Mills TF, Travers D, Biese K, *et al.* Accuracy of the Emergency Severity Index triage instrument for identifying elder emergency department patients receiving an immediate life-saving intervention. *Acad Emerg Med.* 2010; **17**(3): 238–43.

94. Burch VC, Tarr G, Morroni C. Modified early warning score predicts the need for hospital admission and inhospital mortality. *Emerg Med J.* 2008; **25**(10): 674–8.

95. Cei M, Bartolomei C, Mumoli N. In-hospital mortality and morbidity of elderly medical patients can be predicted at admission by the Modified Early Warning Score: a prospective study. *Int J Clin Pract.* 2009; **63**(4): 591–5.

96. Callaway DW, Shapiro NI, Donnino MW, *et al.* Serum lactate and base deficit as predictors of mortality in normotensive elderly blunt trauma patients. *J Trauma.* 2009; **66**(4): 1040–4.

97. Del Portal DA, Shofer F, Mikkelsen ME, *et al.* Emergency department lactate is associated with mortality in older adults admitted with and without infections. *Acad Emerg Med.* 2010; **17**(3): 260–8.

98. Corti M, Guralnik JM, Salive ME, *et al.* Serum albumin level and physical disability as predictors of mortality in older persons. *JAMA.* 1994; **272**(13): 1036–42.

99. Boumendil A, Somme D, Garrouste-Orgeas M, *et al.* Should elderly patients be admitted to the intensive care unit? *Intensive Care Med.* 2007; **33**(7): 1252–62.

100. Ryan D, Conlon N, Phelan D, *et al.* The very elderly in intensive care: admission characteristics and mortality. *Crit Care Resusc.* 2008; **10**(2): 106–10.

101. Somme D, Maillet J, Gisselbrecht M, *et al.* Critically ill old and the oldest-old patients in intensive care: short- and long-term outcomes. *Intensive Care Med.* 2003; **29**(12): 2137–43.

102. De Rooij SE, Abu-Hanna A, Levi M, *et al.* Factors that predict outcome of intensive care treatment in very elderly patients: a review. *Crit Care.* 2005; **9**(4): R307–14.

103. Boumendil A, Maury E, Reinhard I, *et al.* Prognosis of patients aged 80 years and over admitted in medical intensive care unit. *Intensive Care Med.* 2004; **30**(4): 647–54.

104. Rodriguez-Molinero A, Lopez-Dieguez M, Tabuenca AI, *et al.* Physicians' impression on the elders' functionality influences decision making for emergency care. *Am J Emerg Med.* 2010; **28**(7): 757–65.

105. Marang AT, Sikka R. Resuscitation of the elderly. *Emerg Med Clin North Am.* 2006; **24**(2): 261–72.

106. Ip SPS, Leung YF, Ip CY, *et al.* Outcomes of critically ill elderly patients: is high-dependency care for geriatric patients worthwhile? *Crit Care Med.* 1999; **27**(11): 2351–7.

107. National Confidential Enquiry into Patient Outcome and Death (NCEPOD). *Time to Intervene? A review of patients who underwent cardiopulmonary resuscitation as a result of an in-hospital cardiorespiratory arrest.* London: NCEPOD; 2012. Available at: www.ncepod. org.uk/2012cap.htm (accessed 22 January 2013).

108. Nolan JP, Soar J, Perkins GD. Cardiopulmonary resuscitation. *BMJ.* 2012; **345**: 34–40.

109. O'Donnell H, Phillips RS, Wenger N, *et al.* Preferences for cardiopulmonary resuscitation among patients 80 years or older: the views of patients and their physicians. *J Am Med Dir Assoc.* 2003; **4**(3): 139–44.

110. Creditor MC. Hazards of hospitalization of the elderly. *Ann Intern Med.* 1993; **118**(3): 219–23.

111. Kortebein P, Symons TB, Ferrando A, *et al.* Functional impact of 10 days of bed rest in healthy older adults. *J Gerontol A Biol Sci Med Sci.* 2008; **63**(10): 1076–81.

112. Brown CJ, Redden DT, Flood KL, *et al.* The underrecognized epidemic of low mobility during hospitalization of older adults. *J Am Geriatr Soc.* 2009; **57**(9): 1660–5.

113. Zisberg A, Shadmi E, Sinoff G, *et al.* Low mobility during hospitalization and functional decline in older adults. *J Am Geriatr Soc.* 2011; **59**(2): 266–73.

114. Leape LL, Brennan TA, Laird N, *et al.* The nature of adverse events in hospitalized patients: results of the Harvard Medical Practice Study II. *N Engl J Med.* 1991; **324**(6): 377–84.

115. Brennan TA, Leape LL, Laird NM, *et al.* Incidence of adverse events and negligence in

hospitalized patients: results of the Harvard Medical Practice Study I. *N Engl J Med*. 1991; **324**(6): 370–6.

116. Oliver D, Connelly JB, Victor CR, *et al*. Strategies to prevent falls and fractures in hospitals and care homes and effect of cognitive impairment: systematic review and meta-analyses. *BMJ*. 2007; **334**(7584): 82–5.

117. Perry SW, Wu A. Rationale for the use of hypnotic agents in a general hospital. *Ann Intern Med*. 1984: **100**(3): 441–6.

118. O'Reilly R, Rusnak C. The use of sedative-hypnotic drugs in a university teaching hospital. *CMAJ*. 1990; **142**(6): 585–9.

119. Kryger M, Monjan A, Bliwise D, *et al*. Sleep, health, and aging: bridging the gap between science and clinical practice. *Geriatrics*. 2004; **59**(1): 24–30.

120. Flaherty JH. Insomnia among hospitalized older persons. *Clin Geriatr Med*. 2008; **24**(1): 51–67.

121. Glass J, Lanctot KL, Herrmann N, *et al*. Sedative hypnotics in older people with insomnia: meta-analysis of risks and benefits. *BMJ*. 2005; **331**(7526): 1169–75.

122. Young J, Robinson J, Dickinson E. Rehabilitation of older people. *BMJ*. 1998; **316**(7138): 1108–9.

123. Mair A. *Report of Sub-Committee of the Standing Medical Advisory Committee. Scottish Health Service Council on Medical Rehabilitation*. Edinburgh: HMSO; 1972.

124. Calkins DR, Ruberstein LV, Cleary PD. Failure of physicians to recognise functional disability in ambulatory patients. *Ann Intern Med*. 1991; **114**(6): 451–4.

125. Caplan GA, Brown A, Croker WD, *et al*. Risk of admission within 4 weeks of discharge of elderly patients from the emergency department-the DEED study. *Age Ageing*. 1998; **27**(6): 697–702.

126. Caplan GA, Williams AJ, Daly B, *et al*. A randomized, controlled trial of comprehensive geriatric assessment and multidisciplinary intervention after discharge of elderly from the Emergency Department: the DEED II Study. *J Am Geriatr Soc*. 2004; **52**(9): 1417–23.

127. McCusker J, Cardin S, Bellavance F, *et al*. Return to the emergency department among elders: patterns and predictors. *Acad Emerg Med*. 2000; **7**(3): 249–59.

128. Khan SA, Miskelly FG, Platt JS, *et al*. Missed diagnoses amongst elderly patients discharged from an accident and emergency department. *J Accid Emerg Med*. 1996; **13**(4): 256–7.

129. Boyd M, Koziol-McLain J, Yates K, *et al*. Emergency department case-finding for high-risk older adults: the Brief Risk Identification for Geriatrics Health Tool (BRIGHT). *Acad Emerg Med*. 2008; **15**(7): 598–606.

130. McCusker J, Bellavance F, Cardin S, *et al*. Detection of older people at increased risk of adverse health outcomes after an emergency visit: the ISAR screening tool. *J Am Geriatr Soc*. 1999; **47**(10): 1229–37.

131. McCusker J, Verdon J, Tousignant P, *et al*. Rapid emergency department intervention for older people reduces risk of functional decline: results of a multicenter randomized trial. *J Am Geriatr Soc*. 2001; **49**(10): 1272–81.

132. McCusker J, Bellavance F, Cardin S, *et al*. Prediction of hospital utilization among elderly patients during the 6 months after an emergency department visit. *Ann Emerg Med*. 2000; **36**(5): 438–45.

133. Salvi F, Morichi V, Grilli A, *et al*. Predictive validity of the Identification of Seniors at Risk (ISAR) screening tool in elderly patients presenting to two Italian emergency departments. *Aging Clin Exp Res*. 2009; **21**(1): 69–75.

134. Cotter PE, Bhalla VK, Wallis SJ, *et al*. Predicting readmissions: poor performance of the LACE index in an older UK population. *Age Ageing*. 2012; **41**(6): 784–9.

135. Moons P, De Ridder K, Geyskens K, *et al.* Screening for risk of readmission of patients aged 65 years and above after discharge from the emergency department: predictive value of four instruments. *Eur J Emerg Med.* 2007; **14**(6): 315–23.

136. Kansagara D, Englander H, Salanitro A, *et al.* Risk prediction models for hospital readmission: a systematic review. *JAMA.* 2011; **306**(15): 1688–98.

137. Woodford HJ, George J. Intermediate care for older people in the UK. *Clin Med.* 2010; **10**(2): 119–23.

138. Purdy S. *Avoiding Hospital Admissions: what does the research evidence say?* London: The King's Fund; 2010. Available at: www.kingsfund.org.uk/publications/avoiding-hospital-admissions (accessed 22 January 2013).

139. Steventon A, Bardsley M, Billings J, *et al. An Evaluation of the Impact of Community-Based Interventions on Hospital Use.* London: Nuffield Trust; 2011. Available at: www.nuffieldtrust.org.uk/publications/evaluation-impact-community-based-interventions-hospital-use (accessed 22 January 2013).

140. Leong IY, Chan S, Tan B, *et al.* Factors affecting unplanned readmissions from community hospitals to acute hospitals: a prospective observational study. *Ann Acad Med Singapore.* 2009; **38**(2): 113–20.

141. Banks L, Haynes P, Balloch S, *et al. Changes in Communal Provision for Adult Social Care 1991–2001.* York: Joseph Rowntree Foundation; 2006. Available at: www.jrf.org.uk/sites/files/jrf/9781859354865.pdf (accessed 22 January 2013).

142. Office of Fair Trading. *Care Homes for Older People in the UK: a market study.* London: Office of Fair Trading; 2005. Available at: www.oft.gov.uk/shared_oft/reports/consumer_protection/oft780.pdf (accessed 25 January 2013).

CHAPTER 2

Assessment

The frail elderly typically present with multiple problems that have multiple causes. Acute illnesses and decompensated chronic illnesses may present merely as a change in cognitive and functional status. Their assessment needs to be tailored to recognise this. Usually the result is a list of diagnoses or problems, rather than just one. Understanding all of your patient's health and social issues is the key to effective treatment. Assessment of the frail elderly in acute settings can be seen in two parts: the initial evaluation adopts a rapid method to detect immediately life-threatening pathology; the second step, and the ultimate goal during the admission, is to complete a comprehensive geriatric assessment (CGA).

INITIAL RAPID ASSESSMENT

The approach to all severely ill adults, independent of age, should be similar and should target key physiological systems in a systematic fashion. The 'ABCDE' approach is recommended.[1] However, we believe that additional rapid, basic evaluations should be added to this for the frail elderly. We propose an 'ABCDEF' method, with the 'F' standing for Focused Frailty assessment. This process is suitable for when acutely ill patients first arrive in hospital – typically, in the emergency department (ED). The aim is to work through the steps in order and to only move on when problems have been addressed. When possible, any pertinent history should be rapidly gathered along the way.

Airway

Can the patient speak? If so, then his or her airway is patent. Otherwise, check for the absence of breath sounds, or presence of cyanosis or stridor. If any of these are found, then clearly this is an emergency and expert help should be sought. It may require airway intubation. Other, simpler, methods include airway opening techniques, oropharyngeal suction and the use of airway protection devices. The airway of any patient with reduced consciousness is at risk. Laryngoscopy may be difficult because of loose dentition, an inflexible cervical spine (osteoarthritis or atlanto-axial subluxation) or temporomandibular joint disease.[2] Movements of the neck can trigger carotid sinus hypersensitivity, causing bradycardia or syncope (*see* p. 136). Older patients may have loss of airway protective reflexes, which increases the risk of aspiration.[3] The doses of any anaesthetic drugs used may need to be adjusted for the frail elderly.

Breathing

Check oxygen saturations. These should be maintained well above 90% (partial pressure of oxygen in arterial blood >8 kPa), unless the patient is known to have severe chronic obstructive pulmonary disease, where values around 90% (8 kPa) are acceptable. The patient may need high flow oxygen via a re-breathe mask. Check the respiratory rate, which is normally 12–20 per minute. Respiratory rate is a very sensitive marker for acute illness in old age. A very high rate (>30 per minute) is a sign of severe illness. It cannot be sustained for long periods and heralds an abrupt decline in health. A low respiratory rate with low oxygen saturations requires immediate bag and mask ventilation and a call for expert help. Oxygen masks may fit the frail elderly less well due to changes in the facial contour secondary to loss of teeth and bone resorption. In some situations this may be aided by allowing the patient to retain their dentures in place.[3] A rapid chest examination should be performed to detect serious pathology such as a tension pneumothorax or pulmonary oedema. Arterial blood gas sampling may be required.

Circulation

Check the patient's pulse and blood pressure (BP). The usual tachycardic response to hypotension may be absent in those on rate-limiting drugs such as beta-blockers. In states of shock a weak pulse suggests hypovolaemia or cardiac failure, whereas a bounding pulse suggests sepsis. A predominantly low diastolic BP is suggestive of sepsis or anaphylaxis, whereas a narrow pulse pressure suggests hypovolaemia or cardiac failure; however, these are not absolute. Volume loss due to haemorrhage may be concealed (e.g. intrathoracic, abdominal or pelvic), especially after trauma or surgery.

Check the peripheries for colouration, temperature and capillary refill. This latter sign is assessed by pressing on the patient's fingertip held at heart level for 5 seconds. When the pressure is released count the time to return to a normal colour (usually <2 seconds). However, note that reduced capillary refill and extremity temperature may present later in older adults.[2] Listen to the heart sounds, check the jugular venous pressure and look for peripheral oedema. If a urinary catheter is inserted then urine output can be assessed more accurately (this should not be routine care for all elderly patients – *see* p. 90). Oliguria is defined as a urine output <0.5 mL/kg/hour. If a catheter was inserted prior to admission, then note the quantity and quality of any urine in the collection bag. If possible also note the reason for and date of insertion.

Obtain intravenous (iv) access (ideally more than one wide bore cannula in the acutely unwell) and send blood samples to the laboratory for testing, including blood cultures. In severe illness, unless there are signs of fluid overload, it is appropriate to give iv fluids even if the patient is normotensive. However, the frail elderly have a higher risk of overload and smaller fluid boluses (250 mL) are recommended.[2] These can be repeated if no signs of improvement are detected. Aim for a systolic BP >100 mmHg – ideally, to the patient's normal level if this is known. The insertion of a central venous line for monitoring may be required in difficult cases. If signs of fluid overload plus shock are present then seek expert advice on the suitability of inotropes. A raised venous lactate level or unexplained acidosis on arterial blood gas sampling are more sensitive markers of tissue hypo-perfusion.[2]

Disability

Assess the patient's conscious level. This can be rapidly recorded by the AVPU or Glasgow Coma Scale methods. The AVPU scale simply records if the patient is **A**lert, responds to **V**erbal or **P**ainful stimuli, or **U**nresponsive. The Glasgow Coma Scale gives a score between 3 (unresponsive) and 15 (fully alert). It is based on a sum of scores for eye opening (1–4), limb movement (1–6) and verbal response (1–5). In patients with reduced conscious level it is not possible to perform a comprehensive neurological examination. In this situation, the size and reactivity of the pupils, the tone in the limbs and the plantar reflexes are most likely to be helpful. The blood glucose should be checked immediately with a bedside fingerprick test. If possible try to establish if any medications or alcohol have been consumed. This may depend on the presence of someone to give a collateral history.

Exposure

It is traditionally taught to expose as much of the patient as possible to look for additional problems such as hidden injuries or the rash of meningococcal septicaemia. It is not appropriate for ambulance crews to do this in public places. In hospital settings try to respect the dignity of the patient and minimise the risk of heat loss. The frail elderly are at risk of developing pressure areas – particularly over bony prominences such as the heels and sacrum. It is important to record these early in the patient's admission. This can aid the assessment of any change over time and the formulation of an appropriate management plan, including mattress selection. Also, if pressure ulcers are present they may be a source of infection or a sign of previous sub-optimal care that might need to be addressed prior to discharge.

It is important to look at what lies under any bandages, such as those covering leg ulcers. There may be important hidden pathology such as cellulitis. General examination may reveal injuries suggestive of elder abuse (see p. 282).

Frailty

Short of trying to do a complete CGA there are some basic additional components that we believe are an important part of the initial evaluation of the frail elderly. Nationally recommended assessments for all older people in acute settings are to ask about any falls or blackouts in the last year, examine gait and balance, and do a brief cognitive screening test.[4] To this list we would add a rapid evaluation of functional ability, social background and to interview a relative or carer (if available) to establish baseline physical and cognitive function, noting any recent changes.

The essential elements of a short-form CGA that should be completed in the acute setting are:

➤ history – with collaboration from family, carers and/or general practitioner (GP) if necessary
➤ physical examination
➤ cognitive screening test
➤ brief functional or social assessment
➤ gait or balance assessment – especially if considering discharge.

Examples of brief cognitive screening tests that can be performed without any specialised equipment at the patient's bedside include the Six-Item Screener (SIS) and four-question Abbreviated Mental Test (AMT4). These are discussed on page 53. A simple method for assessing gait and balance is the 'get up and go' test (*see* p. 50). Functional ability can be estimated by asking what the patient can normally do at home. For example, can they wash and dress independently, do they do the shopping, cooking and cleaning, or do others assist with these tasks? A simple evaluation of social set-up would include whether they live alone, with others or in a care home. What kind of property do they live in (house, flat or bungalow) and do they have stairs at home, including steps to the front door? It is vital to have this additional information at the start of the patient's spell in an acute setting to be able to understand the extent of their problems and to be able to develop a suitable management plan and estimate prognosis. It need not take long and can be supplemented by more detailed assessments at a later time.

COMPREHENSIVE GERIATRIC ASSESSMENT

CGA is an effective intervention.[5] Its benefits seem to extend to all older patients admitted to hospital.[6] Those receiving CGA are more likely to be alive and living in their own homes a year after admission than control subjects. It seems to work best when delivered by experienced teams in designated geriatric wards. Liaison services that simply make recommendations are less likely to be adhered to and so be successful than direct action from the clinical team delivering care. CGA includes the following items:

➤ medical – including co-morbidities and medication
➤ cognition
➤ mood
➤ nutritional state
➤ functional ability – gait, balance and daily activities
➤ social circumstances – care, finances, home set-up, transport, etc.

In some situations, additional evaluations including formal vision, hearing and chiropody assessments may be required. Clearly, in its complete form this is a time-consuming process that requires the input of many multidisciplinary team members. This is unlikely to be feasible in specialist acute areas such as the ED or medical admissions unit. However, it is not necessary to complete it all at once. The initial components can be completed rapidly in any location. They should be considered mandatory to providing adequate care, especially if the patient is to be discharged without reaching a specialised geriatric unit. A study found that 28% of patients aged over 80 years who were discharged from an ED had missed diagnoses that benefited from intervention.[7] These diagnoses included immobility and dementia. At greatest risk are those who presented with a fall and live alone. Proper evaluation allows for some insight into prognosis. The level of physical function and cognitive status are associated with length of stay and mortality risk.[8]

Of course, assessment in itself is just the start and needs to be linked to action. Interventions may need to be more prolonged than possible in the initial acute setting, but they should start as soon as possible and continue afterwards, either in the patient's own home (e.g. an early supported discharge team) or another location (e.g. a rehabilitation unit).

HISTORY

Taking a history from an older patient is similar to that of younger patients. Good communication skills including open questions and adopting an empathetic style are required. It is not the intention to cover the usual aspects of history taking within this chapter, but instead to highlight specific problems and pitfalls when assessing the frail elderly.

Try to maximise the chances that the patient will be able to give an accurate history. For example, is his or her hearing aid fitted, are his or her ears free of wax and are you using a language the patient understands? Wearing any dentures can make speech clearer. A history collaborated by a carer can be very valuable, but try to have a period free of carers when asking some personal questions, such as on the topic of possible elder abuse (*see* p. 282). Anticipate that there may be several problems, all of which will need to be recorded and evaluated prior to discharge, but some may be prioritised for initial intervention.

Cognitive impairment is common among the acutely admitted frail elderly (*see* p. 105). This may render them unable to give a complete or reliable account of recent events. Also, relevant information about patients' current symptoms and past medical history are often omitted in transfer information for patients being admitted from nursing homes.[9,10] Sometimes the admitting doctor has little initial information to guide them. It is appropriate to record if the patient cannot recall all of the events around the time of admission. However, using the label 'poor historian' to excuse the lack of detail is unacceptable. The effective doctor ensures the patient has the best chance of optimal communication, and asks others if the patient can't tell them (e.g. family, carers, care home staff or GP). This does not have to occur when the patient is first seen if this is the middle of the night, but should occur as soon as practical (i.e. before the morning ward round).

Unhelpful or non-specific language should be discouraged. We suggest avoiding the following terms:

➤ poor historian
➤ social admission
➤ acopia
➤ collapse query cause*
➤ mechanical fall
➤ off legs*
➤ dizziness*
➤ confusion*
➤ ageist labels (e.g. bed-blocker).

It should be noted that several of these terms (marked *) are included in the titles of chapters within this book. Although lacking accuracy, they might be used, prior to evaluation, to describe the patient's presentation (e.g. by someone referring the patient for assessment). The role of the clinician is to move away from these terms towards a differential diagnosis and a subsequent management plan.

Social admissions and 'acopia'

'Social admission' is rarely an accurate term. In the past conditions such as reduced mobility and falls were incorrectly labelled as social problems. Patients do not like coming to hospital unless it is absolutely necessary. Always look for reversible acute conditions that have prevented normal functioning. Patients labelled as having social problems are some of those at highest risk of functional decline or death.[11]

'Acopia' is not a proper word, yet it has come into use by some medics to describe older patients not managing at home, suggesting that there is no acute medical problem.[12] These patients are presenting with a geriatric syndrome (most commonly falls and reduced mobility), and the use of the word acopia reflects only the assessing doctor's failure to recognise this. Thorough evaluation leads to a potentially treatable condition in the vast majority of cases.[13]

A younger person who had been run over by a bus and sustained multiple fractures would not be able to manage at home, but this patient would not be labelled as a 'social admission' or acopia. Just because the very nature of frailty makes patients more prone to the effects of a more minor nudge from pathology does not mean we should belittle their problems or suggest that they are wasting our time.

In one study, 9% of elderly patients (median age, 81 years) presenting to the ED were labelled as social admissions.[14] After medical evaluation, over half of this group were found to have an acute illness, with most of the remainder having chronic conditions. Risk factors for being labelled as a social admission included the failure to measure vital signs, poor recognition of neurological symptoms and atypical presentations of illnesses. Doctors may label patients this way to infer that it is the patient who is causing a problem to the smooth functioning of the healthcare system, rather than acknowledging that the patient's problem is the very reason for existence of the healthcare system.

The specifics of appropriate questioning for common presentations are discussed within the relevant chapters. It is recommended that all frail elderly patients presenting to healthcare services are asked about having had any falls in the last year.[15] A history of two or more falls within the last year should lead to a falls prevention assessment (*see* p. 127).

Pain

Older people have a tendency to underreport pain.[16] When pain is present, ask the patient to define its nature, location and severity. This latter feature can be defined by a simple 0- to 10-point scale, where 0 represents no pain and 10 is the worst pain ever. Those with cognitive impairment may not report pain, but there may be simple visual clues to its presence, for example:

➤ vital signs – tachypnoea, tachycardia, hypertension
➤ appearance – sweating, grimacing, frowning, crying, pacing/wandering
➤ vocalisation – shouting, groaning
➤ mental state – agitated, cognitive decline, irritable, altered sleep pattern.

Paracetamol has very few side effects and is the usual recommended first line therapy in mild/moderate pain.[16] Where this is insufficient to control pain the typical next step in the frail elderly is to add a weak opioid and titrate the dose as required. Non-steroidal anti-inflammatory drugs should usually be avoided in the frail elderly (*see* p. 304). Acute severe pain (e.g. myocardial infarct or hip fracture) is usually best managed by a strong opioid drug.

Medication review

An accurate medication list is essential to provide good care, but older patients are frequently unable to recall this reliably. In a study of people over the age of 65 (mean age, 77 years; mean of 5.9 medications each) presenting to ED, just 43% could name all of their medications, and they got the doses correct 66% of the time.[17] The more medications patients were taking, the less likely they were to be able to name all of them. It is often necessary to call the patient's GP surgery to obtain an accurate list. Of course, this does not mean the patient necessarily takes all of these drugs consistently. With any acute presentation it is important to consider whether the patient's symptoms could be partly or fully explained by an adverse drug reaction. Medications and performing a medication review are discussed in Chapter 11.

Alcohol

Alcohol is more toxic to older people than younger; this is partly due to the reduced proportion of body water and partly due to medication interactions (especially sedatives). Estimates of prevalence vary according to differing diagnostic criteria used. The most commonly used is the CAGE question-naire. Screening tests other than the CAGE are also available, some specifically designed for older patients, but all have limitations.[18,19] Asking about current alcohol intake is probably the best initial screening test in acute settings.

C – Have you ever felt you should **C**ut down on your drinking?

A – Have people ever **A**nnoyed you by criticising your drinking?

G – Have you ever felt **G**uilty about your drinking?

E – Have you ever hand a drink first thing in the morning? (an '**E**ye-opener')

A score of 2 or more is considered positive, suggesting problem drinking.

A prevalence of current alcohol abuse of 12%–14% has been detected in patients aged over 65 presenting to ED (defined as self-reported problem, or CAGE questionnaire positive).[20,21] Another study using Diagnostic and Statistical Manual of Mental Disorders (4th Edition) criteria for alcohol abuse or dependence found a prevalence of 5% in patients aged over 60 presenting to an ED.[22] In hospital in-patients aged 65 and over (median age, 79 years), more than half reported no current alcohol intake, but 9% were positive on the CAGE questionnaire and 7% of admissions were thought to be at least partly related to alcohol intake, with a large majority of these patients being male.[23] Similarly, among geriatric inpatients (mean age, 79 years), around half were current drinkers and 9% had signs of alcohol dependence.[24] However, a UK study judged that only 2% of presentations of patients aged over 70 attending the ED were related to alcohol consumption.[25] A more recent study detected alcohol problems (CAGE positive) in just 1% of patients aged 70 and over on hospital wards.[26]

Some studies have shown an association of alcohol with falls and delirium,[22] but others have not.[20,21,27] Alcohol misuse is associated with psychiatric disorders, especially depression.[22] A consistent finding is that male patients are more commonly affected.[20–24] Some studies have found that those who live alone or who are homeless are at increased risk,[22] but others have not.[21]

The assessment and recording of alcohol use is often suboptimal, being documented on ED charts in just 9% of cases in one series.[21] It is important to evaluate alcohol consumption to appreciate any impact on cognition or falls risk. Although moderate alcohol intake may have a protective effect against the development of dementia, chronic excessive alcohol intake is associated with frontal lobe atrophy and cognitive impairment.[28–30] It also allows for earlier intervention on alcohol withdrawal, vitamin deficiency or malnutrition. Alcohol can exacerbate other conditions including hypertension, arrhythmias, cardiomyopathy, osteoporosis, depression and peripheral neuropathy. High alcohol use may be reduced by brief patient-centred counselling tools.[18]

Social background

Knowing the patient's prior social arrangements is essential for planning discharge and setting rehabilitation goals. The following is a list of some common considerations.

➤ Do they live alone or with others?

➤ Do they live in a private residence (house, flat or bungalow) or a care home (residential or nursing)?

➤ Do they have a care package? If so, how many carers and how often do they come in?

➤ Do they have stairs inside their property, or leading to the front door? If so, do they have a stair lift, is there a downstairs bathroom and would there be space to bring a bed downstairs?

Carer assessment

Carers provide vital support to maintain the frail elderly within their own homes. This can be a physically and mentally challenging role. Some carers are trained staff specifically employed for this task, but many others are untrained and informal providers such as family members or friends. Carer stress can affect their well-being, as well as potentially affecting the person they provide care for. It can trigger hospital or care home admission. Identifying problems allows an opportunity to try and improve the situation. The simple question, 'overall how burdened do you feel?' is a rapid way to screen for problems.[31] Practical solutions may include carer education, providing or increasing an additional formal care package at home, support services (e.g. meals on wheels or transportation), provision of equipment, financial assistance or periods of respite care (in the patient's home, a day centre or a care home).

PHYSICAL EXAMINATION

The principles of good clinical examination in older people are the same as those in younger adults. It is not our intention to describe these in full here. Instead, we wish to highlight the key things to look for in the frail elderly. Given the presence of multiple acute problems and co-morbidities in the frail elderly, it is usually necessary to do a complete physical examination rather than target one or two relevant systems. It is likely that abnormalities will be detected – that is, this is an area of low cost but high gain in clinical medicine.

General examination

Key, but frequently overlooked, areas to examine in the frail elderly include common sites of pressure damage (e.g. sacrum and heels) and skin covered by bandages (e.g. cellulitis around leg ulcers). It should also be noted if there are any injuries that could indicate elder abuse (*see* p. 282). When examining the legs, look for any restrictions in movement. Contractures limiting knee extension by 5 degrees or more are present in two-thirds of nursing home residents (mean age, 83 years; mean contracture, 11 degrees).[32] However, loss of ability to walk may only occur once contractures exceed 30 degrees. Chronic contractures are irreversible. Their presence gives an impression of baseline mobility and future rehabilitation goals. Rectal examination is helpful in assessing non-specific decline or incontinence in the frail elderly (e.g. faecal impaction).

Always see if the patient has a urinary catheter. If present, then try to determine when and why it was inserted. Also, record the quality and quantity of urine in the drainage bag (there is no value in doing a dipstick test, as it will always be abnormal). When checking the BP, consider if a postural test would be helpful (i.e. a measurement when lying down for at least 5 minutes and then serial readings over 3 minutes after standing). A drop of 20 mmHg or more in systolic value, especially if accompanied by symptoms (e.g. light-headedness), may be due to hypovolaemia or autonomic failure and increases the risk of falls and syncope (*see* p. 135).

Neurological signs

Neurological abnormalities are commonly detected in older adults, even those without a known diagnosis of neurological disease.[33] Common examples include reduced ankle jerks and reduced vibration sense in the distal legs – both affecting around 40% of those aged over 85 years. However, these should not be considered as insignificant or 'normal', as such findings are associated with an increased risk of functional or cognitive decline and death.

Tremors are more commonly found in older people. Their assessment should include presence at rest, during actions (e.g. finger–nose movements) and when holding a position (e.g. arms outstretched and fingers spread apart). To reveal subtle resting tremors it is useful to ask the patient to rest their hands upwards on their knees and say the months of the year in reverse order. The key features of common types of tremor are shown in Table 2.1. Bradykinesia can be tested for by asking the patient to rapidly repeat movements such as alternately tapping their index then middle finger on the desk, or opening and closing their fingers into a fist.

TABLE 2.1 Differentiating tremor types

Tremor type	Occurs most commonly	Description	Associated features
Parkinsonian	Rest	Pill-rolling	Bradykinesia and increased tone (see p. 253)
			Usually unilateral onset in idiopathic Parkinson's disease
Essential	Postural/action	Fine	May also affect head, legs and voice
			May have a family history of similar tremors
Cerebellar	Action	Intention	Past-pointing, dysarthria, nystagmus, dysdiadokokinesis and ataxic gait
Physiological	Postural	Fine	May be associated with anxiety, thyrotoxicosis, drug or alcohol withdrawal or medications (e.g. sodium valproate, beta-agonists and lithium)

Visual assessment is also important. Impaired vision has been found in 61% of patients who had sustained a fractured neck of femur.[34] This was most commonly due to cataracts, uncorrected refractive errors and age-related macular degeneration, much of which is potentially treatable. Ensure the patient has their own glasses (or ask a relative to them bring in) and that these have clean lenses. Hearing impairment can be assessed with reasonable accuracy by simple bedside tests such as the ability to hear a whispered voice from 60 cm away.[35] If the patient has a hearing aid, then ensure that it is functioning correctly with working batteries and properly fitted. Look for ear wax and treat with a course of ear drops if detected.

FUNCTIONAL ASSESSMENT

Comparing functional ability at the present time with what is usual for the individual is a key part of assessment. It is also a tool to predict outcomes. A rapid decline in functional ability suggests an underlying disease process. Reduced physical function is a strong predictor of worse outcomes.[36,37] Baseline function is the typical aim for rehabilitation goals and if this is not achieved it may determine a patient's future care needs, yet functional ability is often not assessed in ED settings. In one study of 101 elderly patients (mean age, 82 years) presenting to an ED, 75% of cases had no documentation of any functional abilities.[38]

Basic self-care functional tasks are usually termed activities of daily living and more complex interactions with equipment and the environment termed instrumental activities of daily living. Examples are as follows.

Activities of daily living: bathing, dressing, mobility, continence, feeding.
Instrumental activities of daily living: using the phone, using transport, managing money, shopping, preparing meals, doing housework.

Although more detailed multidisciplinary evaluation may be required during
the stay in hospital, simple screening assessments can be performed at the time
of admission. The most basic evaluation should include enquiring about level
of mobility and usual assistance around the house (e.g. with washing, dressing,
shopping, cooking and cleaning). The level of any support should be quantified
– for example, independent, requiring supervision/prompting, or needing the
assistance of one or two people. Usual continence of both bladder and bowel
should be established, along with any current management strategy. Details
should be corroborated with those who provide assistance. Do things normally
work OK, or were problems apparent before this latest illness? What equipment
or adaptations have previously been provided at home?

Functional ability is best assessed by objective measures. Severe impairments
tend to be detected by clinical judgement, but moderate impairments are poorly
recognised.[39] Self-reported or estimates of functional ability made by family
members or physicians are inaccurate, with a tendency to underestimate problems.[40,41] One commonly used objective assessment scale is the Barthel Index.[42]
Scores are awarded for a range of daily activities including continence, self-care,
mobility and transfers. It ranges from 0 to 20 (sometimes scored as 0–100), with
higher scores suggesting greater functionality and independence. Longer assessment schemes have also been developed but, given the time needed to use them
(i.e. 45 minutes), they are unlikely to be practical in most acute medical settings.[43]
Some service models may use occupational therapists or physiotherapists to
administer functional assessment tools within the ED setting.[44]

The best way to determine a patient's ability to function in their own home
is to assess them at home. This can be done by occupational therapists on home
visits. The type of assessments they make would include ability to get on and off
the toilet, in and out of the bath, prepare drinks and simple meals, and look for
any home hazards such as loose rugs or wires to trip over. They can advise on
and provide or arrange suitable equipment or modifications (see p. 24).

Gait, balance and mobility assessment

Patients are not simply mobile or immobile – there are multiple degrees of mobility. At a basic level this may be the ability to turn in bed, which can reduce the
risk of developing pressure ulcers. The patient may be able to transfer from bed
to chair (or chair to toilet). This may be done independently, with the assistance

of one or two people, or require hoisting. This can have significant implications for discharge planning. Sitting balance is also important (e.g. if planning to use wheelchair or getting the correct seating for home). When able to walk this can be independently, with the assistance of aids (e.g. stick or frame) or with one or two people offering support. These different levels of mobility can be considered as hierarchical – i.e. a patient who can do high level tasks (e.g. walk unaided) will also be able to do lower level tasks (e.g. transfer independently).[45]

Older people can find it hard to stand from low chairs, including toilets. They may need to use a toilet seat raiser device. It is worth watching the patient stand up from sitting. Signs of impaired standing ability include using their arms, the need to shuffle to the edge of the seat and several attempts to rise before succeeding.[45] Patients who fall into chairs when sitting down rather than lowering themselves down are also at risk. The need to get up at night (e.g. nocturia) can affect the discharge of a patient who relies on a carer to assist their transfers and mobility. Some patients rely on holding onto their furniture to get around their home ('furniture walking') rather than using specially designed aids.

A simple assessment of gait and balance is the 'get up and go test'.[46] Here the patient is asked to stand from sitting, walk forwards 3 m, turn around, walk back to the chair and sit down again. The patient can use their normal mobility aid during the assessment. The test can be timed. Longer times (e.g. over 12 seconds) suggest a higher risk of falls. An improvement in time can be used to monitor progress with rehabilitation.

When observing gait look at the patient's steps (note height of foot, length of stride and symmetry), width of stance, reduction in arm swing and any path deviation. Patterns of gait may suggest the underlying pathology – for example, Parkinsonism (loss of arm swing, shuffling steps and stooped posture, possibly with start hesitation, freezing and festination) or cerebrovascular disease (small steps and start hesitation associated with cognitive impairment and urinary incontinence). Subtle gait abnormalities may be seen when asked to do heel–toe walking (also called 'tandem gait'). Rhomberg's test (the ability to maintain standing balance with eyes closed) can be done just after testing gait. A positive result suggests impaired joint position sense, possibly due to peripheral neuropathy. Look for the underlying cause – for example, vitamin B_{12} deficiency. Postural instability may also be assessed (*see* p. 254). Patients with impaired gait or balance should be offered a formal falls risk assessment (*see* p. 127).[15]

COGNITIVE ASSESSMENT

Cognitive impairment has a high prevalence but it is easily overlooked if not specifically tested for (*see* p. 105). However, studies have found low rates of cognitive assessment performed by ED staff. In a group of 319 elderly people (mean age, 76 years), 87% were judged to have had a cognitive assessment that was inadequate to be able to detect delirium.[47] A recent national audit of patients admitted to acute hospitals with dementia found that a standardised mental assessment was carried out in less than half.[48] Assessment is important as deficits are associated with worse outcomes and recognition allows appropriate investigation for reversible causes and effective discharge planning (including capacity assessments). It may also provide some prognostic information regarding recovery from an acute illness.[49]

Quality indicators obtained by consensus agreement for older people presenting to the ED have been defined.[50] These include the following recommendations.

➤ All should have a cognitive assessment performed (unless there is a documented reason why not).

➤ If an abnormality is found, then record if it is acute or chronic.

➤ Consider support and follow-up if discharged home, including assessment to formalise a diagnosis of chronic impairment.

The gold standard for a diagnosis of dementia is a full psychological assessment by a clinical psychologist combined with a full medical assessment including history, examination and investigations, including neuroimaging. Clearly, it is not possible to do this with every older patient but it is reasonable to do a simple cognitive screen combined with a history, examination and focused investigations as part of CGA in all older patients admitted to hospital. In addition, at the time of an acute presentation the patient is likely to have at least a degree of delirium (*see* p. 107), and so the patient's cognitive ability may not accurately reflect his or her true potential. More detailed assessment should wait until a background history has been obtained and delirium has resolved or been excluded.

There are a wide variety of cognitive assessments available to the geriatrician.[51] The ideal test would be brief, sensitive and specific, not require any testing equipment that is not readily available, and be easily remembered to aid routine use during patient assessments. Unfortunately such a test does not currently exist. It is usually necessary to compromise between extent of the testing and the time taken. We recommend that all elderly patients admitted to hospital have a brief cognitive test performed at the time of admission. In those who have abnormalities it is usually necessary to perform a more detailed evaluation later in their stay, when time permits. Some specific assessment tools have also been designed to detect the presence of delirium and these are discussed on page 109. Key cognitive domains are outlined in Table 2.2.

TABLE 2.2 Key cognitive domains

Cognitive domain	Comments
Attention	Ability to focus on a task. It can be simply tested by getting the patient to count backwards from 20 to 1 or to list the months of the year in reverse order. When inattention is present, the rest of the cognitive assessment is hard to interpret.
Memory	Can be classified as short or long term, and semantic (knowledge of the world) or episodic (personal experiences). Simple tests involve giving the patient some information to remember (e.g. a list of objects or an address) and then asking them to repeat it a few minutes later.
Language	Language centres are in the dominant hemisphere (the left in most people). Dysphasia can be expressive (difficulty naming objects) or receptive (difficulty understanding words). Errors may be semantic (a different word in the same category – e.g. pear instead of apple) or phonemic (similar sound – e.g. fox instead of box).
Visuospatial ability	Simple tests include copying interlocking pentagons or the Clock Drawing Test (see p. 55).
Praxis	Apraxia is an inability to perform complex motor tasks despite adequate motor function. For example, dressing apraxia is the inability to get dressed – clothes may be put on in the incorrect way or incorrect order (e.g. pants over trousers). Such deficits may become obvious when assessing functional ability.
Executive function	Includes complex behaviours such as planning and judgement. An example of a simple test is to ask patients to interpret the meanings of proverbs – e.g. 'people in glass houses shouldn't throw stones'.

Prior to assessing cognition it is important to exclude non-confusion problems that limit the ability to perform cognitive tests:
➤ hearing deficits
➤ not speaking the same language
➤ isolated dysphasia (e.g. due to a stroke) – expressive or receptive.

These may have been ruled out during interaction with the patient prior to this stage (e.g. taking the history and doing the physical examination). If in any doubt then get the patient to perform simple tasks in response to verbal commands – for example, touch the bed then point to the ceiling, and to name simple objects (e.g. pen, watch and their component parts – nib, hands and winder).

When taking a history of cognitive impairment explore any problem areas such as forgetfulness, getting lost in familiar environments, difficulty using everyday equipment such as the cooker, managing finances or driving. Another key component is to obtain an account of any changes (and their timescale) from a person who knows the patient (i.e. a friend, relative, carer or GP). This is particularly helpful to distinguish delirium alone from delirium on a background of dementia (*see* p. 106). Tools to formalise the process are available. An example is the Informant Questionnaire on Cognitive Decline in the Elderly, which asks questions about cognitive change over the previous 10 years.[52] Such tests can sometimes be administered over the phone.

Brief screening tests

A really useful brief screening test for use in an emergency care setting is one that can be performed at the patient's bedside in less than 3 minutes. Longer tests, taking around 10 minutes, include the Mini-Mental State Examination (MMSE) and the Montreal Cognitive Assessment (MoCA). These tests offer more coverage of cognitive domains and should be considered during the patient's stay to clarify any detected or suspected deficits. The key properties of commonly used simple tests are shown in Table 2.3. When more detailed evaluations are required it is reasonable to refer the patient to a specialist memory clinic.

TABLE 2.3 Comparison of commonly used simple cognitive tests

Test	Points	Time taken (minutes)	Comments
AMT4	4	1	Rapid to use and requires no equipment
			Limited cognitive domains tested
AMT	10	3	Harder to remember than the AMT4
			Limited cognitive domains tested
SIS	6	2	Rapid to use and requires no equipment
			Limited cognitive domains tested
CDT	Variable	2	Requires pen and paper
			Doesn't test memory
			Less affected by first language
			Many different scoring systems
Mini-Cog	Plus or minus	3	Requires pen and paper
			Adds a memory test to the CDT
			Simply scored as 'positive' or 'negative'
QCS	15	3	Requires some simple calculations to weight the scores
			Limited cognitive domains tested
MMSE	30	10	Requires pen and paper
			Limited cognitive domains tested
MoCA	30	10	Requires pen and printed test sheet (including images)
			Wider range of cognitive domains assessed

Abbreviations: AMT4 = four-question Abbreviated Mental Test, AMT = Abbreviated Mental Test, SIS = Six-Item Screener, CDT = Clock Drawing Test, QCS = Quick Confusion Scale, MMSE = Mini-Mental State Examination, MoCA = Montreal Cognitive Assessment

Mini-Mental State Examination

The MMSE is perhaps the best-known cognitive test. It is a 30-point assessment scale that takes about 10 minutes to perform. Scores of 23 or less for those with education up to high school and of 25 or less for those who underwent higher education are commonly used to indicate significant impairment. The MMSE has both a ceiling and a floor effect, but the main drawback is that it does not have much capacity to test executive function or visuospatial ability which is very important in suspected vascular dementia and dementia with Lewy bodies.

Montreal Cognitive Assessment

The MoCA is also a 30-point assessment scale that takes about 10 minutes to perform. It appears to have a greater sensitivity than the MMSE to detect mild cognitive deficits.[53] It covers a wider range of cognitive domains, including executive and visuospatial ability.

Abbreviated Mental Test Score

The abbreviated mental test score (AMT) is a brief 10-item scale that tests short- and long-term memory and orientation. It also tests attention (counting from 20 to 1) which is important in delirium assessment. A score <8 is the usual cut-off and it takes about 3 minutes to administer. There is also a four-question version of the AMT (AMT4) using the following questions:

1. What year are we in? (1 point)
2. What do we call this place you are in? (1 point)
3. How old are you? (1 point)
4. What is your date of birth? (1 point)

An incorrect answer to any of the four questions suggests the presence of cognitive impairment. It is even quicker to perform and easier for the examiner to remember. Compared to an MMSE score <24, the AMT and AMT4 performed similarly in a population of patients aged 65 or over (mean age, 77 years) attending an ED.[54]

Six-Item Screener

The SIS is also useful in acute assessment. It consists simply of three-word recall and asking the day, month and year. This gives a score between 0 and 6. A score of 4 or less suggests significant cognitive impairment.

➤ Give the patient three objects to remember (e.g. apple, ball, piano) and ask them to repeat them back to ensure they have heard them correctly.
➤ Ask the patient the day of the week. (1 point)
➤ Ask the patient the month. (1 point)

➤ Ask the patient the year. (1 point)

➤ Ask the patient to repeat the three items. (3 points)

The SIS has been used to detect cognitive impairment in older patients in the ED. In a study it was compared with the MMSE (score <24) in 149 elderly patients (mean age 75 years) and found to have a sensitivity of 94% and a specificity of 86%.[55] However, a more recent study of 352 elderly patients (mean age, 77 years) found the sensitivity and specificity (compared to the MMSE <23) to be just 63% and 81%.[56]

Quick Confusion Scale

The Quick Confusion Scale is a six-item test that results in a score between 0 and 15, which has been used to detect cognitive impairment in an ED setting.[57] It consists of memory (5 marks), orientation (6 marks) and attention (4 marks) components. It also does not require the subject to read or write. A score of 11 or below is suggestive of significant cognitive impairment. It takes around 2.5 minutes on average to administer in an ED population aged over 18 years.[57,58] In such a population (mean age, 48 years) it has been shown to have a sensitivity and specificity of 64% and 85% (cut-off, 11 or below) when compared with the MMSE (score 23 or below).[58]

Clock Drawing Test

The Clock Drawing Test (CDT) has been used to screen for cognitive impairment in patients aged over 65 years presenting to the ED.[59] It is an alternative to the language-based tests, and particularly suitable where there are cultural and language issues. The patient is first asked to draw a circle and then put on numbers as though it were a clock face. Finally, they are asked to draw on hands to represent a specific time. The time ten past 11 is typically used, as this tests the patient's capacity to work out that the minute hand should be pointing to the number two rather than ten (an executive function). There are at least 15 different scoring systems for the CDT but the easiest is to score 1 point for each component task (total of 3 points). The CDT takes only 2 minutes to perform and has the advantage of testing visuospatial and executive function.

Mini-Cog

The Mini-Cog test combines a three-word recall test (similar to the SIS) and the CDT. Subjects are classified as having cognitive impairment if they are unable to recall any of the three words or if they recall only one or two words and draw an abnormal clock.

Mental capacity

Mental capacity is a term for a patient's ability to make informed decisions about his or her healthcare and social welfare. Strictly speaking it is not an assessment of cognition, but there is some overlap. An assessment of mental capacity is not a routine part of patient care. It should only be performed when a specific decision has to be made and, wherever possible, this should be done at a time in which the patient is in optimal health.

Capacity is decision specific – that is, lacking capacity on deciding where to live does not automatically mean the patient cannot safely make other decisions about their welfare. In conveying the question whether a person is able to make a decision one should consider whether:

➤ the person has a general understanding of the decision they need to make and only they need to make it

➤ the person has a general understanding of the likely consequence of making or not making the decision

➤ the person is able to understand and 'weigh up' the information relevant to the decision

➤ the person can communicate their decision (e.g. by speech, writing or sign language).

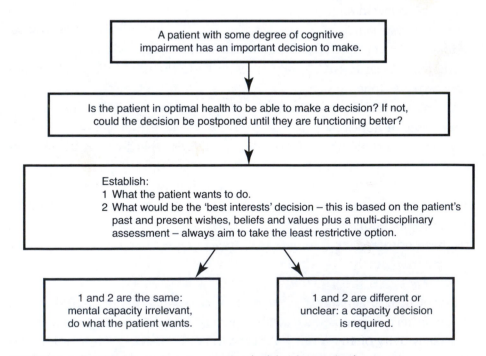

FIGURE 2.1 Establishing when a capacity decision is required

In general, the most likely decision the patient needs to make in an acute ill-ness is the decision to accept treatment in hospital. If the patient does not have capacity, then it may be necessary to treat in his or her best interests, especially if it is an emergency. In terms of place of discharge after hospital treatment, most patients will express a wish to return home and, even if they have limited capacity to make their decision, it can usually be agreed that a trial home discharge with maximum support in place should be the best option.[60] For many decisions the best interests decision and the patient's apparent wishes are the same and capacity is irrelevant (see Figure 2.1). To make a 'best interests' decision it is good practice to consult relatives and carers to help assess the patient's past and present wishes, feelings, beliefs and values.

MOOD ASSESSMENT

Depression is a common co-morbidity in older adults admitted to acute medi-cal services. It is discussed on page 261. Simple screening tests for depression include the Geriatric Depression Scale (GDS). This is available in the original 30-question form and a shortened 15-question version (GDS-15).[61] Of the avail-able depression screening tools, the GDS has the most evidence for efficacy in detecting depression in the hospitalised elderly.[62] The GDS was found to have a sensitivity of 92% and specificity of 89% at a cut-off of 11 compared with psy-chiatric interview in men aged 70 and over presenting to hospital.[63] A cut-off of 6 or more seems suitable for the GDS-15. It is also available in a four-question version that has a reasonably similar performance.[64]

An even shorter alternative is the Patient Health Questionnaire 2.[65] It com-prises two questions:
1. During the last month, have you often been bothered by feeling down, depressed or hopeless?
2. During the last month, have you often been bothered by having little interest or pleasure in doing things?

Answering 'yes' to either question is considered suggestive of depression and should prompt asking three further questions: During the last month have you often been bothered by (1) feelings of worthlessness? (2) poor concentration? (3) thoughts of death? This then should be followed by a comprehensive assess-ment, including a medical assessment and a review of medication.[66] When compared with Diagnostic and Statistical Manual of Mental Disorders (4th Edition) criteria in people aged over 65 years in the community, it was found to have a sensitivity of 100% and specificity of 77% to detect major depression.[67] Compared with the GDS-15, it had a sensitivity of 84% and specificity of 61%

to detect depression in patients aged 70 and over in an ED.[68] This suggests it is a moderately effective screening tool but with low specificity in a hospital setting, and therefore a positive result should always prompt more detailed assessment.

NUTRITIONAL ASSESSMENT

Elderly people are at an increased risk of malnutrition. Around 20%–25% of geriatric inpatients have clear malnutrition, and a further 50% are partially malnourished or at risk.[69] This is due to a combination of factors that may reduce oral intake, changes in bodily composition and the effects of disease (*see* Table 2.4). Protein-energy malnutrition plus immobility results in accelerated rates of muscle loss. This is particularly important in the hospitalised elderly. In order to prevent functional decline it is necessary to ensure both adequate nutritional intake and mobilisation. The early detection of malnutrition is vital. Malnourished patients are at an increased risk of death following hospital admission.[69,70]

TABLE 2.4 Possible reasons for weight loss in the elderly

Factors that reduce oral intake	Dementia
	Depression
	Impaired swallow
	Loss of sense of smell or taste
	Drug side effects (e.g. nausea or dry mouth)
	Reduced access to food (e.g. poor mobility or poverty)
Changes in body composition	Sarcopenia
	Osteoporosis
Effects of disease	Cachexia (e.g. cancer, heart failure or COPD)
	Malabsorption

Abbreviation: COPD = chronic obstructive pulmonary disease

Healthcare staff members are poor at recognising malnutrition based on observation alone.[71] Asking about unintentional weight loss is a simple screening test for malnutrition.[72] Measuring the patient's weight on admission and repeating this during their time in hospital can be a helpful guide. Serum albumin is a poor marker for nutritional status in hospital settings as it tends to fall during severe illnesses such as sepsis or trauma (and as such is an indicator of worse prognosis).[72–74]

Body mass index (BMI) is calculated by dividing the patient's weight in kilograms by their height in metres squared (kg/m^2). Patients with a BMI $<18.5\,kg/m^2$ are considered underweight. The BMI is of limited value when there is oedema, ascites or loss of height due to osteoporotic fractures, and it takes no account of recent weight loss (unless serial measurements are taken). If height cannot be attained (e.g. patients who cannot stand), it can be estimated by measuring ulna length.[75] The role of other anthropometrics, such as skin fold thickness, is unclear. Values such as mid-arm circumference tend to be inaccurate because they require a consistent site of measurement.

A range of nutritional assessment tools has been validated for use in hospitalised patients.[76] Two of the more commonly used are the Malnutrition Universal Screening Tool (MUST) and the Mini Nutritional Assessment (MNA).

The MUST incorporates the BMI plus estimations of recent unintentional weight loss (over the past few months) and the likelihood of reduced oral intake in those who are acutely unwell over the coming five day period (leading to a total score between 0 and 6).[75]

The MNA is a brief screening tool for malnutrition that includes anthropometric measurements (e.g. BMI), dietary assessment and self-reported components (score 0–30, malnutrition defined as <17).[77] It has been found to correlate with nutritional intake of the patient.[78] It is lengthier than the MUST, but a short form (MNA-SF) has been developed (score 0–14, malnutrition defined as <8).[79] When it is not possible to calculate the BMI, calf circumference can be substituted. The MNA is estimated to take 10–15 minutes to complete and the MNA-SF around 4 minutes.[80] Based on MNA scores, the rates of malnutrition in elderly people living in the community (mean age 79) have been found to be 9.5% for men and 5.3% for women.[81] In nursing homes (mean age, 84 years) the respective proportions were 14.4% and 13.5%, and in hospitals (mean age, 82 years) 45.2% and 36.0%, with a large proportion of the rest classified as at risk of malnutrition.

INVESTIGATIONS

Similar to assessing other populations, investigations are usually targeted depending on the clinical features. This can be more challenging in non-specific presentations in the frail elderly. Acute results can also be harder to interpret due to chronic background changes.

Blood tests

Most patients who present acutely unwell to hospital will have basic blood tests performed. Commonly detected abnormalities include hyponatraemia (*see* p. 74), dehydration and anaemia. The higher incidence of diabetes and risk of hypoglycaemia makes testing blood sugar even more important. Many geriatricians consider testing vitamin B_{12}, TSH, calcium and ESR levels as a routine part of care given that abnormalities are sufficiently common and readily correctable.

Some patients with non-specific declines will have had a myocardial infarct that is only apparent by testing troponin levels.

Serum lactate levels can be used as a marker of severe illness (e.g. trauma or sepsis) (*see* p. 177). Blood cultures can allow the earlier detection and targeting of treatment in sepsis. In patients aged over 65 years presenting acutely to hospital, having any of a raised temperature (>38.2°C), hypotension (BP <90 mmHg), raised serum white blood cell count (>18 × 10^9/L), high serum creatinine (>150 umol/L), low serum platelets (<150 × 10^9/L), rigors, vomiting or suspected endocarditis is sufficient to have a reasonable chance of detecting bacteraemia (around 11%, compared with <1% in those without).[82]

Electrocardiogram

ECG recordings are often abnormal in elderly patients. Non-specific presentations can be due to silent myocardial infarcts (*see* p. 226). It is useful to obtain an old ECG whenever possible to allow the identification of new changes.

Urine testing

Urinalysis and urine culture have only limited diagnostic ability in the frail elderly and they should not be performed as part of routine care for unselected patients. This is discussed on page 186.

Chest X-ray

Chest X-rays can be difficult to interpret – for example, because of poor positioning, kyphoscoliosis and poor inspiration (*see* Figure 2.2). They may also miss subtle changes. When compared with high-resolution computed tomography in patients with suspected community-acquired pneumonia, high-resolution computed tomography detected changes in some patients that were not seen on chest X-ray at presentation.[83]

Brain imaging

CT or MRI of the brain can provide valuable diagnostic information in the right situation. The tendency among inexperienced clinicians is to overuse these tests. CT head scans generally have a low yield unless targeted to those with new focal neurological deficits.[84] Their use in the setting of trauma is discussed on page 167 and in the setting of confusion on page 111. They can also be difficult to interpret because of background changes that are commonly seen in the frail elderly, such as white matter lesions (*see* p. 6 and Figure 2.3).

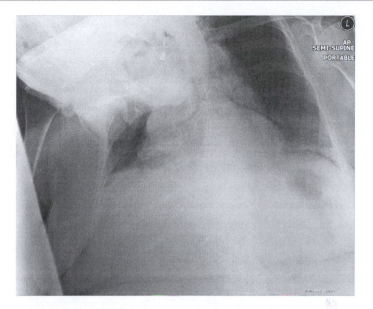

FIGURE 2.2 An example of a difficult to interpret chest X-ray image in a frail elderly patient

Note: The lung fields are incompletely seen because of suboptimal patient positioning (including the patient's overlying edentulous jaw) and a poor inspiration (which is common in those presenting with shortness of breath or cognitive impairment). The film is marked as having been taken with a portable machine, in a semi-supine position and from an anterior–posterior (AP) direction – this is common in acute settings but not ideal for viewing the lungs.

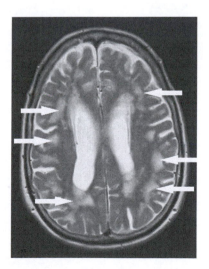

FIGURE 2.3 An MRI brain scan showing extensive white matter lesions (white arrows)

KEY POINTS

- Common diseases often present atypically in the frail elderly and there may be the confounding effects of co-morbidities.
- All assessments should include the essential extras of social, functional and cognitive domains.
- A focused frailty assessment should be completed in the ED as a rapid screen, but the gold standard is GCA completed by a multidisciplinary team.
- A collateral history from someone who knows the patient well is usually very helpful.
- CGA should include the following components: medical (including medication), cognition, mood, nutritional state, functional ability and social circumstances.
- If you do not specifically test all areas then important deficits will be missed and patient care is likely to be suboptimal.
- Quantitative assessment scales are more likely to be accurate than subjective judgements.
- Consider whether presenting features could be due to adverse effects of medications.
- On general examination, look for damage to pressure areas and beneath bandages. Could any injuries give clues to underlying elder abuse?
- Investigations may be harder to interpret in the frail elderly because of background changes from chronic conditions.
- Assessment of frail elderly people is both challenging and rewarding.

REFERENCES

1. American College of Surgeons Committee on Trauma. *Advanced Trauma Life Support for Doctors: instructor course manual.* 6th ed. Chicago, IL: American College of Surgeons; 1997.
2. Marang AT, Sikka R. Resuscitation of the elderly. *Emerg Med Clin N Am.* 2006; **24**(2): 261–72.
3. Buxbaum JL, Schwartz AJ. Perianesthetic considerations for the elderly patient. *Surg Clin North Am.* 1994; **74**(1): 41–58.
4. Department of Health. *Urgent Care Pathways for Older People with Complex Needs.* London: Department of Health; 2007. Available at: www.dh.gov.uk/en/Publicationsandstatistics/Publications/PublicationsPolicyAndGuidance/DH_080135 (accessed 22 January 2013).
5. Stuck AE, Siu AL, Wieland GD, *et al.* Comprehensive geriatric assessment: a meta-analysis of controlled trials. *Lancet.* 1993; **342**(8878): 1032–6.
6. Ellis G, Whitehead MA, Robinson D, *et al.* Comprehensive geriatric assessment for older adults admitted to hospital: meta-analysis of randomised controlled trials. *BMJ.* 2011; **343**: 1034.
7. Khan SA, Miskelly FG, Platt JS, *et al.* Missed diagnoses among elderly patients discharged from an accident and emergency department. *J Accid Emerg Med.* 1996; **13**(4): 256–7.

8. Campbell SE, Seymour DG, Primrose WR. A systematic literature review of factors affecting outcome in older medical patients admitted to hospital. *Age Ageing.* 2004; **33**(2): 110–15.

9. Jones JS, Dwyer PR, White LJ, *et al.* Patient transfer from nursing home to emergency department: outcomes and policy implications. *Acad Emerg Med.* 1997; **4**(9): 908–15.

10. Cwinn MA, Forster AJ, Cwinn AA, *et al.* Prevalence of information gaps for seniors transferred from nursing homes to the emergency department. *CJEM.* 2009; **11**(5): 462–71.

11. Richardson DB. Elderly patients in the emergency department: a prospective study of characteristics and outcome. *Med J Aust.* 1992; **157**(4): 234–9.

12. Obeid JL, Ogle SJ. Acopia: a useful term or not? *Austral J Ageing.* 2000; **19**(4): 195–8.

13. Gonski PN. Acopia: a new DRG? *Med J Aust.* 1997; **167**(8): 421–2.

14. Rutschmann OT, Chevalley T, Zumwald C, *et al.* Pitfalls in the emergency department triage of elderly patients without specific complaints. *Swiss Med Wkly.* 2005; **135**(9–10): 145–50.

15. National Institute for Health and Clinical Excellence. *The Assessment and Prevention of Falls in Older People: NICE guideline 21.* London: NIHCE; 2004. Available at: www.nice.org.uk/CG021 (accessed 22 January 2013).

16. American Geriatrics Society. Pharmacological management of persistent pain in older persons. *J Am Geriatr Soc.* 2009; **57**(8): 1331–47.

17. Chung MK, Bartfield JM. Knowledge of prescription medications among elderly emergency department patients. *Ann Emerg Med.* 2002; **39**(6): 605–8.

18. Culberson JW. Alcohol use in the elderly: beyond the CAGE. Part 2: screening instruments and treatment strategies. *Geriatrics.* 2006; **61**(11): 20–6.

19. O'Connell H, Chin A, Hamilton F, *et al.* A systematic review of the utility of self-report alcohol screening instruments in the elderly. *Int J Geriatr Psychiatry.* 2004; **19**(11): 1074–86.

20. Adams WL, Magruder-Habib K, Trued S, *et al.* Alcohol abuse in elderly emergency department patients. *J Am Geriatr Soc.* 1992; **40**(12): 1236–40.

21. Friedmann PD, Jin L, Karrison T, *et al.* The effect of alcohol abuse on the health status of older adults seen in the emergency department. *Am J Drug Alcohol Abuse.* 1999; **25**(3): 529–42.

22. Onen S, Onen F, Mangeon J, *et al.* Alcohol abuse and dependence in elderly emergency department patients. *Arch Gerontol Geriatr.* 2005; **41**(2): 191–200.

23. Ganry O, Joly J, Queval M, *et al.* Prevalence of alcohol problems among elderly patients in a university hospital. *Addiction.* 2000; **95**(1): 107–13.

24. Lejoyeux M, Delaroque F, McLoughlin M, *et al.* Alcohol dependence among elderly French inpatients. *Am J Geriatr Psychiatry.* 2003; **11**(3): 360–4.

25. van der Pol V, Rodgers H, Aitken P, *et al.* Does alcohol contribute to accident and emergency department attendance in elderly people? *J Accid Emerg Med.* 1996; **13**(4): 258–60.

26. Goldberg SE, Whittamore KH, Harwood RH, *et al.* The prevalence of mental health problems among older adults admitted as an emergency to a general hospital. *Age Ageing.* 2012; **41**(1): 80–6.

27. Nelson DE, Sattin RW, Langlois JA, *et al.* Alcohol as a risk factor for fall injury events among elderly persons living in the community. *J Am Geriatr Soc.* 1992; **40**(7): 658–61.

28. Pfefferbaum A, Sullivan EV, Mathalon DH, *et al.* Frontal lobe volume loss observed with magnetic resonance imaging in older chronic alcoholics. *Alcohol Clin Exp Res.* 1997; **21**(3): 521–9.

29. Thomas VS, Rockwood KJ. Alcohol abuse, cognitive impairment, and mortality among older people. *J Am Geriatr Soc.* 2001; **49**(4): 415–20.

30. Peters R, Peters J, Warner J, *et al.* Alcohol, dementia and cognitive decline in the elderly: a systematic review. *Age Ageing.* 2008; **37**(5): 505–12.

31. Cameron ID, Aggar C, Robinson AL, *et al*. Assessing and helping carers of older people. *BMJ*. 2011; **343**: 630–3.

32. Mollinger LA, Steffen TM. Knee flexion contractures in institutionalized elderly: prevalence, severity, stability, and related variables. *Phys Ther*. 1993; **73**(7): 437–46.

33. Woodford HJ, George J. Neurological and cognitive impairments detected in older people without a diagnosis of neurological or cognitive disease. *Postgrad Med J*. 2011; **87**(1025): 199–206.

34. Squirrell DM, Kenny J, Mawer N, *et al*. Screening for visual impairment in elderly patients with hip fracture: validating a simple bedside test. *Eye (Lond)*. 2005; **19**(1): 55–9.

35. Macphee GJA, Crowther JA, McAlpine CH, *et al*. A simple screening test for hearing impairment in elderly patients. *Age Ageing*. 1988; **17**(5): 347–51.

36. Campbell SE, Seymour DG, Primrose WR, *et al*. A multi-centre European study of factors affecting the discharge destination of older people admitted to hospital: analysis of in-hospital data from the ACME*plus* project. *Age Ageing*. 2005; **34**(5): 467–75.

37. Davis RB, Iezzoni LI, Phillips RS, *et al*. Predicting in-hospital mortality: the importance of functional status information. *Med Care*. 1995; **33**(9): 906–21.

38. Rodriguez-Molinero A, Lopez-Dieguez M, Tabuenca AI, *et al*. Functional assessment of older patients in the emergency department: comparison between standard instruments, medical records and physicians' perceptions. *BMC Geriatr*. 2006: **6**: 1–9.

39. Pinholt EM, Kroenke K, Hanley JF, *et al*. Functional assessment of the elderly: a comparison of standard instruments with clinical judgment. *Arch Intern Med*. 1987; **147**(3): 484–8.

40. Elam JT, Graney MJ, Beaver T, *et al*. Comparison of subjective ratings of function with observed functional ability of frail older persons. *Am J Public Health*. 1991; **81**(9): 1127–30.

41. Calkins DR, Rubenstein LV, Cleary PD, *et al*. Failure of physicians to recognize functional disability in ambulatory patients. *Ann Intern Med*. 1991; **114**(6): 451–4.

42. Mahoney F, Barthel D. Functional evaluation: the Barthel Index. *Md State Med J*. 1965; **14**: 61–5.

43. Veillette N, Demers L, Dutil E, *et al*. Development of a functional status assessment of seniors visiting emergency department. *Arch Gerontol Geriatr*. 2009; **48**(2): 205–12.

44. Lee V, Ross B, Tracy B. Functional assessment of older adults in an emergency department. *Can J Occup Ther*. 2001; **68**(2): 121–9.

45. MacKnight C, Rockwood K. Mobility and balance in the elderly: a guide to bedside assessment. *Postgrad Med*. 1996; **99**(3): 269–76.

46. Podsiadlo D, Richardson S. The timed 'Up & Go': a test of basic functional mobility for frail elderly persons. *J Am Geriatr Soc*. 1991; **39**(2): 142–8.

47. Press Y, Margulin T, Grinshpun Y, *et al*. The diagnosis of delirium among elderly patients presenting to the emergency department of an acute hospital. *Arch Gerontol Geriatr*. 2009; **48**(2): 201–4.

48. Royal College of Psychiatrists. *Report of the National Audit of Dementia Care in General Hospitals*. London: Royal College of Psychiatrists; 2011.

49. Sands LP, Yaffe K, Covinsky K, *et al*. Cognitive screening predicts magnitude of functional recovery from admission to 3 months after discharge in hospitalized elders. *J Gerontol A Biol Sci Med Sci*. 2003; **58**(1): 37–45.

50. Terrell KM, Hustey FM, Hwang U, *et al*. Quality indicators for geriatric emergency care. *Acad Emerg Med*. 2009; **16**(5): 441–9.

51. Woodford HJ, George J. Cognitive assessment in the elderly: a review of clinical methods. *QJM*. 2007; **100**(8): 469–84.

52. Jorm AF, Jacomb PA. The Informant Questionnaire on Cognitive Decline in the Elderly

(IQCODE): sociodemographic correlates, reliability, validity and some norms. *Psychol Med.* 1989; **19**(4): 1015–22.

53. Nasreddine ZS, Phillips NA, Bedirian V, *et al.* The Montreal Cognitive Assessment, MoCA: a brief screening tool for mild cognitive impairment. *J Am Geriatr Soc.* 2005; **53**(4): 695–9.

54. Schofield I, Stott DJ, Tolson D, *et al.* Screening for cognitive impairment in older people attending accident and emergency using the 4-item Abbreviated Mental Test. *Eur J Emerg Med.* 2010; **17**(6): 340–2.

55. Wilber ST, Lofgren SD, Mager TG, *et al.* An evaluation of two screening tools for cognitive impairment in older emergency department patients. *Acad Emerg Med.* 2005; **12**(7): 612–16.

56. Wilber ST, Carpenter CR, Hustey FM. The Six-item Screener to detect cognitive impairment in older emergency department patients. *Acad Emerg Med.* 2008; **15**(7): 613–16.

57. Irons JM, Farace E, Brady WJ, *et al.* Mental status screening of emergency department patients: normative study of the Quick Confusion Scale. *Acad Emerg Med.* 2002; **9**(10): 989–94.

58. Stair TO, Morrissey J, Jaradeh I, *et al.* Validation of the Quick Confusion Scale for mental status screening in the emergency department. *Intern Emerg Med.* 2007; **2**(2): 130–2.

59. Salen P, Heller M, Oller C, *et al.* The impact of routine cognitive screening by using the clock drawing task in the evaluation of elderly patients in the emergency department. *J Emerg Med.* 2009; **37**(1): 8–12.

60. Stewart R, Bartlett P, Harwood RH. Mental capacity assessments and discharge decisions. *Age Ageing.* 2005; **34**(6): 549–50.

61. Sheikh JA, Yesavage JA. Geriatric Depression Scale (GDS): recent findings and development of a shorter version. In: Brink TL, editor. *Clinical Gerontology: a guide to assessment and intervention.* New York, NY: Howarth Press; 1980. pp. 165–73.

62. Dennis M, Kadri A, Coffey J. Depression in older people in the general hospital: a systematic review of screening instruments. *Age Ageing.* 2012; **41**(2): 148–54.

63. Koenig HG, Meador KG, Cohen HJ, *et al.* Self-rated depression scales and screening for major depression in the older hospitalized patient with medical illness. *J Am Geriatr Soc.* 1988; **36**(8): 699–706.

64. Goring H, Baldwin R, Marriott A, *et al.* Validation of short screening tests for depression and cognitive impairment in older medically ill inpatients. *Int J Geriatr Psychiatry.* 2004; **19**(5): 465–71.

65. National Institute for Health and Clinical Excellence. The Treatment and Management of Depression in Adults: NICE guideline 90. London: NIHCE; 2009. Available at: www.nice. org.uk/nicemedia/live/12329/45888/45888.pdf

66. National Institute for Health and Clinical Excellence. Depression in Adults with a Chronic Physical Health Problem: NICE guideline 91. London: NIHCE; 2010. Available at: www. nice.org.uk/CG91

67. Li C, Friedman B, Conwell Y, *et al.* Validity of the Patient Health Questionnaire 2 (PHQ-2) in identifying major depression in older people. *J Am Geriatr Soc.* 2007; **55**(4): 596–602.

68. Hustey FM. The use of a brief depression screen in older emergency department patients. *Acad Emerg Med.* 2005; **12**(9): 905–8.

69. Persson MD, Brismar KE, Katzarski KS, *et al.* Nutritional status using Mini Nutritional Assessment and Subjective Global Assessment predict mortality in geriatric patients. *J Am Geriatr Soc.* 2002; **50**(12): 1996–2002.

70. Liu L, Bopp MM, Roberson PK, *et al.* Undernutrition and risk of mortality in elderly patients within 1 year of hospital discharge. *J Gerontol.* 2002; **57**(11): M741–6.

71. Suominen MH, Sandelin E, Soini H, *et al.* How well do nurses recognize malnutrition in elderly patients? *Eur J Clin Nutr.* 2009; **63**(2): 292–6.

72. Souba WW. Drug therapy: nutritional support. *N Engl J Med.* 1997; **336**: 41–8.

73. Corti M, Guralnik JM, Salive ME, *et al.* Serum albumin level and physical disability as predictors of mortality in older persons. *JAMA.* 1994; **272**(13): 1036–42.

74. Gibbs J, Cull W, Henderson W, *et al.* Preoperative serum albumin level as a predictor of operative mortality and morbidity: results from the National VA Surgical Risk Study. *Arch Surg.* 1999; **134**(1): 36–42.

75. Malnutrition Advisory Group. *Malnutrition Universal Screening Tool.* 2004. www.bapen. org.uk/pdfs/must/must_full.pdf (accessed 22 January 2013).

76. Anthony PS. Nutritional screening tools for hospitalized patients. *Nutr Clin Pract.* 2008; **23**(4): 373–82.

77. Guigoz Y, Vellas B, Garry PJ. Assessing the nutritional status of the elderly: the Mini Nutritional Assessment as part of the geriatric evaluation. *Nutr Rev.* 1996; **54**(1 Pt. 2): S59–65.

78. Vellas B, Guigoz Y, Baumgartner M, *et al.* Relationships between nutritional markers and the Mini-Nutritional Assessment in 155 older persons. *J Am Geriatr Soc.* 2000; **48**(10): 1300–9.

79. Kaiser MJ, Bauer JM, Ramsch C, *et al.* Validation of the Mini Nutritional Assessment short-form (MNA-SF): a practical tool for identification of nutritional status. *J Nutr Health Aging.* 2009; **13**(9): 782–8.

80. Vellas B, Villars H, Abellan G, *et al.* Overview of the MNA: its history and challenges. *J Nutr Health Aging.* 2006; **10**(6): 456–63.

81. Kaiser MJ, Bauer JM, Ramsch C, *et al.* Frequency of malnutrition in older adults: a multinational perspective using the Mini Nutritional Assessment. *J Am Geriatr Soc.* 2010; **58**(9): 1734–8.

82. Shapiro NI, Wolfe RE, Wright SB, *et al.* Who needs a blood culture? A prospectively derived and validated prediction rule. *J Emerg Med.* 2008; **35**(3): 255–64.

83. Syrjala H, Broas M, Suramo I, *et al.* High-resolution computed tomography for the diagnosis of community-acquired pneumonia. *Clin Infect Dis.* 1998; **27**(2): 358–63.

84. Hirano LA, Bogardus ST, Saluja S, *et al.* Clinical yield of computed tomography brain scans in older general medical patients. *J Am Geriatr Soc.* 2006; **54**(4): 587–92.

CHAPTER 3

'Off legs': non-specific functional decline

The purpose of this chapter is to discuss the common causes and potential consequences of non-specific declines in the frail elderly. Although the term 'off legs' has been chosen, non-specific decline could present in other ways, such as 'off food' or simply 'off colour'.

In the past, many elderly patients who were found 'slumped in a chair' in the community have been inappropriately labelled as either having had a stroke or having a urinary tract infection. However, this was more often wrong than right. Appropriate ways to diagnose these two conditions are discussed on pages 207 and 187. Another important factor to consider is whether the patient's presentation could be in part related to his or her medications. Adverse drug reactions are a common reason for hospital admission (*see* p. 298).

ATYPICAL PRESENTATIONS OF DISEASE

The frail elderly frequently present in atypical ways, in that they do not follow the classic textbook descriptions of disease witnessed in younger people. This can be as one of the 'geriatric giants' – falls, confusion, incontinence and immobility.[1] These patterns represent failures of complex functions requiring the integration of multiple systems. Falls and confusion are discussed in their relevant chapters within this book.

There are also many other examples of atypical presentations of diseases in the elderly (*see* Table 3.1), which are also discussed further elsewhere. These differences may be at least partly explained by a higher prevalence of dementia and higher incidence of delirium affecting symptom reporting in the old.[2] One study found that around 40% of frail elderly patients (mean age, 80 years) presented to acute medical services in an atypical way (most commonly with delirium, or non-specific functional decline) and these patients tended to have worse outcomes.[3]

TABLE 3.1 Examples of atypical presentations of common conditions described more frequently in the elderly

Condition	Atypical feature(s)	Cross-reference
Acute coronary syndrome	Absence of chest pain, more likely to present as shortness of breath alone	*See* p. 225
Septicaemia	Absence of pyrexia	*See* p. 176
Urinary tract infection	Absence of urinary tract symptoms, lack of fever	*See* p. 185
Pneumonia	Lack of pleuritic pain, cough and/or fever More likely to have delirium	*See* p. 179
Pulmonary embolus	Absence of pleuritic chest pain and haemoptysis, more commonly present as syncope	*See* p. 235
Perforated peptic ulcer	Absent epigastric pain and tenderness More likely to have shock	*See* p. 157

MALNUTRITION

Malnutrition is associated with worse outcomes. It is estimated that unintentional weight loss of 5% or more over a 1-year period is associated with an increased risk of death.[4] Accepted definitions of malnutrition vary and so the actual prevalence of malnutrition is unknown. It is estimated to affect 5%–10% of elderly adults in the community and 13%–40% of patients acutely admitted to hospital, but it goes unrecognised in around 75% of these cases.[5-7]

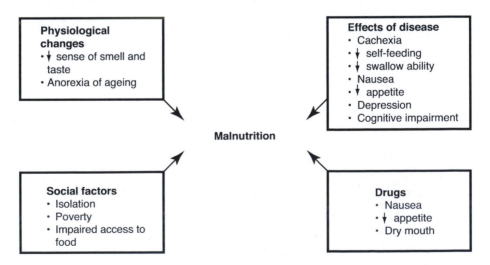

FIGURE 3.1 Causes of malnutrition in the frail elderly

The cause of malnutrition is often multifactorial in the elderly (*see* Figure 3.1). The risk is increased by social isolation, poverty, chronic disease (including cachexia), depression, reduced cognition, poor mobility, poor swallow, and reduced senses of smell and taste, which become commoner. Disease often leads to reduced appetite, self-feeding and swallow ability. Drugs can also cause reduced appetite, nausea, and a dry mouth that can affect swallowing (e.g. anticholinergics). Losing weight during a hospital stay is very common.[6] Many people have a lessened food intake and appetite as they age, often termed the 'anorexia of ageing'. This may explain why around 25% of cases of weight loss have no identifiable cause despite extensive investigation.[4]

Treatment

Hospital care can fall short of acceptable standards regarding nutrition. Common problems include lack of assistance feeding among those who require it, interrupted meal times, lack of specialised diets and poor recording of actual food intake.[8] Effective simple interventions include identifying those patients who require help eating and avoiding doing ward rounds or non-urgent interventions during meal times. Reduced exercise, even if normal nutritional intake is maintained, will result in a reduction in muscle mass. To maintain muscle mass and function it is necessary to promote early mobilisation and the avoidance of 'bed rest'.

Nutritional supplementation does appear to cause a modest degree of weight gain in elderly people at risk of malnutrition, but overall it does not improve mortality rates.[9] However, it does benefit to those who are malnourished. Often there is suboptimal adherence to prescribed supplements, which is likely to be in the range of 15%–50%,[10,11] although even low levels of adherence to supplementation regimens can be associated with significant increases in overall energy intake.[10]

Non-oral enteral feeding is sometimes required for those with reduced oral intake. This is usually via a small-bore nasogastric tube. There is a risk of re-feeding syndrome in those who have gone several days without nutrition, especially if malnourished previously. In this situation the recommencement of feeding can provoke rapid intracellular uptake of potassium, magnesium, calcium and phosphate ions, leading to a fall in serum levels. If untreated, this can cause arrhythmias, neuromuscular dysfunction, confusion and death. The best way to avoid this is to start feeding at a slow rate and to monitor blood tests daily, with replacement of any deficiencies. Percutaneous endoscopic gastrostomy tubes are usually better tolerated than nasogastric tubes but require a minor operation to site them. Total parenteral nutrition is another possible alternative;

however, it has potential harms, high costs, needs to be given via central venous access and the evidence of benefit in the frail elderly is unclear. Enteral nutrition is preferable to the parenteral route whenever possible.[12]

KEY POINTS

- Atypical presentations of disease are common in the elderly and these include non-specific functional declines.
- There are many possible causes, including adverse drug reactions.
- Malnutrition is very common in the hospitalised frail elderly and is often multi-factorial in its aetiology.
- The re-feeding syndrome is a potentially fatal complication of improving nutritional intake. At-risk individuals should restart feeding slowly with close monitoring of serum potassium, magnesium, calcium and phosphate levels.

DEHYDRATION

Elderly people are at an increased risk of dehydration due to reduced fluid intake and increased fluid loss (*see* Figure 3.2). Intake of fluid declines because of reduced thirst sensation and, in some individuals, cognitive impairment. Fluid loss increases secondary to a reduced ability of the kidneys to concentrate urine mediated by reduced aldosterone production and reduced renal response to antidiuretic hormone (ADH), also known as 'vasopressin'. This can be made worse by diuretics or by fever and hyperventilation. The healthy elderly also have a lower proportion of body water to begin with than younger people (*see* p. 3).

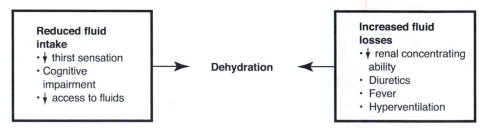

FIGURE 3.2 Common factors leading to dehydration in the frail elderly

Rarely, dehydration will be associated with diabetes insipidus (DI) resulting from reduced ADH activity. This can be due to reduced ADH secretion from the pituitary gland (termed 'neurogenic' or 'central'), which can be provoked by brain trauma, stroke, tumours or infections. DI can also be caused by reduced renal response to ADH (termed 'nephrogenic'). This can be induced by renal disease, lithium, hypokalaemia or hypercalcaemia. DI tends to cause polyuria and polydipsia and the urine osmolality will be low.

Clinical presentation

Features of mild dehydration include dry mouth, tiredness and postural light-headedness. Patients may notice passing small volumes of darkly coloured urine. Dehydration can also lead to constipation (*see* p. 82). Severe dehydration may cause confusion, seizures and reduced consciousness.

Assessment

Clinical signs of dehydration include tachycardia, hypotension, a dry mouth or tongue and a low jugular venous pulse. A low urine output is also a sign of dehydration. In order to excrete the normal daily solute load, a urine output of at least 0.5 mL/kg/hr is required.[13] In acute illness the concentrating ability of the kidney may be impaired, requiring greater urine volumes to maintain a normal balance. Changes in the skin and connective tissues associated with ageing make skin turgor and the appearance of sunken eyes less reliable in determining fluid status in the old. Blood tests are likely to show a raised urea (creatinine may be in the normal range, especially in those with sarcopenia) and haematocrit. The serum sodium concentration may be normal (matched sodium and water losses, e.g. vomiting and diarrhoea), there may be hypernatraemia (water deficit exceeds that of sodium, e.g. fever and reduced oral intake), or hyponatraemia (sodium loss exceeds fluid deficit, e.g. diuretic therapy). A serum sodium concentration >150 mmol/L should always be considered to be due to dehydration in the frail elderly.

Management

Ideally, frail elderly patients will receive adequate hydration to prevent the development of dehydration. Fluids are required both to maintain daily turnover and for the replacement of any excess losses. They can be taken orally or be administered intravenously or subcutaneously. Normal daily losses of fluid are in the region of 1.5–2.5 L per day.[13] 'Insensible' losses such as lung water vapour and sweating can be over 3 L per day in people with febrile illnesses.

Parenteral fluids are available in two main types: (1) crystalloids, which contain low-molecular-weight salts or sugars, and (2) colloids, which contain high-molecular-weight substances (e.g. gelatine, hydroxyethyl starch or albumin). In theory, colloids allow a more sustained expansion of the intravascular volume, but there is no evidence that using colloids for resuscitation improves survival compared with the use of crystalloids.[14] Given they are more expensive, they should not be considered the first-line treatment in the majority of cases. The approximate compositions of commonly used fluids are show in Table 3.2. Dextrose and saline solutions are also available with added potassium (typically 20–40 mmol/L). It is important to try to match the composition of fluid with the deficit that is to be met. When given large volumes of normal saline for fluid resuscitation, the body can struggle to excrete the excess sodium. This poses a risk of hyperchloraemic acidosis and can impair the glomerular filtration rate.

TABLE 3.2 Approximate compositions of commonly used fluids with that of normal bodily plasma for comparison

Type of fluid	Sodium (mmol/L)	Chloride (mmol/L)	Potassium (mmol/L)	Dextrose (mmol/L)	Osmolarity (mOsmol/L)
Plasma	136–145	98–105	3.5–5.0	–	280–300
Normal saline (0.9%)	154	154	–	–	308
Half normal saline (0.45%)	77	77	–	–	154
Dextrose–saline (4%, 0.18%)	30	30	–	223	283
5% Dextrose	–	–	–	280	280
Physiologically balanced solutions (e.g. Hartmann's and Ringer's solutions)	130	110	4–5	–	275
Colloids	145–154	145–154	–	–	290–308

Subcutaneous fluids (hypodermoclysis) can be administered at a rate of up to 1.5 L per 24 hours at a single injection site (this could reach 3 L per day if two sites are used).[15] Suitable sites include the thighs, back, arms and abdominal wall. Typically, normal saline, dextrose–saline or 5% glucose solutions can be used (5% dextrose is more acidic and is more likely to cause skin irritation).[16] Solutions containing potassium at concentrations up to 34 mmol/L have been safely infused but may cause localised irritation.[17] A similar safety and efficacy to iv fluid administration has been reported.[15] Possible adverse effects include localised oedema, erythema, pain and bruising. The benefits include not needing to insert venous cannulae and being less likely to be pulled out by a confused patient (the insertion site can be hidden on the patient's back). This technique is not suitable for severe dehydration or when careful monitoring of intake is required.

ACUTE KIDNEY INJURY

Acute kidney injury (AKI) (previously called acute renal failure) is not clearly defined. It can range in severity from minor changes in renal function up to the requirement for dialysis. It is associated with a three to six times increased risk of death in hospitalised patients.[18] Around 7% of patients develop some degree of renal insufficiency during a hospital admission.[19] It is more common in the elderly and those with pre-existing renal disease.[18-20] Explanations for this include age-related changes of the kidney, a greater number of co-morbidities (e.g. diabetes), greater exposure to potentially harmful medications (polypharmacy), increased risk of dehydration (*see* previous section), urinary obstruction (e.g. prostatic enlargement in men) and a higher prevalence of chronic kidney disease (e.g. secondary to diabetes, hypertension, atherosclerosis or heart failure). A reliance on creatinine levels to estimate renal function is not accurate in the frail elderly because of lower muscle mass related to sarcopenia.

Typical precipitating factors for AKI in the elderly include reduced renal perfusion (e.g. dehydration or cardiac failure), drugs (e.g. non-steroidal anti-inflammatory drugs, gentamicin, angiotensin-converting enzyme inhibitors and diuretics), radiocontrast media, perioperative factors, sepsis and urinary tract obstruction.[19,21] It can also be due to rhabdomyolysis (*see* next section). Cases are often multifactorial in their aetiology. Cardiorenal syndrome is a term for impairment of either cardiac or renal function causing dysfunction in the other system.

The in-hospital mortality for elderly patients with AKI is estimated at 15%–40%.[18] It also carries an increased risk of the future development of chronic kidney disease, and less than half of patients regain their previous renal function after an acute episode.[19,22] It is important to minimise exposure to causative factors in the elderly – i.e. nephrotoxic medications and dehydration.

RHABDOMYOLYSIS

Rhabdomyolysis is the breakdown of striated muscle cells. It can be caused by trauma (typically falling down plus lengthy periods lying on the floor in the frail elderly), prolonged seizures, medications (e.g. statins, antipsychotics (*see* p. 303), drugs with pro-serotinergic effects (*see* p. 260), sedatives and alcohol) or by hyperglycaemic states (*see* p. 266).[23]

Patients may report myalgia and muscular weakness. Diagnosis is based on the finding of very elevated levels of creatine kinase in the blood (typically, >1000 U/L). Urine may appear brown in colour due to containing myoglobin. Urine dipstick tests are usually positive for haemoglobin, even if microscopy does not show any red blood cells due to a false positive result caused by myoglobin.

Myoglobin can precipitate in the kidneys leading to AKI. Muscle cell breakdown also leads to the release of intracellular potassium and phosphate. Blood calcium levels are usually low. Hyperkalaemia and hypocalcaemia can lead to arrhythmias and an ECG should be performed. Such electrolyte disturbances should be managed appropriately (*see* next section).

Renal function should be tested and consideration should be given to inserting a urinary catheter for monitoring urine output. Intravenous (iv) fluids should be prescribed with the aim of maintaining a high urine output (ideally >200 mL/hour). Avoiding the risk of fluid overload may necessitate the insertion of a central line for pressure monitoring, especially in those with a history of heart failure. Severe cases may require temporary renal replacement therapy. In most cases renal function will recover and long-term dialysis is not required.

KEY POINTS

- Frail elderly patients are an increased risk of dehydration.
- Try to select replacement fluids to meet the bodily deficit in fluid and electrolytes.
- Subcutaneous fluid administration can be a safe and effective technique in selected patients.
- The frail elderly are at an increased risk of AKI – it is important to limit exposure to dehydration and nephrotoxic medications.
- A reliance on creatinine levels to estimate renal function is not accurate in the frail elderly because of lower muscle mass related to sarcopenia.
- Rhabdomyolysis can cause AKI – in the frail elderly this is often provoked by falling down and spending a long period lying on the floor.

ELECTROLYTE DISTURBANCES

Sodium

Sodium disorders are common electrolyte disturbances in the acutely ill frail elderly. Advanced age is a risk factor for both hypo- and hypernatraemia.[24]

Hyponatraemia

Hyponatraemia has been found to be present in 15%–30% of acute hospital admissions but is usually mild.[25,26] A serum sodium value to 125 mmol/L or less has been found in 6% of hospitalised elderly medical patients at some stage of their illness.[27] It is associated with worse outcomes.[28]

Clinical features

Mild to moderate hyponatraemia (serum sodium 125–134 mmol/L) is typically asymptomatic but may have subtle effects on gait or cognition in the frail elderly. Mild hyponatraemia (mean value 131 mmol/L) has been associated with a three to four times increased risk of fracture.[29] However, the causality is difficult to establish, as some precipitants of hyponatraemia (e.g. antidepressant drugs) may themselves have effects on cognition and gait. Moderate to severe hyponatraemia (115–124 mmol/L) may provoke nausea, headache and delirium.[25] Severe hyponatraemia (<115 mmol/L) can cause cerebral oedema resulting in seizures or coma, especially if of rapid onset. Symptoms are less profound if the onset is more gradual.

Causes

Hyponatraemia is commonly linked with chest infections, alcohol excess and thiazide diuretics. The mechanism by which alcohol causes hyponatraemia is not well defined and is likely to be due to a diverse range of problems.[30] The stress response to acute illness or surgery can cause sodium and water retention via increased ADH release, elevated catecholamines and activation of the rennin-angiotensin system. It can also be due to inappropriate iv fluid prescription, especially 5% dextrose and dextrose–saline solutions. There are many other potential contributing factors (e.g. chronic proton pump inhibitor drug use) and in the frail elderly it is frequently multifactorial in aetiology. This can make evaluation more challenging. Occasionally it can be confused with pseudo-hyponatraemia due to hyperglycaemia where increased osmolality draws water into the extracellular space. Around 40% of hyponatraemia is secondary to the syndrome of inappropriate antidiuretic hormone (*see* next section) and around 30% is associated with diuretic drug use.[27,29] Key causes can be divided into those associated with a normal intravascular volume of fluid ('euvolaemia'), reduced fluid ('hypovolaemia') or excess fluid ('hypervolaemia').

Euvolaemic hyponatraemia

The main cause of euvolaemic hyponatraemia is the syndrome of inappropriate antidiuretic hormone (SIADH) where elevated levels of ADH subtly increase water retention that leads to low serum sodium levels plus clinical euvolaemia. Other possibilities are hypothyroidism and adrenocortical insufficiency, which need to be excluded before diagnosing SIADH. The common causes of SIADH are shown in Table 3.3. In some cases, no underlying cause is detected (termed idiopathic). This appears to be more common in the elderly, probably because of underlying physiological changes. Some of these patients may have 'reset osmostat syndrome' – here the patient's osmoreceptors have developed a lower threshold to trigger ADH release. Estimates of the frequency of hyponatraemia induced by antidepressants in elderly patients range widely, from 0.5% to 22%.[31,32]

TABLE 3.3 Key causes of the syndrome of inappropriate antidiuretic hormone in the elderly

Cause
Central nervous system disease
Inflammatory lung disease
Cancer (ectopic ADH – e.g. small cell lung cancer, pancreatic cancer, lymphoma)
Drugs: • antidepressants • carbamazepine • less commonly: sodium valproate, ACE inhibitors, and antipsychotics
Idiopathic

Abbreviations: ADH = antidiuretic hormone, ACE = angiotensin-converting enzyme

Hypovolaemic hyponatraemia

Hypovolaemic hyponatraemia is due to excess loss of salt and water typically from the kidney or gastrointestinal tract. It is most frequently due to diuretic drugs, especially thiazides, and may present after the patient has been on the drug for more than a year.[33] It can be due to excessive vomiting or diarrhoea. Bowel purgatives, especially those containing sodium phosphate or magnesium citrate, can also induce profound hyponatraemia in the frail elderly.[34] Polyethylene glycol preparations are probably safer for bowel preparation in this population. Cerebral salt wasting is a term for hyponatraemia due to excessive brain natriuretic factor release, causing urinary sodium and water loss, triggered by a brain insult (e.g. following subarachnoid or intracerebral haemorrhage).

Hypervolaemic hyponatraemia

Hypervolaemic hyponatraemia is seen in some cases of congestive cardiac failure, hepatic cirrhosis, nephrotic syndrome and other low albumin states. The profoundly increased extracellular fluid presents clinically as oedema and ascites. The reduced circulating volume causes the kidneys to conserve water. The amount of total body sodium is elevated but the degree of fluid overload exceeds this. Polydipsia (the oral ingestion of large volumes of water) may also lead to hyponatraemia. This may occur in those with mental health problems, especially if on medications that cause dry mouth. In practice it is a rare cause of hyponatraemia in the frail elderly.

Assessment

The assessment of causation of hyponatraemia begins with a clinical evaluation of fluid status (*see* Figure 3.3). The frequently requested tests of serum and urine osmolality often do not help to distinguish causes of hyponatraemia. Serum osmolality can be estimated by the equation 2× [sodium + potassium] + urea + glucose (with all units as millimoles per litre). It will be low in cases of hyponatraemia unless there are very high values for urea or glucose. Urine osmolality is usually elevated (i.e. greater than the serum value) in all causes of hypovolaemia except polydipsia. Urinary sodium is also often unhelpful, but can be used in cases of hypovolaemia (in patients not on diuretics) to distinguish renal losses (sodium >20 mmol/L) from extrarenal losses (e.g. gastrointestinal tract – sodium <20 mmol/L). However, this may be obvious from the clinical presentation. Urinary sodium is >20 mmol/L in cases of SIADH, and it is typically >40 mmol/L.[35]

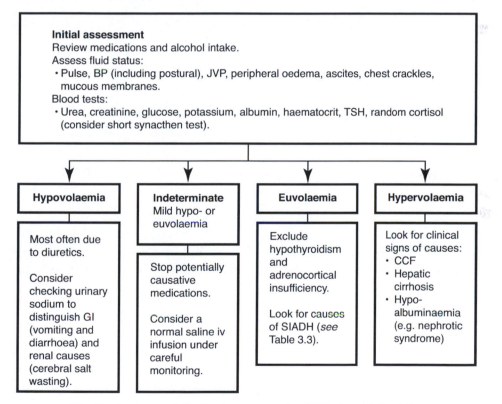

BP = blood pressure, JVP = jugular venous pulse, TSH = thyroid stimulating hormone, GI = gastrointestinal, iv = intravenous, SIADH = syndrome of inappropriate antidiuretic hormone, CCF = congestive cardiac failure.

FIGURE 3.3 The assessment of hyponatraemia in the frail elderly

Before making a diagnosis of SIADH it is necessary to exclude hypothyroidism or adrenocortical insufficiency. This latter problem is usually associated with hyperkalaemia but this is not the case for isolated cortisol deficiency due to hypothalamic-pituitary disease.[25] If there is any doubt then a short synacthen test should be performed.

Clinical assessment may not be able to distinguish some cases of hypovolaemic hyponatraemia from SIADH. In this situation a test infusion of normal saline may be helpful.[36] The plasma sodium concentration typically rises in cases of hypovolaemia, but not SIADH, where instead there is an increase in urinary sodium excretion.

Treatment

The treatment will depend on the underlying cause, and reversible factors should be sought and corrected. The aim is to improve serum sodium levels by no more than 12 mmol/L per 24 hours. This reduces the risk of central pontine myelinolysis – a cause of coma and quadriplegia induced by raid changes in osmolality. If the patient is hypovolaemic then they should be given normal saline. Occasionally, in severe symptomatic cases the very cautious and closely monitored use of hypertonic (3%) saline will be required to correct the sodium deficit. The first-line management of SIADH is fluid restriction (0.8–1.2 L/day).[25] Demeclocycline induces renal tubule resistance to ADH and is a second-line treatment. The vasopressin antagonist tolvaptan may be beneficial in some resistant cases, but its use is currently limited by the high cost of the drug.

Hypernatraemia

Hypernatraemia is typically defined as a serum sodium level >145 mmol/L. Clinical signs of hypernatraemia include irritability, lethargy, muscle twitches, hyperreflexia, hyperpnoea, delirium and coma, but these are only likely to develop with sodium levels >160 mmol/L. It is likely to be associated with evidence of dehydration (e.g. tachycardia and hypotension). It is estimated to have a prevalence of 1%–3% in hospital admissions, with 50% of cases being present at the time of admission and 50% developing during the hospital stay.[37,38] Mortality rates of 40%–60% are reported in the frail elderly, but this is mainly related to underlying causes rather than hypernatraemia itself.[37–39]

Hypernatraemia is very rarely due to excess sodium intake alone, and it is almost always due to reduced body water. This has three causal mechanisms: (1) reduced oral intake, (2) DI (*see* p. 70) or (3) increased fluid losses (e.g. fever). Those with dementia or from nursing homes are at greater risk, which may be partly due to relying on others to obtain adequate oral fluid intake. Those requiring the use of thickened fluids, due to swallowing problems, may find it difficult to drink sufficient fluids. A high oral sodium intake can worsen the problem, which may be due to medications. The World Health Organization recommends an adult sodium intake of no more than 2 g per day, yet eight soluble paracetamol tablets contain 3.4 g of sodium.

The sodium level should be corrected no faster than 10 mmol/L per 24 hours, to avoid the risk of cerebral oedema that can provoke seizures.[40] This is usually best achieved with half normal saline (0.45%) solutions. The volume required to correct the deficit can be estimated by the following equation:

$$\text{Water deficit (L)} = \frac{[\text{sodium}] - 140}{140} \times \text{total body water (L)}$$

(0.5 × weight for elderly man,
0.45 × weight for elderly woman)

The typical recommended aim is to correct half of the water deficit within the first 24 hours of treatment.

Potassium

Hypokalaemia

Hypokalaemia in the frail elderly is usually caused by diuretics (e.g. furosemide or bendroflumethiazide). Occasionally it can be due to dietary deficiency (including being part of the re-feeding syndrome (*see* p. 69)), renal disease or vomiting/diarrhoea. When severe it can lead to generalised muscle weakness. It may also increase the risk of constipation and digoxin toxicity.

Hyperkalaemia

Hyperkalaemia is also commonly caused by drugs, especially potassium-sparing diuretics (e.g. spironalactone or amiloride) and angiotensin-converting enzyme inhibitors. Other possible drug causes include trimethoprim and non-steroidal anti-inflammatory drugs. It can also be induced by acidosis (e.g. renal failure or diabetic ketoacidosis), or by increased release from cells in response to tissue damage (e.g. rhabdomyolysis).

Hyperkalaemia is potentially very dangerous as it increases the risk of cardiac arrhythmias. Assessment includes obtaining an ECG – signs of hyperkalaemia include widening of the QRS complex. Calcium gluconate (e.g. 10 mL of 10% over 5 minutes) can be given to help protect the myocardium. An insulin and glucose infusion can temporarily lower serum potassium levels by causing increased cellular uptake. Longer-term management involves looking for and correcting the underlying cause. Chronic hyperkalaemia secondary to acidosis due to renal failure can be corrected by oral sodium bicarbonate supplementation.

Magnesium

Hypomagnesaemia is more common in the elderly because of lower dietary intake (including the re-feeding syndrome), malabsorption (including chronic diarrhoea), alcoholism, diabetes mellitus and increased renal losses – e.g. renal disease or secondary to diuretic therapy, aminoglycosides or proton pump inhibitors. It often co-exists with hyponatraemia, hypocalcaemia (*see* next section) and hypokalaemia. Hypomagnesaemia has been found to be present in 36% of a cohort of psychogeriatric inpatients (mean age, 78 years).[41] When severe it can cause tremor, ataxia, delirium, muscle cramps, hyperreflexia and seizures. It can also promote cardiac failure and arrhythmias. Mild to moderate deficiency may be corrected by oral supplementation, but symptomatic patients should receive iv magnesium.

Calcium

The normal serum range for calcium is usually quoted as 2.10–2.60 mmol/L, but around half of calcium in the serum is bound to albumin. This latter point means that values need to be adjusted for albumin levels. This is calculated by adding or subtracting 0.02 for every gram that the serum albumin level is below or above 40 g/L, respectively. For example, the corrected calcium value for a patient with a serum calcium value of 1.96 mmol/L and an albumin level of 26 g/L would be 2.24 mmol/L [1.96 + (14 × 0.02)]. Although modern laboratories can measure ionised calcium levels directly.

Hypocalcaemia

Hypocalcaemia in the elderly is most commonly caused by renal failure or vitamin D deficiency (*see* p. 165). Another possibility is hypoparathyroidism. When it develops slowly there are typically no associated symptoms.[42] Occasionally it can present rapidly after parathyroid surgery. It can be associated with rhabdomyolysis. Hypomagnesaemia can also cause hypocalcaemia, as it leads to inhibition of parathyroid hormone (PTH) release. When of more rapid onset or greater severity, patients can develop muscle twitching, spasms, numbness, tetany, seizures and cardiac arrhythmias.

Assessment involves testing blood for levels of calcium, albumin, renal function, vitamin D, PTH, phosphate, alkaline phosphatase and magnesium. Table 3.4 shows the typical pattern of biochemical changes seen in renal failure, vitamin D deficiency and hypoparathyroidism. Symptomatic cases should be treated with iv calcium gluconate. The management of less severe cases should be aimed at correcting the underlying problem (e.g. vitamin D supplementation). If hypomagnesaemia is present, then this should also be treated.

TABLE 3.4 The typical biochemical changes seen in hypocalcaemia caused by renal failure, vitamin D deficiency or hypoparathyroidism

	1,25 hydroxy Vitamin D	PTH	Phosphate	ALP	Creatinine
Renal failure	↓	↑	↑	↑/normal	↑
Vitamin D deficiency	↓	↑	↓/normal	↑/normal	Normal
Hypoparathyroidism	Normal	↓/normal	↑	Normal	Normal

Abbreviations: PTH = parathyroid hormone, ALP = alkaline phosphatase

Hypercalcaemia

Mild hypercalcaemia (up to 2.90 mmol/L) is usually asymptomatic but higher levels lead to polyuria, polydipsia and subsequent dehydration. There may also be constipation, fatigue, generalised weakness and nausea. Severe cases (i.e. >3.50 mmol/L) may lead to vomiting, pancreatitis, delirium and reduced consciousness.

Hyperparathyroidism is the commonest cause of hypercalcaemia, but it is usually mild and asymptomatic.[43] The vast majority of cases are due to parathyroid adenomas. Chronic hyperparathyroidism can lead to the formation of renal calculi and osteoporosis. Another possibility is PTH-related peptide that can be excreted by tumour cells (most often squamous cell carcinomas of the lung, oesophagus or head and neck, or adenocarcinomas of the breast, ovary or kidney).[43] This is the most common form of malignancy-related hypercalcaemia. The other malignancy-related mechanism is via locally invasive lytic bone lesions. Typical causative tumours are multiple myeloma and breast adenocarcinoma. Mild hypercalcaemia can be induced by medications such as calcium and vitamin D supplements or thiazide diuretics. Other causes of hypercalcaemia are rare in the elderly.

In cases of hyperparathyroidism the PTH level will either be elevated or inappropriately within the 'normal' range. Serum phosphate levels are usually depressed in cases of hyperparathyroidism or when due to PTH-related peptide secretion. When hypercalcaemia is related to bone destruction, alkaline phosphatase levels are typically elevated.

Severe or symptomatic hypercalcaemia should be treated by iv normal saline solution to replace the fluid deficit (e.g. 3 L over 24 hours). Once the deficit is corrected, the loop diuretic furosemide can be used to help promote renal calcium loss; iv bisphosphonate infusions (e.g. pamidronate or zoledronate) can be used concurrently with normal saline infusions in severe cases. Other treatment should be directed toward correcting the underlying cause.

KEY POINTS

- Electrolyte abnormalities are common in the frail elderly and can present with a range of non-specific symptoms, which may only be mild if the onset of the electrolyte disturbance is gradual.
- A history and examination are of more value in determining the cause of hyponatraemia than measuring urinary and serum osmolality.
- A serum sodium value of >150 mmol/L suggests dehydration.
- Abnormal sodium levels should be corrected cautiously to reduce the risk of causing harm.
- Electrolyte abnormalities can be part of the re-feeding syndrome.
- Severe hypercalcaemia is caused by hyperparathyroidism or related to malignancy.

CONSTIPATION

Constipation in older people is often precipitated by immobility and dehydration. It can lead to the formation of a mass of hard faeces within the rectum that cannot be easily passed, termed 'faecal impaction'. This can lead to nausea,

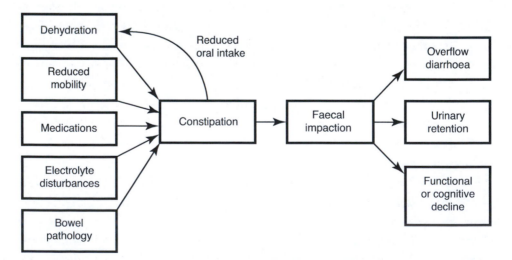

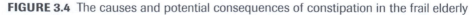

FIGURE 3.4 The causes and potential consequences of constipation in the frail elderly

vomiting, abdominal pain and non-specific functional or cognitive decline. This may result in reduced oral intake and therefore a worsening of the dehydration. The faecal mass can also precipitate overflow diarrhoea and urinary retention, which may lead to incontinence of stool or urine respectively (*see* Figure 3.4). Medications can cause or worsen constipation. Examples include opiates, calcium channel blockers, iron tablets and anticholinergics. Bulk-forming laxatives (e.g. ispaghula husk) can cause faecal impaction if there is insufficient oral fluid intake. Electrolyte disturbances, especially hypokalaemia and hypercalcaemia, can also reduce bowel motility. Bowel disease such as diverticulitis and colonic carcinoma may also cause constipation.

Management

The management of constipation should include correcting dehydration and electrolyte disturbances, reducing or stopping unhelpful medications and improving mobility. It may be necessary to exclude underlying bowel pathology, especially if there is unexplained weight loss or iron deficiency anaemia. In addition, the patient is likely to require laxative medications. There is limited clinical trial evidence to guide best practice.[44,45] Key groups of agents are outlined here.

➤ *Bulking agents* (e.g. ispaghula husk, methylcellulose): can cause faecal impaction in patients who are unable to drink sufficient water.[46] Not typically suitable to treat constipation in the frail elderly.

➤ *Osmotic laxatives* (e.g. lactulose, polyethylene glycol (also called 'macrogol')): lactulose is partially metabolised by bacteria in the large bowel, which can lead to abdominal pain and flatulence. It may also worsen dehydration in those with limited oral intake. Polyethylene glycol solutions do not carry the same risks, but do require the patient to be able to drink large volumes of liquid.

➤ *Stimulant laxatives* (e.g. senna): usually safe and effective in the frail elderly.

➤ *Stool softeners* (e.g. sodium docusate): only limited evidence of efficacy.[47]

➤ *Enemas*: phosphate enemas can cause hyperphosphataemia and hypernatraemia in the frail elderly and are usually best avoided, especially if there is renal impairment.[48] Simple water enemas can be a safer alternative.

➤ *Suppositories* (e.g. glycerol, bisacodyl): unlikely to cause harm but limited evidence of efficacy.

Faecal impaction is usually resolved with a combination of laxatives and enemas. A high-dose polyethylene glycol solution for up to 3 days has been shown to be effective.[49]

INCONTINENCE

Urinary incontinence

Urinary incontinence (UI) is a major cause of morbidity in the frail elderly. A study of community-dwelling adults over the age of 70 years (mean age 77) found that around 19% of women and 9% of men had had an episode of UI in the preceding month.[50] The prevalence of UI in general nursing home patients has been found to be 70%, and it is even more common in those with dementia.[51,52] It is associated with increased risk of functional decline, death, hospitalisation and nursing home placement.[50,53] However, this may be due to its association with cerebral white matter lesions. It is usually of multifactorial causation in older people and this should be reflected in its assessment and management. Appropriate interventions can lessen the impact of the condition, even if it is not possible to provide a cure.

Causes of urinary incontinence

Maintaining continence is a complex process that requires input from multiple bodily systems (*see* Table 3.5). Almost any acute medical illness can precipitate a problem. Ageing itself can be contributory, as bladder contraction is affected by increased collagen deposition, urine-concentrating ability is reduced and a greater proportion of daily urine is formed at night.[54]

TABLE 3.5 Possible factors contributing to urinary incontinence in the elderly

Factor	Examples of pathological processes or unhelpful elements	Affect on continence
Mobility	Neurological disorder (e.g. stroke or Parkinson's disease), arthritis, general functional decline (multiple possible causations)	Unable to access toileting facilities
Cognition	Delirium or dementia	Disinhibition or reduced geographic awareness impairing getting to the toilet appropriately
Sensation	Brain or spinal cord lesions	Reduced awareness of the need to pass urine
Bladder contraction	Brain lesions (e.g. stroke), spinal cord lesions, bladder nerve lesions (e.g. diabetic neuropathy), detrusor muscle overactivity and increased collagen deposition secondary to ageing	May be overactive leading to inappropriate contractions or underactive leading to retention then subsequent overflow of urine
Bladder outflow tract	Benign prostatic hyperplasia, pelvic floor disorders	May be obstructed leading to overflow or prone to leakage in times of pelvic floor stress

Factor	Examples of pathological processes or unhelpful elements	Affect on continence
Environment	Lack of accessible toilet (e.g. stairs), difficulty removing clothes quickly (e.g. arthritis)	Impaired access to toilet
Urine quality and quantity	Diuretics, diabetes, hypercalcaemia, caffeine or alcohol intake, reduced urine-concentrating ability associated with ageing	Polyuria
Nocturia	Peripheral oedema (e.g. heart failure, calcium channel blockers)	Reabsorption of fluid when lying down can increase nocturnal urine formation

Subtypes of urinary incontinence

The following section describes the commonly recognised subtypes of UI, but many cases in the frail elderly have multiple underlying factors and are termed of 'mixed' aetiology.

Urge

Overactive bladder is defined as urinary urgency, with or without incontinence, usually with increased daytime frequency and nocturia. It is more common in older age.[55] Overactive bladder is associated with falls, which may be due to rushing to toilet or perhaps its association with cerebral white matter lesions that are also linked to gait disturbances. Urge UI is due to inappropriate strong contractions of the bladder. This gives the sensation of bladder fullness and the urgent need to pass urine. It is the commonest cause of UI in the institution-alised elderly.[56] Urge UI can be due to a bladder (detrusor) muscle problem, a peripheral nerve or an upper motor neuron lesion affecting the bladder nerves. In the elderly, urge UI is associated with cerebral white matter lesions.[57] This may explain the link between urge UI and cognitive impairment. It is likely to have a different pathological basis in older people compared with younger people. In the elderly it may not truly be 'overactive bladder', but more a case of 'underactive brain'.

Stress

Stress UI is caused by an ineffective bladder outflow tract. Usually it occurs in women and is related to a pelvic floor problem impairing sphincter function. It can occur in men following prostate surgery. Typically, there is leakage of urine following episodes of increased intra-abdominal pressure, such as after cough-ing, sneezing or on postural change. It can be provoked by alpha-adrenergic blocking medications (e.g. prazosin or doxazosin) that impair the sympathetic nerves supplying the bladder neck and urethral smooth muscle.

Overflow

Overflow UI can be caused by an underactive bladder or a blocked bladder outlet tract. The former can be due to lesions of the spinal cord (e.g. multiple sclerosis) or peripheral nerves (e.g. diabetic neuropathy), or it can be due to medications (e.g. anticholinergics). Outflow obstruction is often due to constipation or to prostatic hyperplasia in older men. With any of these causes there tends to be a continuous loss of small amounts of urine. Post-voiding bladder scans will demonstrate large volumes or urine within the bladder (i.e. >200 mL). Rectal examination may reveal the underlying cause.

Functional

Functional UI is a term used to group together factors outside the urinary tract and its innervation that lead to incontinence. Typically, it relates to cognitive, mobility and environmental factors that limit the ability to access appropriate toileting facilities. These are common components in the frail elderly.

Assessment

History

Almost any acute illness can precipitate a functional decline in the frail elderly, and this could provoke UI. This would include UTI; however, there is tendency to overdiagnose UTI (*see* p. 184). Symptoms of duration longer than 1 week are unlikely to be due to UTI. Multiple different causations are likely to co-exist in the frail elderly. It is useful to ask questions to try to identify the predominant subtype of UI. For example:

➤ Do you get the sudden desire to pass water and have to rush to the toilet?
➤ Do you ever leak urine when you cough or sneeze?
➤ Do you constantly leak small amounts of urine?
➤ When you pass water is there a good flow of urine?
➤ How many times do you have to get up during the night to pass water?

The frequency and an estimate of the amount of urine lost may give clues to the cause. This can be aided by the use of a bladder diary, i.e. a recording of frequency and volume. Also, ask how UI is affecting the patient's life and what is their current coping strategy? Have there been associated falls and have they stopped going out? Easily reversible causes should be looked for. These include UTI (e.g. acute onset and associated with dysuria), medications (*see* Table 3.6)[58] and constipation.

TABLE 3.6 Medications that can induce urinary incontinence (UI)

Type of medication	Comments
Anticholinergics (*see* p. 302)	Impair bladder contraction leading to urine retention and possible overflow
	May also affect cognition or mobility
Alpha-adrenergic blockers	Can provoke stress incontinence via urethral sphincter relaxation
Cholinesterase inhibitors	Pro-cholinergic action can provoke urge UI
Sedating medications	For example, benzodiazepines, antipsychotics or opiates
	Can reduce awareness of the need to pass water or impair mobility to the toilet
Constipating medications	For example, calcium channel blockers, anticholinergics or opiates
	May precipitate urinary retention and possible overflow
Oestrogens	Previously thought to be helpful in reducing UI, these drugs have now been associated with an increased risk[58]

Nocturia (getting up at night to pass urine) should be asked about. It needs to be established if the patient does need to get up to pass water or if they simply were awake and decided to get up (i.e. insomnia). It may be induced by other co-morbidities (e.g. the reabsorption of peripheral oedema when lying flat), or it can be a symptom of overactive bladder.

The past medical history may reveal other contributory conditions (e.g. diabetes). It is important to assess social and functional factors that may limit access to toileting facilities. The amount and type of fluids taken should be ascertained, particularly caffeine and alcohol.

Examination

Examination should be thorough, incorporating the elements of comprehensive geriatric assessment (see p. 46). In particular, abdominal examination may reveal a distended bladder or faecally loaded colon. Rectal examination may detect faecal impaction and give an indication of prostate size. Other key elements are the neurological system (including mobility) and cognition. A patient smelling of urine has a combination of UI and reduced personal hygiene. It is not a specific sign of UTI, and when UTI is suspected as an underlying cause it should be diagnosed as discussed on page 187.

Investigations

Blood tests should exclude diabetes and hypercalcaemia. A post-voiding bladder scan should be performed. In older people a residual volume >200 mL suggests urinary retention. Urodynamic studies are sometimes used in the assessment of UI. These include a number of tests that measure urine flow rate and pressures within the bladder and rectum in response to water instilled into the bladder. They are not routinely performed, but they may be appropriate in selected cases under the guidance of specialists, typically when surgical intervention is being considered. They are not suitable for those with cognitive impairment severe enough to make the patient unable to comply with the tests.

Treatment

The multi-factorial nature of incontinence in the frail means that management is typically multifaceted, involving several members of the multidisciplinary team. The process is supported by goal-setting, careful bladder charting and regular review. Specialist nurse continence advisers are also available to help with management strategies. Continence should be promoted while in hospital. Patients should be encouraged and assisted to use toilets or commodes whenever possible. It is inexcusable to tell a patient just to be incontinent in his or her sheets because it is easier to clean the patient up than assist him or her to the toilet, yet there are many reports of this happening. Simple environmental adaptations include bedside commodes or bottles. Clothing with either elasticised or Velcro fasteners can aid rapid toilet access.

Pelvic floor exercises

Pelvic floor muscle training has been used to treat stress, urge and mixed stress–urge incontinence subtypes. It is only suitable for women without significant cognitive impairment. They also need to be highly motivated, as the exercises need to be repeated 30–200 times per day, lifelong. It can produce early benefits, but these may not be maintained.[59]

Bladder training

In bladder training, individuals are taught to control their bladder activity and gradually increase the time interval between micturitions, typically commencing at 30- to 60-minute gaps and extending these by 30 minutes each week. The aim is for 3-hour gaps between toilet visits without UI. It is only suitable for people without significant cognitive impairment. It has been shown to be effective, with a similar size of effect to pelvic floor exercises.[60,61]

Prompted voiding

Prompted voiding is a non-pharmacological option for patients with UI plus cognitive impairment. The patient is asked if he or she would like to go to the toilet at regular intervals during the day (e.g. 2-hourly). It has been used with some success to reduce frequency of UI in nursing home populations, but is not a cure.[62,63] An alternative is 'scheduled toileting'. Here a pattern of taking the patient to the toilet is adopted with regular, pre-specified intervals (e.g. 2-hourly) or planned to coincide with the individual's toileting habit.

Anticholinergic drugs for urge incontinence

Anticholinergic drugs used in the treatment of urge UI act at muscarinic receptors that can be found in bladder muscle. Available drugs include oxybutynin, tolterodine, tropsium, solifencin and darifenacin. A meta-analysis of studies using anticholinergic drugs for overactive bladder found that symptoms were significantly improved compared to placebo, but the effect size was small (0.5 fewer episodes of UI per day).[64] This may be of questionable clinical significance, particularly if the person continues to need to use containment aids such as pads.

Anticholinergic drugs have many potential adverse effects in the frail elderly (*see* p. 302) but dry mouth and constipation are the most commonly reported (affecting around 10%–30%).[55] Perhaps of greater concern is their association with cognitive deterioration and delirium.[65–68] It has been suggested that some anticholinergics may cause fewer cognitive side effects than others, possibly by being less lipophilic and thus less likely to cross the blood–brain barrier, or by being more specific inhibitors of the muscarinic receptors found in bladders (M3) rather than those located in brain tissue (M1 and M2). However, there is currently no robust evidence to support these ideas. There is evidence that anticholinergic drugs can affect brain function even in elderly patients with normal cognition and there are insufficient trial data to assess the safety in those with cognitive impairment.[55,69] Additionally, there is a lack of evidence of efficacy in this latter group.[51,70,71] This may reflect a different or mixed aetiology (i.e. functional or related to brain lesions) rather than overactive bladder in this population.

Given the small clinical benefits seen in the frail elderly and the large potential to cause harm, anticholinergic drugs are not suitable for widespread use. They may be beneficial in some individuals who have urge UI without cognitive impairment, but these two conditions commonly co-exist. They should probably be reserved for cautious use in patients at low risk of harm who fail to respond to non-pharmacological measures.

Surgery for stress incontinence

A variety of surgical procedures have been used in the treatment of stress UI. These include colposuspension that elevates the tissues that surround the lower bladder and upper urethra, which can be performed laparoscopically. Less invasive procedures include the use of tension-free vaginal tape, which probably promotes continence by inducing some urethral kinking.[72]

Containment

Urinary catheters

Urinary catheters are certainly not the first-line management of UI. They are associated with numerous problems, including blockage, infection (*see* p. 188) and interference with sexual activity. Urinary catheters have been found to be inserted in 14% of hospital inpatients aged over 70 years without a good indication,[73] and up to 23% of nursing home residents seen in the ED have a urinary catheter inserted (in addition to 7% with a chronic catheter already *in situ*).[74] Such patients have a greater risk of death and longer average lengths of stay. But occasionally a catheter will be the most appropriate intervention for a particular patient. Such situations may include urinary retention with overflow, times when all other options have failed, patient preference or the need to protect ulcerated skin from further damage.

Good practice in catheter insertion includes recording the reason and urine volume drained within the patient's records. There should also be a plan to remove it if not intended to be permanent. If inserted due to urinary retention (with overflow incontinence), then an underlying cause for the retention should be sought, and constipation should be treated. Consider prostatic enlargement in men – it may be appropriate to try commencing alpha-blocker drugs prior to a trial of catheter withdrawal. Using a catheter with a smaller lumen (larger-bore tubes can impair sphincter closure around them) or the concomitant use of bladder relaxing medication can reduce bypassing of catheters. Mobile patients use a portable 300 mL leg bag. The patient, or his or her carers, will need appropriate education to look after the catheter. In some situations, input from district nurses will be required.

The intermittent passage of a catheter to drain a full bladder is an alternative to having a permanent indwelling device. This is usually self-administered, but it could be performed by a carer. It is associated with a lower infection rate than indwelling devices and has other advantages such as preservation of sexual function, but is not suitable for all. Condom-like external catheters are also available. Their main disadvantage is the difficulty retaining them in position. They may also be associated with skin irritation.

Pads

Typically, body-worn disposable pads are used. Alternatively, bed pads, which are a form of absorbent sheet placed beneath the patient, can be used, but these can impair the correct function of pressure relieving devices or become wrinkled beneath the patient, increasing the risk of pressure damage to skin.

Faecal incontinence

The prevalence of faecal incontinence (FI) varies depending on the population studied and the definition employed. Among community-dwelling people over the age of 65, 3%–7% report either difficulty controlling their bowels or occasional stool leakage.[75,76] The prevalence may be as high as 12% of those aged over 75 years living in their own home.[77] In nursing home populations, the prevalence is around 60%.[52] In this situation it typically co-exists with UI, poor mobility and cognitive impairment. This latter association may be partly related to decreased awareness of the need to defaecate or the presence of disinhibited behaviour. In many cases it is associated with chronic constipation or diarrhoea.[75,77] Diarrhoea can occur as 'overflow' of liquid stools around impacted faeces or secondary to autonomic neuropathy associated with diabetes or Parkinson's disease. A new onset of diarrhoea in a healthcare setting should always raise suspicion of *Clostridium difficile* infection (*see* p. 189). It can also be caused by drugs such as laxatives, proton pump inhibitors, erythromycin and cholinesterase inhibitors. Chronic diarrhoea may also be due to an underlying pathological process such as colonic carcinoma, inflammatory bowel disease, coeliac disease or small bowel bacterial overgrowth. There may be impairment of normal sphincter function seen more commonly in older age.[78] FI increases the risk of nursing home placement.[79]

Assessment

The frequency and consistency of the stools should be established by the use of a stool chart while in hospital (i.e. the Bristol Stool Scale – a visual rating system with scores ranging from 1 (firm) to 7 (watery)). This will help detect any underlying diarrhoea or constipation. Rectal examination can exclude faecal impaction. Cognition and the patient's awareness of the incontinent episodes should be established. There may be mobility or environmental factors that prevent the patient accessing the toilet in time. A stool sample may be appropriate to exclude *C. difficile*. If an underlying bowel disease is suspected then targeted investigations may be necessary. Colonoscopy should be considered if there is a history of change in bowel habit, especially if associated with weight loss or rectal bleeding. When FI is associated with constipation this should be assessed and managed appropriately (*see* p. 82). Medications should be reviewed, including looking for those that may provoke diarrhoea.

Treatment

Treatment should try to improve any associated diarrhoea or constipation. Polyethylene glycol has been shown to be useful in the treatment of faecal impaction.[49] When FI is associated with chronic non-infective diarrhoea, then antimotility agents (e.g. loperamide or codeine) can be tried. Regular toileting at times when the passage of stools is more likely (e.g. following meals) can promote bowel continence.[80] Another option is the alternate use of constipating drugs and enemas – for example, on a thrice-weekly basis. If the patient is aware of the need to pass stools but unable to access the toilet, then simple environmental modifications such as a bedside commode may help. In the frail elderly many cases of FI will persist despite intervention. In this situation containment with pads is the current best option.

KEY POINTS

- Constipation in the frail elderly is usually due to a combination of reduced mobility, dehydration, medications, electrolyte disturbances and bowel pathology.
- Treatment is likely to require laxatives but should also include looking for reversible underlying causes.
- UI in the frail elderly is often multifactorial including problems related to medications and their environment.
- Acute incontinence is likely to be due to problems not related to the urinary tract – look for modifiable risk factors.
- UI is rarely due to UTI.
- Anticholinergic drugs have only limited efficacy and a high probability of causing harm in the frail elderly.
- It is rarely appropriate to use catheters to manage UI.
- In patients with FI look for any underlying diarrhoea or constipation.

PRESSURE ULCERS

Pressure ulcers (PUs) can also be called 'pressure sores', 'bedsores' or 'decubitus ulcers'. They are defined as localised areas of tissue damage resulting from direct pressure on the skin or from shearing forces causing mechanical stress to the tissues. They typically develop in areas of skin overlying a bony prominence that restricts capillary blood flow, resulting in tissue hypoxia, necrosis and breakdown. Ischaemia is likely to develop if the normal capillary pressure of 12–33 mmHg is exceeded for long enough.[81] This process is worsened by a reduction in the natural padding provided by subcutaneous fat associated with poor nutrition. Increased skin moisture also contributes to the development of PU by increasing friction, and also by altering skin integrity through maceration, compromising the natural barrier to infection. PUs occur most commonly on the lower half of the body, particularly over the sacrum (43%), greater trochanter (12%), heel (11%), ischial tuberosities (5%) and lateral malleolus (6%). Risk factors include advanced age, reduced conscious level, immobility, sensory impairment, vascular disease, malnutrition and dehydration.

PUs are described by the European Pressure Ulcer Advisory Panel classification system as four grades (Table 3.7), but progression of the lesions does not always follow this linear pattern.[82]

TABLE 3.7 The grading of pressure ulcers

Grade	Description
1	Non-blanchable erythema of intact skin
2	Partial thickness skin loss
	The ulcer is superficial and presents clinically as an abrasion or blister
3	Full thickness skin loss, including damage to or necrosis of the subcutaneous tissue
4	Extensive destruction, tissue necrosis or damage to muscle, bone or supporting tissues with or without full skin loss

Most PUs arise in hospital, where the prevalence among inpatients is around 3%–14%.[83] Only a fifth develop at home and a further fifth in nursing homes. Seventy per cent of PUs occur in patients aged over 70. PUs are also more commonly seen in patients who have delirium.[84] They result in a fivefold increase in mortality, and the in-hospital mortality of this group is around 25%.[83] It is estimated that a grade four ulcer can cost over £10 000.[85] PUs are often considered to be a ward or nursing problem, but all doctors have a crucial role in preventing and treating them. At the time of admission, the site and stage of any pressure damage should be recorded. The monitoring of progression may be aided by the use of photographs. PUs can indicate an unmet care need that should be addressed prior to discharge.

Prevention

Prevention is dependent on good medical and nursing care. Older patients are at particular risk and attention to hydration, nutrition and skin care is very important immediately on admission. These patients should not be kept waiting on trolleys with no pressure support systems, allowed to become dehydrated and without analgesia. PU formation has been known to occur after time intervals as short as 2 hours. Those with a fractured neck of femur are especially vulnerable, especially in the first few days of admission.[86] Older patients should be mobilised as soon as possible (early mobilisation) rather than merely sat out in a chair (early angulation), which continues to put the patient at risk of PUs. Frequently repositioning of the patient who is restricted to their bed can also reduce his or her risk.

High-risk patients should be identified with the help of one of the prediction scores (e.g. Waterlow or Braden score), to which the doctor should contribute by alerting the nurses to the predisposing medical conditions – for example, diabetes, renal impairment, heart failure, anaemia and peripheral vascular disease.[87,88] Conventional risk scores, however, have a low predictive value, and the National Institute for Health and Clinical Excellence recommends that provision of pressure-relieving devices should be based on an overall assessment of the individual patient, rather than being totally reliant on a risk score.[88,89] Pressure-relieving devices include mattress overlays, special foam mattresses, alternating pressure mattresses and flotation beds.[81] The aim of these devices is to provide equal pressure over the largest possible area, thereby eliminating point pressures and tissue distortion. Alternating pressure systems work by relieving the pressure under different parts of the body in a sequential and cyclical manner. Considerations are availability, ease of use, patient comfort and cost. Unfortunately, there are few randomised controlled trials in the literature comparing different pressure-relieving devices.[81] However, one large randomised study did find that alternating pressure overlays and alternating pressure mattresses were equally effective, although the patients tended to prefer the mattresses.[90]

Treatment

The main principles of treatment are to treat the patient's underlying medical conditions, to relieve pressure, to provide adequate pain control, to ensure adequate protein and calorie intake and to allow the wound to repair by removing any necrotic tissue that may delay healing. The use of zinc and vitamin C supplements, although often used, are not of proven benefit and antibiotics should only be used if there are clinical signs of infection.[91] The National Institute for Health and Clinical Excellence recommends that all patients with grade three or four PUs should be treated with an alternating pressure system.[92] It may be necessary to treat associated infection, which should be suspected if there is surrounding erythema or the characteristic odour of anaerobic organisms. Swabs taken from wounds will always identify bacterial growth and are often unhelpful. Surgical debridement is occasionally suitable for grade three or four ulcers in patients suitable to undergo an operation.

ACCIDENTAL HYPOTHERMIA

Accidental hypothermia is defined as an unintentional fall in core temperature below 35°C. It can be classified as mild (32.2°C –35°C), moderate (32.1°C–28°C) and severe (<28°C). It is primarily a problem of older people, and older patients admitted to hospital with hypothermia have a mortality of over 70%.[93] Normal heat loss occurs through five mechanisms: (1) radiation to the environment (around 55%), (2) evaporation (20%), (3) convection (12%), (4) respiration (10%) and (5) conduction (3%).[94] The hypothalamus controls two body mechanisms of heat conservation: shivering thermogenesis and non-shivering thermogenesis. The first is the heat gain through shivering and the second consists of an increase in metabolic rate. Older people are vulnerable, as their homeostatic capability may decline with age.[95] They are likely to have reduced hypothalamic function, reduced basal metabolic rate (related to sarcopenia) and impaired vasoconstriction ability. Elderly non-ambulatory patients may develop hypothermia at relatively mild cold temperatures, especially if they fall and lie on the floor. Additional factors include reduced heat generation through mobility, which can be made worse by the use of drugs (e.g. antipsychotics) or alcohol. More prevalent endocrine disorders, such as hypothyroidism, may further reduce basal metabolic rate.

Pathophysiology

Initially, heart rate, cardiac output and blood pressure rise, but with decreasing temperature these then decline. Arrhythmias may occur, typically a sinus bradycardia or slow atrial fibrillation then, at very low temperatures, ventricular fibrillation (VF) and asystole. The risk of precipitating VF by tracheal intubation has probably been overstated in the past and relates to lack of pre-oxygenation.[96] In severe hypothermia, VF is extremely resistant to electrical cardioversion and prolonged cardiac resuscitation may be necessary until the patient is sufficiently re-warmed.[96,97] There is no place for prophylactic anti-arrhythmic treatment.[96] The ECG in moderate or severe hypothermia may show a J wave, which is a positive deflection at the ST segment (*see* Figure 3.5).

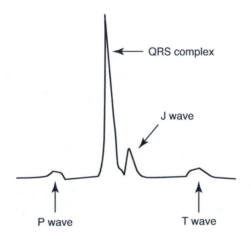

FIGURE 3.5 The appearance of a J wave on ECG

Hypothermia impairs renal concentrating ability and causes a 'cold diuresis', but subsequent acute tubular necrosis may result in a drop in urine output due to poor renal perfusion and possible rhabdomyolysis (*see* p. 73). In mild hypothermia there is an initial tachypnoea followed by a reduction in minute volume and reduced oxygen consumption. Bronchospasm may occur. As the temperature falls to moderate levels of hypothermia, protective airway reflexes are lost and this predisposes to aspiration pneumonia. A direct cooling effect depresses respiratory drive and in severe hypothermia hypoventilation and apnoea can develop. There is a left shift of the oxyhaemoglobin dissociation curve in response to falling temperature which can result in tissue hypoxia.[96] Acidosis can be both respiratory (due to raised partial pressure of carbon dioxide) or metabolic (due to lactic acidosis). The reduced oxygen delivery to the tissues is compensated to some extent by decline in oxygen demand. Both hypokalaemia (due to impairment of the sodium-potassium pump) and hyperkalaemia (due to acidosis) may be present. Hypothermia often causes pancreatitis, which is found at autopsy in 20%–30% of cases.[96] Cold directly inhibits the enzymatic reactions of both intrinsic and extrinsic pathways of the clotting cascade and hence a coagulopathy can develop. The neurological effects of cold are initially mild confusion and amnesia. As the temperature drops, apathy, impaired judgement and paradoxical undressing may occur. Importantly, patients with hypothermia usually do not realise that they are cold, and neither may their carers, and hence it is important to have a low index of suspicion.

Management

As with all older patients presenting to hospital, a full history, including a collateral history and physical examination, is crucial. Temperature should be taken with a low reading tympanic thermometer. Any wet clothing should be removed and the patients covered with blankets. Intubation for airway protection may be required. It is important to consider underlying causes for hypothermia, particularly sepsis, drugs and alcohol, and hypoadrenalism or hypopituitarism. Sometimes hypothermia can mask a cerebral injury – for example, after head trauma that is common in alcohol-dependent patients. A full set of screening investigations should be undertaken (Table 3.8).

TABLE 3.8 Investigations in accidental hypothermia

Investigation
Blood tests:
• electrolytes, urea, creatinine
• liver function tests
• glucose
• amylase
• creatine kinase
• serum lactate
• random cortisol
• thyroid function tests
• full blood count
• clotting screen
• blood cultures
• arterial blood gases
ECG
Chest X-ray

Management is generally supportive with fluid and electrolyte replacement along with re-warming. Sepsis is common in older patients with hypothermia and thought to be a precipitating factor in up to 80% of cases,[98] although it can be difficult to detect because the classic clinical features are not present. It is justified to give broad-spectrum antibiotics if you suspect sepsis, even if the source is not initially obvious. Also older patients who are malnourished, or have a history of alcohol abuse, may be thiamine deficient. There is a risk of developing Wernicke's encephalopathy during re-warming if thiamine deficiency remains uncorrected. Therefore, iv thiamine should be given as routine.[97] Passive re-warming by using warm blankets is sufficient for patients with a body temperature >32°C. Active re-warming methods should be considered for patients with a temperature of 32°C or below – most usually, forced air re-warming blankets (*see* Figure 3.6). Correction should be at the rate of 0.5°C per hour in older people as too rapid re-warming may precipitate arrhythmias and also result in 're-warming acidosis' as pooled lactic acid from the peripheries enters the central circulation.[96] 'Re-warming shock' may also occur because of peripheral vasodilatation causing venous pooling.

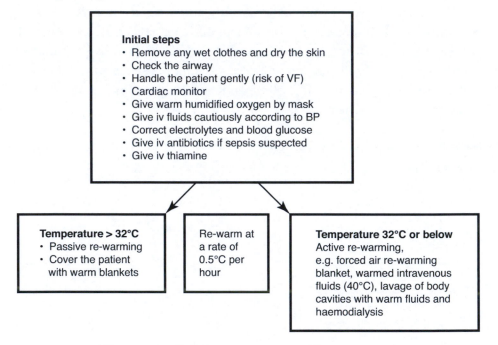

VF = ventricular fibrillation, iv = intravenous, BP = blood pressure.

FIGURE 3.6 The management of hypothermia

Prognosis

The lowest initial temperature recorded in an adult who survived was 13.7°C; this justifies the adage that a patient is not 'dead' until 'warm and dead', and resuscitation may need to continue until the core temperature is at least 30°C.[97] The prognosis of hypothermia depends on the underlying precipitant or cause. Unfortunately, in older people this is often severe sepsis, which has a high mortality when presenting with hypothermia.[98,99]

Prevention

Doctors, nurses and therapists should advise frail older patients on how to keep warm in winter. Older people who are isolated are particularly vulnerable and should be advised to eat well, keep mobile, dress in warm clothes with several layers and wear a hat. A room thermometer in the house is also a good idea.

KEY POINTS

- Always have a high index of suspicion for hypothermia in older people, and routinely measure temperature with a low-reading tympanic thermometer.
- Be alert for an underlying cause for hypothermia (e.g. head injury, hypothyroidism, sepsis, drugs or alcohol).
- Be aware of the complications of too rapid re-warming – acidosis and shock. The patient with severe hypothermia may get worse before they get better.
- Consider broad-spectrum antibiotics if there is any evidence of sepsis.
- The frail elderly are at risk of thiamine deficiency and iv supplementation should be given.
- Institute preventative strategies before discharge for older people who present with hypothermia – e.g. advise about keeping warm, provide a home thermometer, consider a social work referral and provision of a care alarm.

REFERENCES

1. Isaacs B. *The Challenge of Geriatric Medicine*. Oxford: Oxford University Press; 1992.
2. Johnson JC, Jayadevappa R, Baccash PD, *et al*. Nonspecific presentation of pneumonia in hospitalized older people: age effect or dementia? *J Am Geriatr Soc*. 2000; **48**(10): 1316–20.
3. Jarrett PG, Rockwood K, Carver D, *et al*. Illness presentation in elderly patients. *Arch Intern Med*. 1995; **155**(10): 1060–4.
4. Alibhai S, Greenwood C, Payette H. An approach to the management of unintentional weight loss in elderly people. *CMAJ*. 2005; **172**(6): 773–80.
5. McWhirter JP, Pennington CR. Incidence and recognition of malnutrition in hospital. *BMJ*. 1994; **308**(6934): 945–8.
6. Kelly IE, Tessier S, Cahill A, *et al*. Still hungry in hospital: identifying malnutrition in acute hospital admissions. *Q J Med*. 2000; **93**(2): 93–8.
7. Milne AC, Potter J, Vivanti A, *et al*. Protein and energy supplementation in elderly people at risk from malnutrition. Cochrane Database Syst Rev. 2009; 2: CD003288.
8. Care Quality Commission. *Dignity and Nutrition Inspection Programme*. Newcastle upon Tyne: Care Quality Commission; 2011. Available at: www.cqc.org.uk/public/reports-surveys-and-reviews/themes-inspections/dignity-and-nutrition-older-people (accessed 23 January 2013).
9. Milne AC, Potter J, Vivanti A, *et al*. Protein and energy supplementation in elderly people at risk from malnutrition. Cochrane Database Syst Rev. 2009; 2: CD003288.

10. Lawson RM, Doshi MK, Ingoe LE, *et al.* Compliance of orthopaedic patients with postoperative oral nutritional supplementation. *Clin Nutr.* 2000; **19**(3): 171–5.

11. Botella-Carretero JI, Iglesias B, Balsa JA, *et al.* Perioperative oral nutritional supplements in normally or mildly undernourished geriatric patients submitted to surgery for hip fracture: a randomized clinical trial. *Clin Nutr.* 2010; **29**(5): 574–9.

12. Zaloga GP. Parenteral nutrition in adult inpatients with functioning gastrointestinal tracts: assessment of outcomes. *Lancet.* 2006; **367**(9516): 1101–11.

13. Leach R. Fluid management on hospital medical wards. *Clin Med.* 2010; **10**(6): 611–15.

14. Perel P, Roberts I. Colloids versus crystalloids for fluid resuscitation in critically ill patients. Cochrane Database Syst Rev. 2011; 3: CD000567.

15. Remington R, Hultman T. Hypodermoclysis to treat dehydration: a review of the evidence. *J Am Geriatr Soc.* 2007; **55**(12): 2051–5.

16. Barua P, Bhowmick BK. Hypodermoclysis: a victim of historical prejudice. *Age Ageing.* 2005; **34**(3): 215–17.

17. Rochon PA, Gill SS, Litner J, *et al.* A systematic review of the evidence for hypodermoclysis to treat dehydration in older people. *J Gerontol.* 1997; **52**(3): M169–76.

18. Coca SG. Acute kidney injury in elderly persons. *Am J Kidney Dis.* 2010; **56**(1): 122–31.

19. Nash K, Hafeez A, Hou S. Hospital-acquired renal insufficiency. *Am J Kidney Dis.* 2002; **39**(5): 930–6.

20. Yilmaz R, Erdem Y. Acute kidney injury in the elderly population. *Int Urol Nephrol.* 2010; **42**(1): 259–71.

21. Chronopoulos A, Cruz DN, Ronco C. Hospital-acquired acute kidney injury in the elderly. *Nat Rev Nephrol.* 2010; **6**(3): 141–9.

22. Amdur RL, Chawla LS, Amodeo S, *et al.* Outcomes following diagnosis of acute renal failure in U.S. veterans: focus on acute tubular necrosis. *Kidney Int.* 2009; **76**(10): 1089–97.

23. Cervellin G, Comelli I, Lippi G. Rhabdomyolysis: historical background, clinical, diagnostic and therapeutic features. *Clin Chem Lab Med.* 2010; **48**(6): 749–56.

24. Hawkins RC. Age and gender as risk factors for hyponatremia and hypernatremia. *Clin Chim Acta.* 2003; **337**(1–2): 169–72.

25. Thompson CJ, Crowley RK. Hyponatraemia. *J R Coll Physicians Edinb.* 2009; **39**: 154–7.

26. Ball SG. Hyponatraemia. *J R Coll Physicians Edinb.* 2010; **40**(3): 240–5.

27. Shapiro DS, Sonnenblick M, Galperin I, *et al.* Severe hyponatraemia in elderly hospitalized patients: prevalence, aetiology and outcome. *Intern Med J.* 2010; **40**(8): 574–80.

28. Wald R, Jaber BL, Price LL, *et al.* Impact of hospital-associated hyponatremia on selected outcomes. *Arch Intern Med.* 2010; **170**(3): 294–302.

29. Kengne FG, Andres C, Sattar L, *et al.* Mild hyponatremia and risk of fracture in the ambulatory elderly. *Q J Med.* 2008; **101**(7): 583–8.

30. Liamis GL, Milionis HJ, Rizos EC, *et al.* Mechanisms of hyponatraemia in alcohol patients. *Alcohol Alcoholism.* 2000; **35**(6): 612–16.

31. Wilkinson TJ, Begg EJ, Winter AC, *et al.* Incidence and risk factors for hyponatraemia following treatment with fluoxetine or paroxetine in elderly people. *Br J Clin Pharmacol.* 1999; **47**(2): 211–17.

32. Wee R, Lim WK. Selective serotonin re-uptake inhibitors (SSRIs) and hyponatraemia in the elderly. *Int J Geriatr Psychiatry.* 2004; **19**(6): 590–1.

33. Sharabi Y, Illan R, Kamari Y, *et al.* Diuretic induced hyponatraemia in elderly hypertensive women. *J Hum Hypertens.* 2002; **16**(9): 631–5.

34. Frizelle FA, Colls BM. Hyponatremia and seizures after bowel preparation: report of three cases. *Dis Colon Rectum.* 2005; **48**(2): 393–6.

35. Miller M. Hyponatremia and arginine vasopressin dysregulation: mechanisms, clinical consequences, and management. *J Am Geriatr Soc.* 2006; **54**(2): 345–53.
36. Musch W, Decaux G. Utility and limitations of biochemical parameters in the evaluation of hyponatremia in the elderly. *Int Urol Nephrol.* 2001; **32**(3): 475–93.
37. Borra SI, Beredo R, Kleinfeld M. Hypernatremia in the aging: causes, manifestations, and outcome. *J Nat Med Assoc.* 1995; **87**(3): 220–4.
38. Liamis G, Tsimihodimos V, Doumas M. Clinical and laboratory characteristics of hypernatraemia in an internal medicine clinic. *Nephrol Dial Transplant.* 2008; **23**(1): 136–43.
39. Chassagne P, Druesne L, Capet C, *et al.* Clinical presentation of hypernatremia in elderly patients: a case control study. *J Am Geriatr Soc.* 2006; **54**(8): 1225–30.
40. Adrogue HJ, Madias NE. Hyernatremia. *N Engl J Med.* 2000; **342**(20): 1493–9.
41. Arinzon Z, Peisakh A, Schrire S, *et al.* Prevalence of hypomagnesemia (HM) in geriatric long-term care (LTC) setting. *Arch Gerontol Geriatr.* 2010; **51**(1): 36–40.
42. Cooper MS, Gittoes NJL. Diagnosis and management of hypocalcaemia. *BMJ.* 2008; **336**(7656): 1298–302.
43. Inzucchi SE. Understanding hypercalcemia: its metabolic basis, signs, and symptoms. *Postgrad Med.* 2004; **115**(4): 69–76.
44. Petticrew M, Watt I, Brand M. What's the 'best buy' for treatment of constipation? Results from a systematic review of the efficacy and comparative efficacy of laxatives in the elderly. *Br J Gen Pract.* 1999; **49**(442): 387–93.
45. Ram Kumar D, Rao SSC. Efficacy and safety of traditional medical therapies for chronic constipation: systematic review. *Am J Gastroent.* 2005; **100**(4): 936–71.
46. Xing JH, Soffer EE. Adverse effects of laxatives. *Dis Colon Rectum.* 2001; **44**(8): 1201–9.
47. Hurdon V, Viola R, Schroder C. How useful is docusate in patients at risk for constipation? A systematic review of the evidence in the chronically ill. *J Pain Symptom Manage.* 2000; **19**(2): 130–6.
48. Mendoza J, Legido J, Rubio S, *et al.* Systematic review: the adverse effects of sodium phosphate enema. *Aliment Pharmacol Ther.* 2007; **26**(1): 9–20.
49. Culbert P, Gillett H, Ferguson A. Highly effective oral therapy (polyethylene glycol/electrolyte solution) for faecal impaction and severe constipation. *Clin Drug Invest.* 1998; **16**(5): 355–60.
50. Holroyd-Leduc JM, Mehta KM, Covinsky KE. Urinary incontinence and its association with death, nursing home admission, and functional decline. *J Am Geriatr Soc.* 2004; **52**(5): 712–18.
51. Skelly J, Flint AJ. Urinary incontinence associated with dementia. *J Am Geriatr Soc.* 1995; **43**(3): 286–94.
52. Chiang L, Ouslander J, Schnelle J, *et al.* Dually incontinent nursing home residents: clinical characteristics and treatment differences. *J Am Geriatr Soc.* 2000; **48**(6): 673–6.
53. Thom DH, Haan MN, Van Den Eeden SK. Medically recognized urinary incontinence and risks of hospitalization, nursing home admission and mortality. *Age Ageing.* 1997; **26**(5): 367–74.
54. Kirkland JL, Lye M, Levy DW, *et al.* Patterns of urine flow and electrolyte excretion in healthy elderly people. *BMJ.* 1983; **287**(6406): 1665–7.
55. Wagg A, Verdejo C, Molander U. Review of cognitive impairment with antimuscarinic agents in elderly patients with overactive bladder. *Int J Clin Pract.* 2010; **64**(9): 1279–86.
56. Resnick NM, Yalla SV, Laurino E. The pathophysiology of urinary incontinence among institutionalized elderly persons. *N Engl J Med.* 1989; **320**(1): 1–7.
57. Poggesi A, Pracucci G, Chabriat H, *et al.* Urinary complaints in nondisabled elderly people

with age-related white matter changes: the Leukoaraiosis And DISability (LADIS) Study. *J Am Geriatr Soc.* 2008; **56**(9): 1638–43.

58. Ruby CM, Hanlon JT, Boudreau RM, *et al.* The effect of medication use on urinary incontinence in community-dwelling elderly women. *J Am Geriatr Soc.* 2010; **58**(9): 1715–20.

59. Bo K, Kvarstein B, Nygaard I. Lower urinary tract symptoms and pelvic floor muscle exercise adherence after 15 years. *Obst Gyn.* 2005; **105**(5 Pt. 1): 999–1005.

60. Fantl JA, Wyman JF, McClish DK, *et al.* Efficacy of bladder training in older women with urinary incontinence. *JAMA.* 1991; **265**(5): 609–13.

61. Wyman JF, Fantl JA, McClish DK, *et al.* Comparative efficacy of behavioral interventions in the management of female urinary incontinence. *Am J Obstet Gynecol.* 1998; **179**(4): 999–1007.

62. Hu T, Igou JF, Kaltreider L, *et al.* A clinical trial of a behavioural therapy to reduce urinary incontinence in nursing homes: outcome and implications. *JAMA.* 1989; **261**(18): 2656–62.

63. Ouslander JG, Schnelle JF, Uman G, *et al.* Predictors of successful prompted voiding among incontinent nursing home residents. *JAMA.* 1995; **273**(17): 1366–70.

64. Nabi G, Cody JD, Ellis G, *et al.* Anticholinergic drugs versus placebo for overactive bladder syndrome in adults. Cochrane Database Syst Rev. 2006; 4: CD003781.

65. Donnellan CA, Fook L, McDonald P, *et al.* Oxybutynin and cognitive dysfunction. *BMJ.* 1997; **315**(7119): 1363–4.

66. Edwards KR, O'Connor JT. Risk of delirium with concomitant use of tolterodine and acetylcholinesterase inhibitors. *J Am Geriatr Soc.* 2002; **50**(6): 1165–6.

67. Tsao JW, Heilman KM. Transient memory impairment and hallucinations associated with tolterodine use. *N Engl J Med.* 2003; **349**(23): 2274–5.

68. Ancelin ML, Artero S, Portet F, *et al.* Non-degenerative mild cognitive impairment in elderly people and use of anticholinergic drugs: longitudinal cohort study. *BMJ.* 2006; **332**(7539): 445–9.

69. Paquette A, Gou P, Tannenbaum C. Systematic review and meta-analysis: do clinical trials testing antimuscarinic agents for overactive bladder adequately measure central nervous system adverse events? *J Am Geriatr Soc.* 2011; **59**(7): 1332–9.

70. Griffiths DJ, McCracken PN, Harrison GM, *et al.* Urge incontinence in elderly people: factors predicting the severity of urine loss before and after pharmacological treatment. *Neurourol Urodyn.* 1996; **15**(1): 53–7.

71. Lackner TE, Wyman JF, McCarthy TC, *et al.* Efficacy of oral extended-release oxybutynin in cognitively impaired older nursing home residents with urge urinary incontinence: a randomized placebo-controlled trial. *J Am Med Dir Assoc.* 2011; **12**(9): 639–47.

72. Atherton MJ, Stanton SL. The tension-free vaginal tape reviewed: an evidence-based review from inception to current status. *BJOG.* 2005; **112**(5): 534–46.

73. Holroyd-Leduc JM, Sen S, Bertenthal D, *et al.* The relationship of indwelling urinary catheters to death, length of hospital stay, functional decline, and nursing home admission in hospitalized older medical patients. *J Am Geriatr Soc.* 2007; **55**(2): 227–33.

74. Ackermann RJ, Kemle KA, Vogel RL, *et al.* Emergency department use by nursing home residents. *Ann Emerg Med.* 1998; **31**(6): 749–57.

75. Talley NJ, O'Keefe EA, Zinsmeister AR, *et al.* Prevalence of gastrointestinal symptoms in the elderly: a population-based study. *Gastroenterol.* 1992; **102**(3): 895–901.

76. Edwards NI, Jones D. The prevalence of faecal incontinence in older people living at home. *Age Ageing.* 2001; **30**(6): 503–7.

77. Goode PS, Burgio KL, Halli AD, *et al.* Prevalence and correlates of fecal incontinence in community-dwelling older adults. *J Am Geriatr Soc.* 2005; **53**(4): 629–35.

78. Barrett JA, Brocklehurst JC, Kiff ES, *et al.* Anal function in geriatric patients with faecal incontinence. *Gut.* 1989; **30**(9): 1244–51.

79. Grover M, Busby-Whitehead J, Palmer MH, *et al.* Survey of geriatricians on the effect of fecal incontinence on nursing home referral. *J Am Geriatr Soc.* 2010; **58**(6): 1058–62.

80. Hinninghofen H, Enck P. Fecal incontinence: evaluation and treatment. *Gastr Clin North Am.* 2003; **32**(2): 685–706.

81. Young JB. Everyday aids and appliances: aids to prevent pressure sores. *BMJ.* 1990; **300**(6730): 1002–4.

82. Parish LC, Witkowski JA. Controversies about the decubitus ulcer. *Dermatol Clin.* 2004; **22**(1): 87–91.

83. Grey JE, Enoch S, Harding KG. ABC of wound healing: pressure ulcers. *BMJ.* 2006; **332**(7539): 472–5.

84. American Psychiatric Association. Practice guideline for the treatment of patients with delirium. *Am J Psychiatry.* 1999; **156**(5 Suppl.): 1–20.

85. Bennett G, Dealey C, Posnett J. The cost of pressure ulcers in the UK. *Age Ageing.* 2004; **33**(3): 230–5.

86. Versluysen M. How elderly patients with femoral fractures develop pressure sores in hospital. *BMJ.* 1986; **292**(6531): 1311–13.

87. Waterlow J. Pressure sores: a risk assessment card. *Nurs Times.* 1985; **81**(48): 49–55.

88. Braden BJ, Bergstrom N. Predictive validity of the Braden scale for pressure sore risk in a nursing home population. *Res Nurs Health.* 1994; **17**(6): 459–70.

89. Schoonhoven L, Haalboom JRE, Bousema MT, *et al.* Prospective cohort study of routine use of risk assessment scales for prediction of pressure ulcers. *BMJ.* 2002; **325**(7368): 797–81.

90. Nixon J, Cranny G, Iglesias C, *et al.* Randomised controlled trial of alternating pressure mattresses compared with alternating pressure overlays for the prevention of pressure ulcers: PRESSURE trial. *BMJ.* 2006; **332**(7555): 1413.

91. Langer G, Schloemer G, Knerr A, *et al.* Nutritional interventions for preventing and treating pressure ulcers. Cochrane Database Syst Rev. 2003; 4: CD003216.

92. Royal College of Nursing and National Institute for Health and Clinical Excellence. *The Management of Pressure Ulcers in Primary and Secondary Care: a clinical practice guideline.* London: NIHCE; 2005. Available at: www.nice.org.uk/nicemedia/pdf/CG029fullguideline. pdf (accessed 24 January 2013).

93. Muszkat M, Durst RM, Ben-Yehuda A. Factors associated with mortality among elderly patients with hypothermia. *Am J Med.* 2002; **113**(3): 234–7.

94. Caroselli C, Gabrieli A, Pisani A, *et al.* Hypothermia: an under-estimated risk. *Intern Emerg Med.* 2009; **4**(3): 227–30.

95. Epstein E, Anna K. Accidental hypothermia. *BMJ.* 2006; **332**(7543): 706–9.

96. Mallet ML. Pathophysiology of accidental hypothermia. *Q J Med.* 2002; **95**(12): 775–85.

97. McCullough L, Arora S. Diagnosis and treatment of hypothermia. *Am Fam Physician.* 2004; **70**(12): 2325–32.

98. Darowski A, Najim Z, Weinberg JR, *et al.* Hypothermia and infection in elderly patients admitted to hospital. *Age Ageing.* 1991; **20**(2): 100–6.

99. Tiruvoipati R, Ong K, Gangopadhyay H, *et al.* Hypothermia predicts mortality in critically ill elderly patients with sepsis. *BMC Geriatr.* 2010; **10**: 70–4.

CHAPTER 4

Confusion

Confusion is an important problem in acute hospitals in several ways. First, it is a common reason for elderly people to present to services, where a rapid assessment and treatment plan is necessary to aid speedy recovery and reduce the risk of complications. Second, many cases that present differently will be complicated by co-existent confusion. This will have implications both within the acute hospital (e.g. capacity to consent and risk of complications such as falls) and on discharge (e.g. functional ability, concordance with medications and driving). It is also of prognostic significance. Patients with cognitive impairment have worse outcomes (more functional dependence, higher mortality and higher institutionalisation rates) and longer lengths of stay than non-confused patients.[1,2]

Cognitive impairment (acute or chronic) has been found to have a prevalence of 27%–40% in patients aged 65 and over presenting to an emergency department (ED),[3–7] with rates higher in the oldest, probably affecting in excess of 50% of those aged over 85 years.[3] On hospital wards the prevalence in patients over 65 (mean age, 75 years) has been found to be 22% (being 31% on medical wards and 7% on surgical wards).[8] For patients aged 70 and over (mean age, 85 years) on hospital wards a prevalence of 50% has been found.[9] The cognitively impaired are more likely to reside in nursing homes (NHs). Up to 75% of care home residents have dementia.[10]

However, despite the high prevalence, a study found that only 28% of older patients with cognitive impairment had any documentation of this in their ED records, just 18% were referred on for further evaluation, and 37% of patients with delirium were discharged home.[5] A UK dementia audit found that just 43% of patients with known dementia had a cognitive assessment performed at the time of hospital admission.[11] Another study found that less than half of patients with dementia in hospital had previously been diagnosed.[12] Such a failure to recognise this serious health problem is unacceptable. Patients with undetected delirium in the ED are more likely to die in the 6 months after discharge than those whose delirium is detected.[13]

Initial assessment should exclude non-confusion disorders such as dysphasia and deafness. The key causes of cognitive impairment in the frail elderly are delirium and dementia. However, there is much overlap and they commonly co-exist. Occasionally depression can resemble either delirium or dementia (*see* p. 261).

DELIRIUM, DEMENTIA OR BOTH?

There are similarities (e.g. memory impairment) and differences (e.g. speed of onset) between delirium and dementia. Patients with delirium superimposed on dementia are difficult to distinguish clinically from patients with delirium alone.[14] Patients with dementia alone tend to have less impairment of attention and orientation, and they tend to have less alteration of motor activity, affective lability and thought process abnormalities. The development of delirium in patients with dementia is suggested by rapid worsening in cognition, fluctuations in mental status and an altered level of consciousness. As having dementia and developing an acute illness are both risk factors for delirium, it is not surprising that many patients with dementia acutely admitted to hospital will also develop delirium. Table 4.1 compares the key clinical features of these conditions. An elderly patient presenting to medical services with new or worsened confusion should be assumed to have delirium, with or without background dementia, until proven otherwise.

TABLE 4.1 A comparison of the key clinical features of delirium, dementia and a combination of the two

Variable	Delirium	Dementia	Delirium and dementia together
Onset	Rapid (hours/ days)	Gradually progressive (weeks/months)	Abrupt decline on background deficit
Course	Fluctuating	Slow decline	Fluctuating
Impaired short-term memory and visuospatial skills	+	+	+
Reduced attention	+	−	+
Hallucinations or delusions	+	−	+
Psychomotor change (activation or retardation)	+	−	+
Sleep disturbance	+	−	+

Note: + = common, − = uncommon

DELIRIUM

> ### Less helpful terms
>
> Delirium has traditionally been described as a 'clouding of consciousness' coupled with an 'intact sensorium'. However, many people find these terms hard to define or confusing, and so we advise against this definition.
>
> *Clouding of consciousness*: a reduced perception or comprehension of the environment and impaired reaction to external stimuli.
>
> *Intact sensorium*: no impairment of ability to perceive and understand information from the sensory systems.

Clinical features

Delirium is the medical term for an acute confusional state (sometimes called a 'toxic confusional state'). It is due to a metabolic imbalance causing a global impairment of cognitive function. It has three key clinical characteristics:
1. Cognitive impairment – particularly affecting attention
2. Rapid onset
3. Fluctuating severity.

Delirium has a prevalence of around 7%–10% in patients over the age of 65 presenting to an ED,[4,6,15,16] and a prevalence of 16%–18% in elderly patients admitted to an acute medical unit.[17,18] However, only around 28%–35% of cases are detected by the initial assessing doctors.[15,18] A further proportion will go on to develop delirium while in hospital (2%–25%).[17,19,20] Around 13% of patients aged over 65 years develop delirium post-operatively, and this figure rises to 28%–40% following surgery for acute hip fracture.[21-23] The prevalence in a medical intensive therapy unit setting may be as high as 72% in patients aged 65 and over.[24] A further proportion of older patients admitted to hospital will experience a mild reversible cognitive decline that does not fit the diagnostic criteria for delirium.[25] Delirium is not recognised by ED physicians in around 76%–83% of cases and is not initially recognised by the admitting physician in 71% of cases.[16,26] This is unsurprising, given that cognitive assessment is performed in just 29% of older patients admitted to medical units, and often not with formal assessment tools.[17]

Delirium has been described as hypoactive, hyperactive and mixed forms. These variants are usually seen in roughly equal numbers in older hospitalised patients (hypoactive, 24%–29%; hyperactive, 21%–30%; and mixed, 43%–46%).[27,28]

Those with the hypoactive form are less alert with reduced psychomotor activity, and may appear depressed (withdrawn and tearful) or sedated. These cases are more likely to be missed, yet in some studies more common (92% in one study in an ED setting, 71% following surgery for hip fracture).[16,22] These patients tend to have a lower prevalence of delusions and hallucinations, and fewer fluctuations in symptoms.[27] Some studies have found these patients are more likely to develop pressure ulcers, have longer lengths of stay and show higher mortality rates.[28,29] This may be because the hypoactive form presents more commonly in severely ill patients, such as in medical intensive therapy unit settings, where a purely hyperactive form is rare.[24] However, a different study has associated lesser severity and better outcomes with this variant.[22]

Hyperactive cases show increased psychomotor activity and appear anxious or agitated. They may display disruptive behaviours such as wandering, shouting and aggression. This makes them more likely to be recognised by medical staff. They are also more likely to experience falls and be prescribed antipsychotic medications.[28,29] The mixed variety shows a combination of the above subtypes at different stages of their illness.

Causes of delirium

Delirium usually occurs in susceptible individuals exposed to precipitating circumstances. The more frail the individual, the more minor the insult required to provoke it. Typically there are a number of both underlying risk factors and likely precipitants in any delirious elderly individual (*see* Table 4.2).[16,17,19,20,30–32]

Acute illness is a common precipitant, especially if diagnosed with infection, or severe illnesses.[16,17,19] Medical literature is full of case reports of almost every known condition precipitating delirium. The one condition that we do not believe ever causes delirium is a transient ischaemic attack (*see* p. 207), yet this very specific condition is often wrongly blamed for non-specific presentations in the elderly. Unfortunately, hospitalisation itself also increases the risk of delirium because of the disorienting effect of multiple room changes, or lack of a clock, watch or reading glasses.[31] Additionally, many cases are iatrogenic because of medications or the insertion of urinary catheters.[20] Medications with anticholinergic effects (*see* p. 302) are associated with more severe delirium symptoms.[33] Lower rates of use of benzodiazepines are associated with lower rates of delirium.[34] Drug causes include quinolone antibiotics in susceptible individuals.[35]

TABLE 4.2 Patient-related risk factors and some common precipitants for delirium

At-risk patient characteristics	Precipitants
Advanced age	Acute illness
Dementia	Drugs (especially anticholinergics, sedatives and opiates)
Polypharmacy	Electrolyte disturbances
Functional impairment (including residing in nursing homes)	Alcohol (intoxication or withdrawal)
Visual or hearing impairment	Hospitalisation (especially if multiple room moves and lack of orientation aids)
Malnutrition	Urinary catheterisation
Co-morbidities (e.g. heart failure)	Perioperative period
	Dehydration
	Constipation

Diagnosis

There are two stages to the diagnosis of delirium: first, recognising the presence of the clinical syndrome of delirium, and second, defining the precipitants. The former of these two steps requires performing a cognitive assessment and obtaining a corroborating history.

To reliably detect cognitive impairment an assessment of cognition has to be performed in all acutely unwell frail elderly patients (*see* p. 50). Whether this is a rapid screening test or a more detailed evaluation will depend on the clinical situation and available time. In terms of the pattern of impairment, delirium most commonly affects attention (97%), although deficits in short-term memory (88%), visuospatial ability (87%) and orientation (76%) are also often associated.[36] Patients are likely to score poorly on any cognitive test, but remember that the severity may fluctuate. It frequently causes disturbance in the sleep–wake cycle (97%), and less frequently perceptual disturbances/hallucinations (50%) or delusions (31%).[36] The tendency to be worse at night ('sun-downing') can make the patient appear fine during the daily ward round, only to cause havoc for the overnight staff. Simple bedside tests for attention include the ability to count backwards from 20 to 1 or to list the months of the year in reverse order.

Our recommendation is that cognitive impairment in any patient acutely admitted to hospital is initially assumed to be at least partly due to delirium. However, there are a number of tests that have been specifically designed to try to detect delirium.[37] Perhaps the best known is the Confusion Assessment Method (CAM). This is based on the Diagnostic and Statistical Manual of Mental Disorders (3rd Edition, Revised) criteria and can be completed in less than 5 minutes.[38] A CAM for the intensive care unit is also available that does not require the patient to make any verbal responses (i.e. can be used with ventilated patients).[39] For a positive result on the CAM test the patient must have evidence of both items A and B, plus either C or D from the following list:

A – Acute confusion with a fluctuating pattern
B – Inattention
C – Disorganised speech
D – Altered level of consciousness

Alternatively, the Delirium Rating Scale performs similarly to the CAM in elderly hospital inpatients.[40] Perhaps the simplest test is the Single Question in Delirium, where the relative or carer is asked: 'do you think [patient's name] has been more confused recently?'[41] Compared with a psychiatrist interview in a cohort of oncology patients, the Single Question in Delirium was more sensitive than the CAM (80% vs 40%) but it was less specific (71% vs 92%). It may have a role as a rapid screening tool.

After identifying acute cognitive impairment, the primary aim is to identify any reversible or modifiable factors (i.e. knowing the patient is old is of no practical help). The process of comprehensive geriatric assessment should lead to the identification of acute illnesses and potentially causative medications. Seek out evidence for alcohol use, dehydration, constipation or urinary catheterisation. Performing appropriate investigations will support this process.

Investigations
We have already said that almost every illness can provoke delirium in the frail elderly, but there is no need to try to exclude all possible diagnoses at the start. Begin with the simplest tests, as these are most likely to be helpful.

Blood tests
A range of blood tests should be performed in all cases. These should look to exclude commonly recognised causes of delirium – hyponatraemia, hypercalcaemia, hyper or hypoglycaemia, dehydration (urea) and sepsis (white cell count and C-reactive protein). Troponin evaluation should be done if there is an abnormal ECG, or unexplained chest pain, shortness of breath or tachycardia.

Chest X-ray
A chest X-ray should be obtained in all acutely confused elderly patients to look for signs of pneumonia.

Electrocardiogram

An ECG may show signs of occult myocardial infarct or arrhythmia.

Urine tests

Urine tests are usually unhelpful in diagnosing delirium due to the high prevalence of asymptomatic bacteriuria (*see* p. 186). They will always be abnormal in those with long-term urinary catheters.

Arterial blood gas

We do not recommend routinely performing arterial blood gas sampling in acutely confused patients, as it can be distressing and it can possibly worsen confusion. It may be useful in those with low oxygen saturations detected by pulse oximetry.

Head CT scan

CT scans are often requested in older adults presenting with confusion, but in the absence of focal neurological signs or an impaired conscious level they only infrequently demonstrate a significant acute lesion.[42] A study looked at the results of CT scans performed on 106 patients over the age of 70 years (mean age, 83 years) with acute confusion in the ED.[43] They found an acute abnormality on 14% of the scans (the vast majority being acute stroke, intracerebral haemorrhage or subarachnoid haemorrhage). Neurological examination was abnormal in all but one of these patients, this patient having presented with a fall. Interestingly, 12% of patients had no documented neurological examination prior to a CT scan being requested.

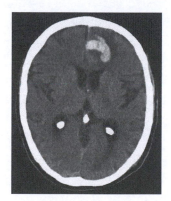

FIGURE 4.1 The brain CT scan of an elderly man who presented with confusion that his family reported was of very rapid onset – an acute intracerebral bleed (white) with some surrounding oedema (dark grey) is seen in his left frontal lobe

However, occasionally a sudden onset of confusion without focal neurological signs can be caused by stroke (*see* Figure 4.1). We recommend that CT scans are only considered a first-line test if there is evidence of a recent head injury, focal neurological deficit or falling consciousness. Otherwise, it is best to concentrate on other tests initially and consider CT scanning if they fail to provide an answer.

Lumbar puncture

A lumbar puncture is rarely helpful in diagnosing the cause of delirium. It may be considered in selected cases if other diagnostic tests have failed to provide an answer in the presence of persisting symptoms (e.g. cerebral vasculitis).

Electroencephalography

Rarely delirium can be provoked by non-convulsive status epilepticus (*see* p. 140). This can be diagnosed by electroencephalography changes.

Treatment

Simply recognising delirium is not enough; a specific management plan is required. Yet, a study that systematically detected delirium did not find that it altered ED physicians' plans of care, with 26% of delirious patients being discharged from the ED.[6] Identify and, where possible, correct underlying risk factors and precipitants of the syndrome. Bear in mind that there are likely to be multiple potentially contributing factors in the frail elderly. The initial treatment is similar for all causes.

Medical illness

The process of comprehensive geriatric assessment supported by relevant investigations should allow the detection of any acute reversible illness. Be sure to assess for evidence of alcohol misuse, dehydration and constipation. Avoid urinary catheterisation unless essential. If a catheter is inserted, then formulate a plan for early withdrawal (e.g. if retention due to constipation, then remove once bowels open). Nutritional status should be assessed and appropriate interventions considered.

Medications

Wherever possible reduce or discontinue potentially causative medications, especially those with anticholinergic properties (*see* Tables 4.3 and 11.3). If there is a compelling need then any initially withheld medications could be cautiously reintroduced once the delirium episode has settled. Reducing polypharmacy will reduce the chance of future delirium.

TABLE 4.3 Examples of changes to consider for potentially causative medications

Stop or withhold	Caution or reduce dose	Cannot stop
Bladder anticholinergics (e.g. oxybutynin, tolterodine or solifenacin)	Opiates – consider pain control	Benzodiazepines (if long-term use) – may be able to slowly reduce at a later date
Antidepressants	Antipsychotics – consider reduction or discontinuation in hypoactive cases	

Sensory impairment

Patients with hearing impairment should be assessed for earwax or the need for a hearing aid. Any aids should be fitted and supplied with a functioning battery. Those with visual acuity problems should be provided with appropriate clean glasses.

Care environment

The ideal environment for the management of acutely confused patients is a specialised delirium unit. However, such units are not available for all patients and the key elements of good care are frequently provided on specialised elderly wards.

A suitable environment would ensure good communication with patient and relatives, orientating stimuli (clocks and calendars), familiar objects from home (e.g. photos), consistency of staff, a simplified space (ideally a side room to control noise and light levels) and low-level lighting at night to reduce the misinterpretation of stimuli. Models of detection and intervention based on liaison services seem to be less effective.[44]

Psychosis and aggression

Some patients with hyperactive or mixed-type delirium will have episodes of challenging behaviour that will put themselves or others at risk of harm. The first line of management is to try to treat the underlying causes, as described earlier. Second, a non-pharmacological approach is advised. Staff should adopt a calm and non-confrontational manner. The last resort is to use sedating or antipsychotic medications. When this is necessary we advise using small doses of haloperidol, which can be given orally (initially 0.5 mg), intramuscularly or intravenously (both initially 1 mg). Patients with either Parkinson's disease or dementia with Lewy bodies should not receive antipsychotic drugs. In these patients, and those with delirium due to alcohol withdrawal, benzodiazepines are a better choice. Lorazepam can be given orally (initially 0.5 mg), intramuscularly or intravenously (both initially 1 mg). Any form of physical restraint is likely to worsen agitation and should be avoided.

Prevention

Evidence suggests that around a third of cases of delirium could be prevented by a multi-component intervention consisting of cognitive reorientation (e.g. clocks and calendars), treatment of dehydration and infection, encouragement of mobility, attention to sensory impairment (e.g. glasses and hearing aids), adequate nutrition and sleep hygiene.[45] Many would consider this to be good-quality basic medical and nursing care.

Prognosis

Delirium should not be considered a benign and fully reversible condition. Mortality rates at 6 months are higher in older patients who present to the ED with delirium than those who do not have delirium (37% vs 14%).[46] Episodes of delirium appear to be associated with an increased risk of future cognitive impairment, perhaps by accelerating the rate of cognitive decline in those with background dementia.[47-49] In many older people the cognitive impact of delirium can be prolonged. Around 45% still have evidence of delirium at the time of discharge, and this figure slowly falls to 21% at 6 months.[50]

Delirium is associated with longer lengths of stay, higher rates of discharge to NHs and more deaths.[22,51] Patients without background dementia have a higher mortality rate and appear to do worse cognitively and functionally than those who did not have delirium up to a year after the episode.[47,52,53] Delirium occurring in people with dementia increases their risk of being transferred to a care home.[52] Those with a longer duration of delirium seem to have worse survival rates and long-term cognitive and functional outcomes.[54-56]

KEY POINTS

- Cognitive impairment affects around 30% of patients aged over 65 and 50% of patients aged over 85 years presenting to acute medical services.
- Those with cognitive impairment have worse outcomes.
- If you do not routinely test cognitive status in all frail elderly patients, many cases will go unrecognised.
- Confusion is usually due to delirium, dementia or both.
- An elderly patient presenting to medical services with new or worsened confusion should be assumed to have delirium, with or without background dementia, until proven otherwise.
- Patients with delirium may be hyper- or hypoactive.
- There are typically multiple causes for delirium in the frail elderly – look for and correct as many as possible.

- Pharmacological intervention should be considered a last resort in the management of psychosis and aggression.
- Delirium in the frail elderly may take a long time to resolve and many will be left with residual cognitive impairment at the time of hospital discharge.

DEMENTIA

Dementia is a chronic progressive neurodegenerative disorder that impairs cognitive function and is severe enough to affect functional ability. The pattern of cognitive loss varies between individuals and different underlying causes (*see* Table 4.4). It affects very few people below the age of 65, but the community prevalence rises rapidly with advancing age, affecting more than a third of people over the age of 85 years (*see* Figure 4.2).[57-59] The prevalence among hospital inpatients is higher, being 42% in patients aged 70 and over, rising from 23% of those aged 70–79, 48% of those aged 80–89, and 66% of those aged 90+.[12]

The commonest cause is said to be Alzheimer's disease, followed by vascular dementia (VaD). However, autopsy studies have suggested that many cases have mixed vascular and Alzheimer's-type pathology.[60,61] These conditions account for over 90% of cases of dementia in the frail elderly. Occasionally, older patients present with either Lewy body or fronto-temporal dementia types. Less common diagnoses include alcohol-related dementia (history of chronic alcohol excess) and Creutzfeldt–Jakob disease (more rapid onset with myoclonic jerks). Brain imaging (CT or MRI) is recommended in the initial evaluation of patients with dementia. This will identify a few patients with alternative diagnoses (e.g. brain tumours, subdural haematomas or normal pressure hydrocephalus) but also helps identify vascular lesions or focal atrophy that may indicate the subtype of dementia (e.g. medial temporal lobe atrophy in Alzheimer's disease).

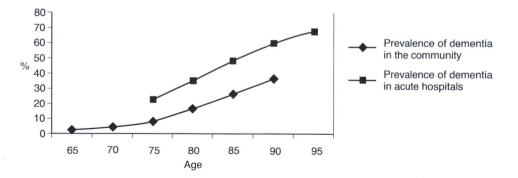

FIGURE 4.2 The prevalence of dementia in community and acute hospital settings (data based on references 12, 57–59)

Two recent studies have looked at the reasons for people with dementia to be admitted to hospital.[62,63] Table 4.5 shows the commonest recorded reasons, accounting for around half of admissions in each study. Differences between the data are likely to reflect variance in the coding of presentations. As most fractured hips occur secondary to falls, it shows the importance of this problem to those with dementia. We suspect that the many of those labelled as urinary tract infection will have been misdiagnosed (*see* p. 184). It is interesting to see the large number of patients ultimately given vague 'diagnoses' such as senility and collapse.

TABLE 4.4 Key features of the commonest types of dementia

	Alzheimer's disease	Vascular dementia	Dementia with Lewy bodies	Frontotemporal dementia
Key clinical features	Gradual onset of progressive decline initially of short-term memory, but also affecting language and visuospatial ability	More rapid or 'step-wise' decline in cognition Vascular risk factors Lesions seen on brain imaging	Fluctuating cognitive impairment associated with Parkinsonism, visual hallucinations or delusions	Impaired executive function, changes in personality May have a family history of this condition

TABLE 4.5 The most common reasons for patients with dementia to be admitted to hospital (according to the Alzheimer's Society's[62] DEMHOS study and Natalwala *et al.*[63])

Reason for admission	DEMHOS (%)	Natalwala *et al.* (%)
Fall	14	–
Hip fracture	12	7
Urinary tract infection	9	5
Chest infection	7	14
Cerebrovascular event	7	2
Dementia or delirium	–	9
Syncope or collapse	–	4
Senility	–	4
Dehydration	–	3

Improving the quality of care while in hospital

In the UK, many carers report that hospitalisation has adverse effects on both physical and cognitive function, and 77% are dissatisfied with the overall quality of dementia care provided.[62] A common complaint was lack of adequate assistance with nutrition and hydration. The patient's relatives or carers can help improve care quality. They may be able to provide information on individual preferences such as preferred foods and the way the person would like to be addressed.[64] They may also bring in familiar objects, such as photographs. Psychiatric liaison services may be able to help manage challenging behaviours.

Prognosis

Admission to hospital of people aged over 65 years (mean age, 75 years) without baseline dementia is associated with an increased risk of subsequent development of dementia (hazard ratio, 1.4; 95% confidence interval, 1.1–1.7).[65] Some of this difference may be explained by a higher prevalence of chronic disease in those admitted to hospital (e.g. diabetes and stroke). Among NH residents with advanced dementia (severe cognitive and functional impairment), mortality rates are around 25% at 6 months, with a median survival of 1.3 years.[66] Patients aged over 70 with end-stage dementia have poorer 6-month mortality rates than non-demented patients following admission for hip fracture (55% vs 12%) or pneumonia (53% vs 13%).[67] Overall, around 18% of patients aged over 70 with dementia will die during their hospital admission.[12] Episodes of infection, or reduced oral intake and swallowing ability are poor prognostic indicators.[66] The placement of feeding tubes does not seem to improve survival rates.[68] Around a third of patients with dementia are admitted from care homes and two-thirds from private residences.[62] At discharge 42% will go to a care home and just 36% a private residence (some will go to intermediate care and some will not survive their admission). Given the progressive nature of dementia, it is important to consider quality of life and advance care planning. Some patients will be best served by a palliative approach to their acute illness.

Challenging behaviour in dementia

Challenging behaviour is a term that has been adapted from the field of learning disability.[69] It can occur in any mental health problem, but is particularly common in dementia and it may precipitate hospital admission. The term covers agitation, aggression, wandering, shouting and disinhibition (including sexual). The management and treatment depends on the underlying cause. In finding the potential cause, it is first of all important to define as accurately as possible the behaviour. For example, aggression may be verbal or physical, or both. If physical, it may be towards staff or other patients and there may be obvious precipitating factors, such as when personal space is invaded. Similarly, wandering may be aimless or an attempt to leave, or simply looking for a carer or relative. It is important to consider the behaviour from the point of view of the patient.

Challenging behaviour may be an attempt by the patient to express an unmet need which could be physiological – for example, hunger or thirst – or psychological. It can be a manifestation of pain, distress or suffering. Possible causes of behavioural and psychological symptoms of dementia are listed in Table 4.6. Pain, breathlessness or constipation can affect behaviour, either directly or indirectly, as part of delirium. Sleep deprivation, environmental change and medication are particularly common causes of behavioural disturbances in hospital. In patients with dementia, even very minor infections, a new drug prescription or suddenly stopping a long-standing drug prescription (e.g. an antidepressant) can be enough to provoke delirium. Alcohol withdrawal delirium ('delirium tremens') should always be considered in any sudden change of mental state. There are two main approaches to the treatment of challenging behaviour – non-pharmacological and pharmacological. Non-pharmacological methods should always be tried first. The use of sedation, particularly with antipsychotics, should only be the very last resort and only when the behaviour puts patients at risk to themselves or others. Also, remember that many behavioural disturbances in dementia resolve spontaneously with time.[70]

TABLE 4.6 Causes of challenging behaviour in dementia (e.g. wandering, agitation, aggression, shouting and screaming)

Problem	Examples
Unmet physical needs	Pain, hunger, thirst, sleep deprivation
Unmet psychological needs	Fear, anxiety and need for reassurance
Delusions	'I am being imprisoned in someone else's home'
Hallucinations	'I can see insects/animals in the room about to attack me'
Depression	Fear, anxiety and need for reassurance
Delirium	Alcohol withdrawal
	Medications (e.g. opiates and anticholinergic drugs)
	Infection
	Constipation
	Electrolyte disorders
	May be multiple contributing factors and lead to delusions and visual hallucinations
Previous established innate behaviour patterns	Wandering in the night due to previous established pattern of leaving home to work a night shift
	(Get to know your patient's background and previous lifestyle)

Non-pharmacological management

The best management of disturbed behaviour is not drugs or physical restraint, but to seek to respond to the patient's unmet physical and psychological needs. A common framework for assessment and treatment is the ABC method,[71] where 'A' stands for the antecedent or trigger (what was happening before the challenging behaviour, who was present, and when and where did it occur?), 'B' is for the behaviour (describe exactly what, be specific – what form did it take, how long did it last?) and 'C' is for the consequence of the behaviour (was there any positive reinforcement that could encourage a repeated pattern?). Careful analysis using this approach may discover the root cause and enable the cycle to be broken. For example, aggressive behaviour may be precipitated by a carer invading the person's personal space without warning or reassurance when the patient has poor vision and hearing. Wandering behaviour may be ingrained as a result of a lifetime's habit of taking the dog for a walk immediately after breakfast.

Sometimes problem behaviour can be prevented by getting relatives to visit and help with open visiting. Patients with delirium particularly may have heightened awareness and become more frightened and anxious because they pick up any anxiety or irritation on the part of the medical and nursing staff unwittingly expressed by tone of voice or body language. It is important to always be calm and reassuring. The National Institute for Health and Clinical Excellence recommends several non-pharmacological approaches to management such as aromatherapy and music therapy, which may help.[72] There is no clear evidence of efficacy for any methods for reducing wandering.[73]

Pharmacological management

Pharmacological intervention with antipsychotic or sedating drugs for challenging behaviour in dementia should only be considered for extreme distress or risk of harm to others.[62] Evidence for efficacy is mainly limited to the treatment of psychosis and aggression (*see* p. 303). A Cochrane review of atypical antipsychotics in the management of dementia showed only a modest benefit from olanzapine and risperidone with an increased risk of extrapyramidal side effects and cerebrovascular events.[74] Risperidone is the only antipsychotic licensed for people with dementia and should only be used as the last resort in small doses, reviewed regularly and ideally not given for longer than 12 weeks.[70] Overall 28% of patients with dementia in the UK currently receive antipsychotic drugs during a hospital admission.[11] Some are already taking these drugs (30% of those in NHs, 14% from private residences) and a further 12% are commenced on these drugs while in hospital. These figures suggest that practice could be improved. Occasionally benzodiazepines (e.g. lorazepam) may be indicated for people unsuitable for antipsychotic drugs (e.g. those with dementia with Lewy bodies).

Depression is very common in dementia and may contribute to behavioural problems, especially if persistent. A trial of an antidepressant may be warranted. Pain is often missed in dementia and may not be expressed in conventional ways, especially in the advanced stages. It is important to recognise non-verbal ways in which a patient with dementia may express pain – for example by grimacing, flushing, guarding the painful area, appearing restless or agitated or not sleeping. Patients are often assessed when lying or sitting, but the pain may sometimes be only present on movement. Regular analgesia (e.g. paracetamol with or without weak opioids) can improve agitation due to pain.[75] Although cholinesterase inhibitors may slow the decline in cognitive function, the benefit in challenging behaviour is only small.[69] They may improve depressive symptoms, such as apathy and anxiety, but not agitation or aggression.[76] Cholinesterase inhibitors may reduce psychiatric symptoms in some patients with dementia with Lewy bodies.[77]

KEY POINTS

- Dementia is highly prevalent among the hospitalised frail elderly.
- The most common causes of dementia are Alzheimer's disease, cerebrovascular disease or a combination of these two.
- Care quality can be improved by careful attention to nutrition and hydration, involving the relatives/carers, and psychiatric liaison services.
- Consider the patient's prognosis and advance care planning.
- When dealing with troublesome behaviour (e.g. wandering, agitation, aggression, shouting), try to define it as precisely as possible and look for precipitating factors (e.g. pain and delirium).
- Treat any underlying causes – for example, stop causative medications and treat infection.
- Use non-pharmacological methods first – for example, improving the environment, such as moving to a side ward/single room, one-to-one nursing or ask relatives or carers to sit with the patient.
- Pharmacological methods (e.g. antipsychotics) are the last resort. Use low doses and review frequently.
- Discuss possible causes with the carers/relatives and explain the adopted approach.

REFERENCES

1. Joray S, Wietlisbach V, Bula CJ. Cognitive impairment in elderly medical inpatients: detection and associated six-month outcomes. *Am J Geriatr Psychiatry*. 2004; **12**(6): 639–47.
2. Royal College of Psychiatrists. *Who Cares Wins*. London: Royal College of Psychiatrists; 2005. Available at: www.rcpsych.ac.uk/PDF/WhoCaresWins.pdf (accessed 23 January 2013).

3. Gerson LW, Counsell SR, Fontanarosa PB, *et al.* Case finding for cognitive impairment in elderly emergency department patients. *Ann Emerg Med.* 1994; **23**(4): 813–17.

4. Naughton BJ, Moran MB, Kadah H, *et al.* Delirium and other cognitive impairment in older adults in an emergency department. *Ann Emerg Med.* 1995; **25**(6): 751–5.

5. Hustey FM, Meldon SW. The prevalence and documentation of impaired mental status in elderly emergency department patients. *Ann Emerg Med.* 2002; **39**(3): 248–53.

6. Hustey FM, Meldon SW, Smith MA, *et al.* The effect of mental status screening on the care of elderly emergency department patients. *Ann Emerg Med.* 2003; **41**(5): 678–84.

7. Wilber ST, Carpenter CR, Hustey FM. The Six-Item Screener to detect cognitive impairment in older emergency department patients. *Acad Emerg Med.* 2008; **15**(7): 613–16.

8. Hickey A, Clinch D, Groarke EP. Prevalence of cognitive impairment in the hospitalized elderly. *Int J Geriatr Psychiatry.* 1997; **12**(1): 27–33.

9. Goldberg SE, Whittamore KH, Harwood RH, *et al.* The prevalence of mental health problems among older adults admitted as an emergency to a general hospital. *Age Ageing.* 2012; **41**(1): 80–6.

10. Department of Health. *Living Well with Dementia: a national dementia strategy.* London: Department of Health; 2009.

11. Royal College of Psychiatrists. *Report of the National Audit of Dementia Care in General Hospitals 2011.* Young J, Hood C, Woolley R, Gandesha A, Souza R, editors. London: Healthcare Quality Improvement Partnership; 2011. Available at: www.rcpsych.ac.uk/pdf/ NATIONAL%20REPORT%20-%20Full%20Report%201201122.pdf (accessed 23 January 2013).

12. Sampson EL, Blanchard MR, Jones L, *et al.* Dementia in the acute hospital: prospective cohort study of prevalence and mortality. *Br J Psychiatry.* 2009; **195**(1): 61–6.

13. Kakuma R, Galbaud du Fort G, Arsenault L, *et al.* Delirium in older emergency department patients discharged home: effect on survival. *J Am Geriatr Soc.* 2003; **51**(4): 443–50.

14. Meagher DJ, Leonard M, Donnelly S, *et al.* A comparison of neuropsychiatric and cognitive profiles in delirium, dementia, co-morbid delirium-dementia and cognitively intact controls. *J Neurol Neurosurg Psychiatry.* 2010; **81**(8): 876–81.

15. Elie M, Rousseau F, Cole M, *et al.* Prevalence and detection of delirium in elderly emergency department patients. *CMAJ.* 2000; **163**(8): 977–81.

16. Han JH, Zimmerman EE, Cutler N, *et al.* Delirium in older emergency department patients: recognition, risk factors, and psychomotor subtypes. *Acad Emerg Med.* 2009; **16**(3): 193–200.

17. Iseli RK, Brand C, Telford M, *et al.* Delirium in elderly general medical inpatients: a prospective study. *Intern Med J.* 2007; **37**(12): 806–11.

18. Collins N, Blanchard MR, Tookman A, *et al.* Detection of delirium in the acute hospital. *Age Ageing.* 2010; **39**(1): 131–5.

19. Inouye SK, Viscoli CM, Horwitz RI, *et al.* A predictive model for delirium in hospitalized elderly medical patients based on admission characteristics. *Ann Intern Med.* 1993; **119**(6): 474–81.

20. Inouye SK, Charpentier PA. Precipitating factors for delirium in hospitalized elderly persons: predictive model and interrelationship with baseline vulnerability. *JAMA.* 1996; **275**: 852–7.

21. Ansaloni L, Catena F, Chattat R, *et al.* Risk factors and incidence of postoperative delirium in elderly patients after elective and emergency surgery. *Br J Surg.* 2010; **97**(2): 273–80.

22. Marcantonio E, Ta T, Duthie E, *et al.* Delirium severity and psychomotor types: their relationship with outcomes after hip fracture repair. *J Am Geriatr Soc.* 2002; **50**(5): 850–7.

23. Edland A, Lundstrom M, Lundstrom G, *et al.* Clinical profile of delirium in patients treated for femoral neck fractures. *Dement Geriatr Cogn Disord.* 1999; **10**(5): 325–9.

24. Peterson JF, Pun BT, Dittus RS, *et al.* Delirium and its motoric subtypes: a study of 614 critically ill patients. *J Am Geriatr Soc.* 2006; **54**(3): 479–84.

25. Inouye SK, Zhang Y, Han L, *et al.* Recoverable cognitive dysfunction at hospital admission in older persons during acute illness. *J Gen Intern Med.* 2006; **21**(12): 1276–81.

26. Lewis LM, Miller DK, Morley JE, *et al.* Unrecognised delirium in ED geriatric patients. *Am J Emerg Med.* 1995; **13**(2): 142–5.

27. Meagher DJ, O'Hanlon D, O'Mahony E, *et al.* Relationship between symptoms and motoric subtype of delirium. *J Neuropsychiatry Clin Neurosci.* 2000; **12**(1): 51–6.

28. O'Keeffe ST, Lavan JN. Clinical significance of delirium subtypes in older people. *Age Ageing.* 1999; **28**(2): 115–19.

29. Kiely DK, Jones RN, Bergmann MA, *et al.* Association between psychomotor activity delirium subtypes and mortality among newly admitted postacute facility patients. *J Gerontol.* 2007; **62**(2): 174–9.

30. Elie M, Cole MG, Primeau FJ, *et al.* Delirium risk factors in elderly hospitalized patients. *J Gen Intern Med.* 1998; **13**(3): 204–12.

31. McCusker J, Cole M, Abrahamowicz M, *et al.* Environmental risk factors for delirium in hospitalized older people. *J Am Geriatr Soc.* 2001; **49**(10): 1327–34.

32. Onen S, Onen F, Mangeon J, *et al.* Alcohol abuse and dependence in elderly emergency department patients. *Arch Gerontol Geriatr.* 2005; **41**(2): 191–200.

33. Han L, McCusker J, Cole M, *et al.* Use of medications with anticholinergic effect predicts clinical severity of delirium symptoms in older medical inpatients. *Arch Intern Med.* 2001; **161**(8): 1099–105.

34. Naughton BJ, Saltzman S, Ramadan F, *et al.* A multifactorial intervention to reduce prevalence of delirium and shorten hospital length of stay. *J Am Geriatr Soc.* 2005; **53**(1): 18–23.

35. Hakko E, Mete B, Ozaras R, *et al.* Levofloxacin-induced delirium. *Clin Neurol Neurosurg.* 2005; **107**(2): 158–9.

36. Meagher DJ, Moran M, Raju B, *et al.* Phenomenology of delirium: assessment of 100 adult cases using standardised measures. *Br J Psychiatry.* 2007; **190**: 135–41.

37. Pompei P, Foreman M, Cassel CK, *et al.* Detecting delirium among hospitalized older patients. *Arch Intern Med.* 1995, **155**(3): 301–7.

38. Inouye SK, van Dyck CH, Alessi CA, *et al.* Clarifying confusion: the Confusion Assessment Method. *Ann Intern Med.* 1990; **113**(12): 941–8.

39. Ely EW, Margolin R, Francis J, *et al.* Evaluation of delirium in critically ill patients: validation of the Confusion Assessment Method for the Intensive Care Unit (CAM-ICU). *Crit Care Med.* 2001; **29**(7): 1370–9.

40. Adamis D, Treloar A, MacDonald AJD, *et al.* Concurrent validity of two instruments (the Confusion Assessment Method and the Delirium Rating Scale) in the detection of delirium among older medical inpatients. *Age Ageing.* 2005; **34**(1): 72–83.

41. Sands MB, Dantoc BP, Hartshorn A, *et al.* Single Question in Delirium (SQiD): testing its efficacy against psychiatrist interview, the Confusion Assessment Method and the Memorial Delirium Assessment Scale. *Palliat Med.* 2010; **24**(6): 561–5.

42. Naughton BJ, Moran M, Ghaly Y, *et al.* Computed tomography scanning and delirium in elder patients. *Acad Emerg Med.* 1997; **4**(12): 1107–10.

43. Hardy JE, Brennan N. Computerized tomography of the brain for elderly patients presenting to the emergency department with acute confusion. *Emerg Med Australas.* 2008; **20**(5): 420–4.

44. Cole MG, McCusker J, Bellavance F, *et al.* Systematic detection and multidisciplinary care of delirium in older medical inpatients: a randomized trial. *CMAJ.* 2002; 167: 753–9.

45. National Institute for Health and Clinical Excellence. Delirium: diagnosis, prevention and management. Clinical guideline 103. London: NIHCE; 2010. Available at: www.nice.org. uk/nicemedia/live/13060/49908/49908.pdf (accessed 23 January 2013).

46. Han JH, Shintani A, Eden S, *et al.* Delirium in the emergency department: an independent predictor of death within 6 months. *Ann Emerg Med.* 2010; **56**(3): 244–52.

47. Rockwood K, Cosway S, Carver D, *et al.* The risk of dementia and death after delirium. *Age Ageing.* 1999; **28**(6): 551–6.

48. Jackson JC, Gordon SM, Hart RP, *et al.* The association between delirium and cognitive decline: a review of the empirical literature. *Neuropsychol Rev.* 2004; **14**(2): 87–98.

49. Fong TG, Jones RN, Shi P, *et al.* Delirium accelerates cognitive decline in Alzheimer disease. *Neurology.* 2009; **72**(18): 1570–5.

50. Cole MG, Ciampi A, Belzile E, *et al.* Persistent delirium in older hospital patients: a systematic review of frequency and prognosis. *Age Ageing.* 2009; **38**(1): 19–26.

51. Siddiqi N, House AO, Holmes JD. Occurrence and outcome of delirium in medical in-patients: a systematic literature review. *Age Ageing.* 2006; **35**(4): 350–64.

52. McCusker J, Cole M, Dendukuri N, *et al.* Delirium in older medical inpatients and subsequent cognitive and functional status: a prospective study. *CMAJ.* 2001; **165**(5): 575–83.

53. McCusker J, Cole M, Abrahamowicz M, *et al.* Delirium predicts 12-month mortality. *Arch Intern Med.* 2002; **162**(4): 457–63.

54. McAvay GJ, Van Ness PH, Bogardus ST, *et al.* Older adults discharged from the hospital with delirium: 1-year outcomes. *J Am Geriatr Soc.* 2006; **54**(8): 1245–50.

55. Kiely DK, Marcantonio ER, Inouye SK, *et al.* Persistent delirium predicts greater mortality. *J Am Geriatr Soc.* 2009; **57**(1): 55–61.

56. Girard TD, Jackson JC, Pandharipande PP, *et al.* Delirium as a predictor of long-term cognitive impairment in survivors of critical illness. *Crit Care Med.* 2010; **38**(7): 1513–20.

57. Rocca WA, Bonaiuto S, Lippi A, *et al.* Prevalence of clinically diagnosed Alzheimer's disease and other dementing disorders: a door-to-door survey in Appignano, Macerata Province, Italy. *Neurology.* 1990; **40**(4): 626–31.

58. Skoog I, Nilsson L, Palmertz B, *et al.* A population-based study of dementia in 85-year-olds. *N Engl J Med.* 1993; **328**(3): 153–8.

59. Lobo A, Launer LJ, Fratiglioni L, *et al.* Prevalence of dementia and major subtypes in Europe: a collaborative study of population-based cohorts. *Neurology.* 2000; **54** (Suppl. 5): S4–9.

60. Zekry D, Hauw J, Gold G. Mixed dementia: epidemiology, diagnosis and treatment. *J Am Geriatr Soc.* 2002; **50**(8): 1431–8.

61. Snowdon DA, Greiner LH, Mortimer JA, *et al.* Brain infarction and the clinical expression of Alzheimer disease: the Nun Study. *JAMA.* 1997; **277**(10): 813–17.

62. Alzheimer's Society. *Counting the Cost: caring for people with dementia on hospital wards.* London: Alzheimer's Society; 2009. Available at: www.alzheimers.org.uk/site/scripts/down load.php?fileID=787 (accessed 23 January 2013).

63. Natalwala A, Potluri R, Uppal H, *et al.* Reasons for hospital admissions in dementia patients in Birmingham, UK, during 2002–2007. *Dement Geriatr Cogn Disord.* 2008; **26**(6): 499–505.

64. Alzheimer's Society. *Care on a Hospital Ward.* London: Alzheimer's Society; 2011. Available at: www.alzheimers.org.uk/site/scripts/documents_info.php?documentID=118 (accessed 23 January 2013).

65. Ehlenbach WJ, Hough CL, Crane PK, *et al.* Association between acute care and critical illness hospitalization and cognitive function in older adults. *JAMA.* 2010; **303**(8): 763–70.

66. Mitchell SL, Teno JM, Kiely DK, *et al.* The clinical course of advanced dementia. *N Engl J Med.* 2009; **361**(16): 1529–38.

67. Morrison RS, Siu AL. Survival in end-stage dementia following acute illness. *JAMA.* 2000; **284**(1): 47–52.

68. Meier DE, Ahronheim JC, Morris J, *et al.* High short-term mortality in hospitalized patients with advanced dementia: lack of benefit of tube feeding. *Arch Intern Med.* 2001; **161**(4): 594–9.

69. Krishnamoorthy A, Anderson D. Managing challenging behaviour in older adults with dementia. *Prog Neurol Psychiatry.* 2011; **15**(3): 20–7.

70. Alzheimer's Society. *Optimising Treatment and Care for People with Behavioural and Psychological Symptoms of Dementia: a best practice guide for health and social care professionals.* London: Alzheimer's Society; 2011. Available at: www.alzheimers.org.uk/site/scripts/download_info.php?fileID=1163 (accessed 23 January 2013).

71. Stokes G. *Challenging Behaviour in Dementia: a person-centred approach.* Milton Keynes: Speechmark; 2000.

72. National Collaborating Centre for Mental Health. Dementia: a NICE–SCIE guideline on supporting people with dementia and their carers in health andsocial care. London: NICE; 2007. Available at: www.nice.org.uk/nicemedia/pdf/CG42Dementiafinal.pdf (accessed 23 January 2013).

73. Robinson L, Hutchings D, Dickinson HO, *et al.* Effectiveness and acceptability of non-pharmacological interventions to reduce wandering in dementia: a systematic review. *Int J Geriatr Psychiatry.* 2007; **22**(1): 9–22.

74. Ballard CG, Waite J. The effectiveness of atypical antipsychotics for aggression and psychosis in Alzheimer's disease. Cochrane Database Syst Rev. 2006; 1: CD003476.

75. Husebo BS, Ballard C, Sandvik R, *et al.* Efficacy of treating pain to reduce behavioural disturbances in residents of nursing homes with dementia: cluster randomised clinical trial. *BMJ.* 2011; **343**: d4065.

76. Howard RJ, Juszczak E, Ballard CG, *et al.* Donepezil for the treatment of agitation in Alzheimer's disease. *N Engl J Med.* 2007; **357**(14): 1382–92.

77. McKeith I, Del Ser T, Spano P, *et al.* Efficacy of rivastigmine in dementia with Lewy bodies: a randomised double-blind, placebo-controlled international study. *Lancet.* 2000; **356**(9247): 2031–6.

CHAPTER 5

'Collapse query cause': falls and blackouts

Although we have used the term 'collapse query cause' in the title of this chapter, we do not consider it suitable for clinicians to use. A collapse is an undefined event that is usually, but not always, used to describe either a fall or blackout. It is little different to saying the patient is unwell. The first step in evaluation is to define this presentation more accurately. It is of no help to complete an assessment still being only able to say there has been a 'collapse query cause'. This may be suitable for an unqualified witness of events, but not a healthcare professional. Falls and blackouts are symptoms, not diagnoses. The effective clinician searches for the underlying causes – and the frail elderly typically have several, although fortunately many of these are remediable. In addition, those who fall or have blackouts are at risk of fractures and so consideration should also be given to the detection and treatment of both injuries and osteoporosis.

The key difference between a fall and a blackout is whether there was a transient loss of consciousness. However, this distinction can be difficult in the absence of a reliable eyewitness account. Around 30% of older adults with syncope have amnesia for loss of consciousness.[1]

FALLS

The risk of falling and subsequent admission to hospital both increase with advancing age.[2] It is estimated that around 30% of people aged over 65 fall each year.[3] In studies of people aged over 65 presenting to the emergency department (ED), 7%–44% of attendances are because of falls.[4-6] The wide variation in reported rates may be partly explained by some events being classified as syncope (*see* p. 132), and some as trauma when injuries are sustained (e.g. hip fracture). In one study, 26% of events classified as falls were associated with loss of consciousness.[4] Patients aged over 65 presenting to the ED following a fall have an average age of about 79 years, approximately 70% have sustained an injury, with half of these patients having a fracture (most often neck of femur, but wrist, head of humerus and pelvis are also common).[7] Even patients who are discharged directly home from ED often have sustained some form of injury, with a third having a fracture.[8] Around 60% of patients are admitted to hospital.[7]

Fallers, especially those who have sustained a fracture, are at high risk of future functional decline.[8,9] If untreated, around 50% will go on to have a further fall in the following year.[5] The majority of falls in older adults occur within their own home.[8] A fall in an older person without an obvious external precipitating factor (e.g. knocked down by a car or during a period of heavy ice) should be seen as a marker of frailty and an opportunity for assessment and intervention. Falling can trigger a cycle of decline. It can result in either injury or 'fear of falling' that can further impair gait and balance. Reduced mobility promotes muscle and bone loss, which increases the risk of recurrent falls and fractures (*see* Figure 5.1).

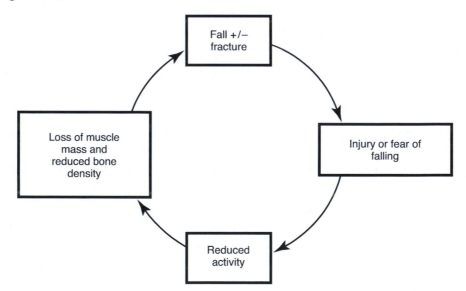

FIGURE 5.1 The negative cycle that can be provoked by falling over

Many elderly patients do not present to hospitals following falling. A study found that around 38% of older people assessed by ambulance crews in their own homes after a fall are not transferred to hospital.[10] The commonest reasons were lack of injury (44%) and patient refusal (19%). The non-transferred patients tended to be older and have greater impairments in mobility. It would seem logical that this group should be referred to falls assessment services. However, a review of patients aged over 70 (mean age 81 years) who presented to ED with a fall, but were not admitted, found that only one of 63 patients was referred to a falls service for assessment, 32% were referred for primary care follow-up and 24% for physiotherapy input.[11] In the 18 months after first presentation, 44% of the women reported a further fall. The development of good communication between services with agreed referral pathways are necessary to optimise care and reduce the risk of recurrence.

A history of previous falls is a strong predictor of future falls, particularly if occurring indoors or the patient was unable to get up off the floor.[12,13] Presently, around 60% of fallers attending an ED have fallen in the previous year.[8] Simply treating any injuries sustained and not looking for the underlying causes is poor management and is destined to fail.

Assessment

The assessment of falls starts with a detailed history of the fall event. When and where did it occur? Were there any preceding symptoms or precipitating factors? Was there a period of reduced consciousness? It is useful to ask the patient if they remember the moment of impact with the ground. The type of injuries sustained may also give clues. Significant facial bruising suggests a blackout with loss of the normal protective reflexes (e.g. putting out a hand), whereas a wrist or clavicle fracture shows that protective reflexes were preserved. An eyewitness account, where available, is very useful. Have they sustained any injuries? Were they able to get up off the floor or did they require assistance? Did they spend a long time lying down, unable to get up (risk of hypothermia, pneumonia and rhabdomyolysis)? It is good practice to ask about any history of falls, but remember there may be amnesia for previous events. One study found that 13%–32% of older people could not recall having fallen when asked between 3 and 12 months later.[14] Unsurprisingly this was more common in those with cognitive impairment, which is detected in 26%–34% of elderly fallers.[4,5] Any reported prior falls should be evaluated to search for a common pattern or precipitant. A history of background functional and social status is also required.

'Mechanical fall' is an unhelpful term. All falls are due to a loss of the mechanism of structural supports that resist the effects of gravity. Nobody wants to fall over and a fall should not be belittled. Approximately half of patients attribute their fall to a slip or trip.[5] However, the patient's recollection may be inaccurate. People in good health rarely trip over. Typically there are multiple contributory causes to falls in the frail elderly and a thorough evaluation seeks out these causes (*see* p. 128).

Clinical examination should include assessments of gait and balance, cognition, neurological system (including visual acuity), cardiovascular (particularly looking for signs of aortic stenosis or orthostatic hypotension (*see* p. 135)) and footwear. A musculoskeletal exam should look for sustained injuries, particularly hip and pelvis fractures or external signs of head injury that could point towards an occult intracerebral lesion such as a subdural haematoma (*see* p. 168). There should also be functional assessments, the consideration of home environmental hazards and inquiry into fear of falling. Other multidisciplinary team members may perform more detailed assessments to support and inform the initial process.

Causes of falls

Broadly speaking the causes of falls in the elderly can be divided into acute illness, chronic conditions affecting gait and balance, the effects of medications and environmental hazards. Problems in several of these categories may be present in any individual. A study of patients aged over 65 (mean age, 77 years) without cognitive impairment presenting to the ED following a fall, who also had a history of previous falls, found a mean number of five risk factors per patient.[15] The commonest problems were balance (93% of subjects), gait (80%), implicated medications (53%), environmental hazards (48%) and visual impairment (27%).

The four key groups of causes of falls are outlined as follows.

1. Acute illness

As stated previously, almost any illness in the frail elderly can present as an acute functional or cognitive decline, including falling over. However, we would warn against labelling falls as a transient ischaemic attack (*see* p. 208) or the over-diagnosis of urinary tract infection (*see* p. 185). All patients should receive a comprehensive evaluation.

2. Chronic conditions

Chronic conditions that affect gait and balance are associated with falling. Patients complaining of multiple stumbles, reduced balance, dizziness or gait impairment are at increased risk.[12,16] Clues to significant balance problems include the inability to cut own toenails or stand on one leg for 5 seconds.[17,18] There is a wide spectrum of conditions that can affect gait and balance. These include osteoarthritis, peripheral neuropathy, visual impairment, lower limb weakness, and foot and ankle problems (e.g. overgrown toenails, reduced power or sensation, pain, reduced flexibility or hallux valgus deformity).[19–21] Unsuitable footwear may be a factor (i.e. anything without a flat sole). Chronic neurological conditions (e.g. stroke and Parkinson's disease), cognitive impairment and depression are also associated with falls.[18] Bifocal glasses can affect depth perception and ideally should be changed to single focal lenses when walking, especially on staircases.[22]

Vitamin D is mainly derived from the action of sunlight on the skin with smaller amounts coming from dietary intake. Elderly people with reduced mobility and subsequent reduced sunlight exposure, often coupled with a diet low in vitamin D, are at high risk of deficiency. Based on a serum 25-hydroxy vitamin D level <25 nmol/L in people over the age of 65 years living in the UK, 10%–15% who live in private residences and around 30% of those residing in residential care are deficient.[23] However, even at levels <50 nmol/L there is evidence of increased parathyroid hormone levels and bone resorption.[24] Using this value, around 55% and 80% of those aged over 65 in private homes or residential care, respectively, are classed as deficient.[23] Deficiency in vitamin D is associated with both proximal myopathy and falls.[25] It may lead to osteomalacia and an increased risk of fracture (see p. 165). Vitamin D supplementation in care home settings has been found to lower rates of falls, but not fractures.[26] Those with severe deficiency (<25 nmol/L plus symptoms) are likely to require initial high-dose supplementation to replenish body stores (e.g. colecalciferol 10 000 IU per day for 8–12 weeks) followed by maintenance therapy (e.g. colecalciferol 800–2000 IU per day).

3. Drugs

A thorough review of medication (including concordance) and history of alcohol intake is essential. Around 80% of elderly fallers attending ED are on four or more regular medications.[8] Psychotropic drugs (antipsychotics, sedatives and antidepressants) have been found to be associated with an increased risk of falls in older people in two studies (odds ratio (OR), 1.47 [95% confidence interval (CI), 1.24–1.74]; OR, 1.73 [95% CI, 1.52–1.97]).[27,28] The effect may be even more pronounced if combined with alcohol. Logically, drugs that can precipitate drops in blood pressure (BP) (e.g. orthostatic hypotension), or those that affect heart rhythm, would be likely to increase the risk of falls. However, this is not strongly supported by currently available clinical trial evidence. A systematic review found limited evidence for a role of digoxin (OR, 1.22; 95% CI, 1.05–1.42) and diuretics (OR, 1.08; 95% CI, 1.02–1.16), but not other antihypertensive drugs.[29]

4. Environmental hazards

Environmental hazards are commonly found in the homes of elderly people.[30] Simple interventions include ensuring adequately lit staircases, double rails on stairs, rails to help get up from the bath or toilet, appropriately heighted bed and chair (possibly raiser-recliner), and the removal of any trailing wires or loose rugs.

Investigations

Basic investigations to look for an acute illness should be performed as outlined in Chapter 2. An ECG should be performed in all patients to exclude cardiac arrhythmia and associated risk factors (e.g. previous cardiac disease or prolonged QT interval). 24-hour ECG recordings are rarely useful in the investigation of falls and should not be performed routinely. A review of 228 older patients (128 following falls and 100 controls; mean age, 76 years) who had 24-hour ECG recording performed found abnormalities were detected in 49% of fallers and 41% of controls (relative risk, 1.2; 95% CI, 0.9–1.6).[31] No type of arrhythmia was more common in fallers.

CT scanning

A study that looked at the results of CT head scans performed on 404 elderly fallers (mean age, 83 years) presenting to an ED, without focal neurological signs, found a rate of intracranial bleeding of 12% (approximately 70% of these due to subdural haematoma, 15% subarachnoid and 15% intraparenchymal).[32] In this department, over 90% of elderly fallers received head CT scans. The only variables associated with an increased risk of blood seen on CT scanning were evidence of head trauma and living in their own home. The use of warfarin was not associated with an increased risk of bleeding. These data suggest that clinicians should have a low threshold for performing head CT scans on frail elderly fallers with any evidence of a head injury or changed mental status, and always if there are new focal neurological signs.

Treatment

Sometimes the focus in the ED is to treat any injuries sustained and discharge the patient, if safely mobile, without intervention to address the underlying causes for falling. This exposes the patient to risk of future harm. Numerous clinical guidelines for falls management have been developed, but creating them alone does not appear to be effective.[33,34] There is a need for a good working partnership between acute services and falls programmes, with clear and easily accessible referral pathways. Given the causes are typically multiple, a multifactorial approach is usually warranted. Initial physiotherapy and OT assessments can often be performed in acute care settings.

When a multidisciplinary intervention has been applied to older adults presenting to ED with falls, a marked reduction in the risk of falling over the following year has been found (OR, 0.39; 95% CI, 0.23–0.66).[5] However, other studies have shown less dramatic results. A multifactorial intervention for elderly patients who had attended ED after a fall resulted in a 36% reduction in number of falls in a 1-year follow-up period, but no difference in the number of people falling.[15] Meta-analyses of multifactorial interventions for community-dwelling fallers have suggested around a 25% reduction in number of falls, but also no reduction in the number of fallers or fall-related injuries.[3,35] Multifactorial interventions used in hospital settings have been associated with a reduced rate of falls (rate ratio, 0.69; 95% CI, 0.49–0.96) and risk of falling (relative risk, 0.73; 95% CI, 0.56–0.96).[36] However, this type of programme is ineffective for elderly people with cognitive impairment.[37]

Treatments that aim to improve strength and balance either through group sessions, individual exercise programmes or t'ai chi seem effective in reducing falls (rate ratio reduction around 30%).[3] However, it may take weeks to months for a benefit and so if commenced in hospital there is a need to consider ongoing input after discharge. Medication reviews including the gradual withdrawal of psychotropic drugs can also reduce the risk of falling.[3] Cutting back any medication that is associated with an increased risk of falls has been shown to improve cardiovascular homeostasis.[38] Home hazard assessment and intervention can be an effective way to reduce future falls if targeted at high-risk populations.[39]

Falls are similar to other geriatric syndromes in that they are due to a combination of many problems that vary from individual to individual and there is no single curative treatment. Patients who fall are most likely to benefit if comprehensive geriatric assessment is performed effectively and the underlying causes are identified; then an individual treatment plan and outcome goals can be developed.

Preventing falls while in hospital

Falls are a recognised complication of hospital admission (*see* p. 20). Steps should be taken to minimise the risk. These include basic good quality care such as identifying those with cognitive impairment and poor nutritional status, and then intervening appropriately. Hospital environments should consider floor surfaces (including freedom from clutter), lighting levels, clear signage for toilets and the ability of staff to observe at-risk patients. Four basic steps have been suggested: (1) ask all patients if they have had a recent fall, (2) avoid psychotropic medications, (3) ensure the patients have suitable footwear and (4) place call bells within easy sight and reach.[40]

- Collapse is a vague term. Falls and blackouts are presentations. Avoid the terms 'mechanical fall' or 'simple trip'. Always look for underlying diagnoses.
- Patients who have fallen or who are at risk of falling should undergo a falls evaluation.
- An accurate history of events is very important, but this can be hampered by amnesia for falls or for unconsciousness. Try to get a witness account.
- Look for causes of falls from the four common categories: (1) acute illnesses, (2) chronic conditions affecting gait and balance, (3) the effects of medications and (4) environmental hazards. Typically, there are multiple contributing factors in the frail elderly.
- Vitamin D deficiency is common in the frail elderly and can increase the risk of falls.
- A multifactorial intervention programme is usually warranted. This may be best delivered by referral to a specialist falls service.
- It is important to take steps to reduce the risk of patients falling while in hospital.

BLACKOUTS

Blackouts are episodes of transient loss of consciousness lasting for just seconds to minutes. They can occur following head trauma (i.e. concussion), but when non-traumatic they are usually caused by syncope or seizures (epilepsy). Other causes of reduced consciousness (e.g. drug overdoses or major strokes) are not transient. Transient ischaemic attacks do not cause loss of consciousness (*see* p. 208).

SYNCOPE

Syncope is caused by transient global cerebral hypoperfusion leading to loss of consciousness with a rapid spontaneous recovery. The duration of unconsciousness is typically seconds to minutes, but it can be difficult for witnesses to accurately recall this. Some patients complain of fatigue for several hours following the event. Approximately 1%–3% of adults presenting to an ED have had syncope.[41,42] In around 50%–70% of cases the underlying diagnosis can be detected by initial evaluation (i.e. history, examination and ECG).[41,43] Other patients may require specialist investigations. Approximately 70% have a non-cardiac cause, 10% a cardiac cause and 20% remain undiagnosed (including those with incomplete testing).[41] Occasionally patients presenting acutely with syncope have an underlying pulmonary embolus or occult haemorrhage.

Evaluation involves getting as much history of the event as possible. From the patient this will include the location, time and activity at the time of onset. Ask about any preceding symptoms and how the patient felt after the event. A witness history is very useful when available. This can provide information about the appearance of the patient, duration of the event, any seizure activity and around the time of recovery. Medications should be carefully reviewed as these often contribute to syncope in the elderly. When diagnosing syncope it is important to distinguish between cardiac and non-cardiac causes. These are compared in Table 5.1.[44] Presyncopal autonomic symptoms suggest a non-cardiac cause, but are not always present.[45] Syncope can affect the driving ability of those who still drive and relevant regulations should be consulted.[46] In the absence of focal neurological signs or a presentation suggesting seizures, electroencephalography (EEG) and CT brain scans are rarely helpful.[43]

TABLE 5.1 A comparison of the classic features of cardiac and non-cardiac syncope that may be detected

Cardiac	Non-cardiac
Onset during exercise or when supine	Presyncopal autonomic symptoms:
Abnormal baseline ECG	• nausea
History of heart disease	• sweating (diaphoresis)
Preceding palpitations or shortness of breath	• light-headedness
No autonomic prodrome	• blurred vision
Cardiac murmur	Onset after prolonged standing or on postural change

Cardiac syncope

Although less common than non-cardiac causes, a cardiac aetiology is more often found in older than younger people.[41] It is also associated with a worse prognosis than other causes.[47] They are most often due to arrhythmias (also *see* p. 231), but other possibilities include aortic stenosis. Cardiac syncope is more likely in the presence of a history of cardiac disease or an abnormal ECG.[48] Onset is often at a time of physical exertion due to either an ischaemia-triggered arrhythmia (e.g. ventricular tachycardia) or impaired cardiac output secondary to aortic stenosis. Bradyarrhythmias (e.g. complete heart block) may induce syncope unrelated to either posture or exertion (e.g. when lying or sitting down). There may be a history of palpitations or shortness of breath prior to the onset.[45]

Decision aids have been proposed to try and identify patients at higher risk of adverse outcomes, including those with cardiac syncope, in an ED setting. For example the San Francisco Syncope Rule, which is based on the presence of any of a history of heart failure, a haematocrit <30%, an abnormal ECG, a history of shortness of breath or an initial systolic BP <90 mmHg. For these criteria, a meta-analysis found pooled estimates of sensitivity of 87% and specificity of 52%.[49] To date, there is little evidence of efficacy in the frail elderly and so the clinical usefulness of such decision aids is unclear.

Asking about previous cardiac disease, auscultating the heart and performing an ECG are the key steps in looking for a cardiac cause. Medications should be reviewed, including checking for any drugs that could prolong the QT interval (*see* Table 5.2) and cholinesterase inhibitors (risk of complete heart block). The effects of these drugs can be additive. Often older people are already taking a drug that prolongs the QT interval and are inadvertently prescribed an additional agent (e.g. an antibiotic on top of an antidepressant). Prolonged ambulatory ECG recording (24- to 72-hour durations) can sometimes be used to detect the cause of syncope in those with paroxysmal, but frequent, symptoms. However, if the baseline ECG is normal there is only a very small chance of detecting a relevant problem.[41] Implantable loop recorders are also available that have battery lives of more than a year. There is some evidence of a useful role in selected elderly patients with ongoing symptoms and no diagnosis despite an extensive work-up.[50]

TABLE 5.2 Commonly used drugs that can prolong the QT interval on an electrocardiogram

Antibiotics	Anti-arrhythmics	Antidepressants	Antipsychotics	Antifungals
Azithromycin	Amiodarone	Amitriptyline	(Examples, all have potential)	Ketoconazole
Clarithromycin	Sotalol	Dosulepin	Haloperidol	
Erythromycin		Doxepin	Risperidone	
Moxifloxacin		Imipramine		
		Citalopram		

Less than 2% of cases of syncope are due to aortic stenosis.[41,51] Echocardiography is only likely to provide diagnostic information in those with a history of cardiac disease, a murmur or an abnormal ECG.[51] An exercise test or stress echocardiography should be considered for patients with symptoms that were induced by exertion. Coronary angiography may be indicated for those with suspected ischaemic heart disease. Cardiac electrophysiology studies may be suitable for the identification and potential treatment of underlying cardiac arrhythmias.

Treatment
Treatment should try to address the underlying cause. Unhelpful medications should be withdrawn if possible. Patients with recurrent ventricular tachycardia

may require an implantable defibrillator. Revascularisation may be appropriate for ischaemia-induced arrhythmias. Pacemaker insertion may be useful for those with symptomatic bradyarrhythmias. Patients with aortic stenosis may be candidates for valve replacement surgery. Those who cannot undergo major surgery might be considered for transcatheter aortic valve implantation.

Non-cardiac syncope

The large majority of non-cardiac syncope is due to what is termed 'reflex' (or 'neurally mediated') syncope. This incorporates vasovagal, orthostatic, situational and carotid sinus forms of syncope.[52] In these conditions, syncope is usually preceded by feeling light-headed (or 'woozy'), hot, sweaty and nauseous. Witnesses may describe a pale appearance.

Vasovagal syncope

Vasovagal syncope or 'fainting' can be precipitated by episodes of prolonged standing (e.g. waiting at a bus stop) or emotional stress (e.g. seeing blood or needles in some individuals). During normal standing there is a gravity-driven tendency for fluid to accumulate in the legs. This is usually compensated for by a peripheral vasoconstriction, which is mediated by the vagus and parasympathetic nervous systems.

It is usually diagnosed based on history of the event. However, in unclear cases a head-up tilt test may be required. Here a patient is positioned on a specialised table at 70 degrees (i.e. nearly vertical) while attached to continual pulse and BP monitoring devices. This is continued for up to 40 minutes or the development of symptoms. A positive test will show a fall in BP with reduced consciousness – this typically occurs after around 20 minutes of testing.

Situational syncope

Certain situations can induce syncope in susceptible individuals. These include coughing, micturition, defecation and post-prandial (after eating). Some medications can also induce syncope, the classic example being glyceryl trinitrate spray use for angina ('GTN syncope'). A post-prandial reduction in systolic BP of 25 mmHg occurring 30–60 minutes after eating has been described in elderly people.[53] The diagnosis is made by an accurate history of activities around the syncopal event.

Orthostatic hypotension

Orthostatic hypotension (OH) is the underlying cause of around 12% of syncope occurring in people aged over 65 years presenting to an ED.[54] It is defined as a drop of 20 mmHg in systolic BP or 10 mmHg in diastolic BP within 3 minutes of standing.[55] But this can be either symptomatic or asymptomatic. Typical symptoms are light-headedness, blurred vision and/or nausea. The relevance of asymptomatic falls in BP is unclear. There are limitations to bedside testing for this problem including poor technique, missing the drop in BP and due to OH not universally being present every time a patient stands. A more sensitive method is simply to ask the patient if they feel light-headed on standing.

When changing from sitting to standing, around 500 mL of blood pools in the lower extremities because of the effects of gravity. If unchecked this would reduce venous return to the heart and cause a fall in cardiac output. It is usually compensated for by baroreceptors triggering increased peripheral vascular resistance (i.e. vasoconstriction) and an increased heart rate. Ageing is associated with reduced baroreceptor activity, reduced autonomic nervous activity, increased risk of dehydration (impaired salt retention), and ventricular stiffness (reduced diastolic filling). All of these changes increase the risk of OH. In addition, co-morbidities in older patients play a significant role. More medications are taken that have either anticholinergic properties (e.g. for overactive bladder) or that cause vasodilatation (e.g. many antihypertensives and anti-anginals). Alcohol intake and volume depletion (e.g. diuretics, vomiting and diarrhea) can also contribute. Autonomic neuropathy is associated with Parkinson's disease and diabetes, which impairs the normal BP corrective reflex. OH is present in around 50% of those with PD because of both associated autonomic neuropathy and the side effects of drug treatment.[56]

Carotid sinus hypersensitivity

The carotid sinus is a dilatation of the internal carotid artery that contains baroreceptors. Carotid sinus hypersensitivity is a condition of abnormal activity of this nervous system, which results in inappropriate falls in heart rate, BP or both. These are termed cardio-inhibitory, vasodepressor or mixed subtypes accordingly. It is diagnosed by carotid sinus massage performed while the patient's heart rate and BP are monitored.

Treatment

Non-pharmacological

Patient education about the cause and ways to minimise symptoms is very important. They should be advised about avoiding triggers (e.g. prolonged standing, hot rooms and volume depletion). The early recognition of warning signs (e.g. light-headedness, sweating and nausea) and then taking evasive action (e.g. sitting or more preferably lying down) can be effective. Physical countermanoeuvres such as gripping the hands and tensing the arms can also terminate the syndrome.[52] In cases of situational syncope it may be appropriate to correct an underlying problem such as treatment for a chronic cough. Eating more frequent but smaller meals may lessen post-prandial hypotension. It had previously been advocated that raising the head of the patient's bed by 5–10 degrees could improve OH symptoms, but a recent study failed to find any benefit.[57] In addition, this technique would make the patient's bed uneven, which may increase the risk of falling when sitting on the edge of the bed. The cardio-inhibitory subtype of carotid sinus hypersensitivity can be effectively treated by cardiac pacemaker insertion.

Medication review

The ongoing need for potentially causative drugs should be reviewed. Drugs associated with syncope include antihypertensives, vasodilators, anticholinergics and anti-Parkinsonians. Diuretics and nitrates seem to be particularly implicated.[54] Despite this known association, current medication lists were found to not be recorded in 33% of patients presenting to an ED with syncope or near-syncope.[58] In addition, medications lists that were recorded were often incomplete.

Pharmacological

Fludrocortisone and midodrine have been used with anecdotal success in the treatment of syncope, but robust trial evidence is lacking.[52] Fludrocortisone is a mineralocorticoid that causes sodium and water retention, and it is taken once a day. Midodrine is an alpha-agonist that has to be taken three times a day. Both drugs may cause supine hypertension and increase the risk of stroke and heart failure. Fludrocortisone can cause fluid retention and peripheral oedema. It is contraindicated in patients with cardiac impairment. Midodrine may cause urinary retention in elderly men. These drugs should only be used by specialists and with ongoing careful review of the patient.

KEY POINTS

- Transient loss of consciousness is most commonly caused by syncope.
- In the majority of cases, history, physical examination and ECG can establish the underlying cause of syncope.
- Cardiac causes of syncope are less common but are associated with a worse prognosis – suggestive features include an onset on exertion or at rest, a history of heart disease, a cardiac murmur or an abnormal ECG.

- Non-cardiac syncope is likely to occur on postural change or after prolonged standing. Autonomic symptoms are usually associated.
- Syncope is often precipitated by medications.

EPILEPSY

The prevalence of epilepsy rises with age and is diagnosed in around 0.8% of those over age 85 years.[59] In the elderly, idiopathic epilepsy is rare and it usually occurs secondary to underlying structural brain changes. Seizures secondary to stroke account for 30%–40% of cases.[60] Around 10%–20% of patients with advanced dementia will have at least one seizure and these are believed to account for 10%–20% of epilepsies in the old.[61,62] Other causes include brain tumours, subdural haematomas, drugs, alcohol and metabolic disturbances (*see* Table 5.3).

TABLE 5.3 Secondary causes of seizures seen in the frail elderly

Secondary cause
Cerebrovascular disease
Brain tumours (primary or secondary)
Neurodegenerative disease (e.g. Alzheimer's disease)
Head injury, including subdural haematoma
Drugs: antidepressants, antipsychotics, theophylline, quinolone antibiotics, baclofen
Withdrawal: alcohol, benzodiazepines
Metabolic: hypoglycaemia, hypoxia, hyponatraemia, hypocalcaemia, hypomagnesaemia

Seizures can be focal (localised symptoms) or generalised (affecting most of the brain). Examples of generalised seizures include tonic–clonic episodes and absences. Focal seizures can be 'simple' (no change in consciousness) or associated with altered mental function or consciousness (previously called 'complex partial seizures' but recently renamed 'focal dyscognitive seizures'). Focal seizures can also become secondarily generalised – for example, localised symptoms followed by a tonic–clonic seizure. In older adults, around 70% of seizures are of focal onset, with or without secondary generalisation.[60] A significant difference from younger patients is the duration of the post-ictal phase, which in the elderly can last much longer – from several hours to multiple days.[63] Around 30% of acute seizures in the elderly present as status epilepticus (*see* p. 140).[62] The presentation of epilepsy in the frail elderly may be vague and can present as confusion, unexplained falls, blackouts or focal neurological signs.

A major differential diagnosis is syncope; these conditions are compared in

Table 5.4. A witness history is extremely valuable for assessment. Relevant blood tests, brain imaging and an ECG should be performed. MRI is more likely to detect subtle structural abnormalities than CT scanning and is the recommended imaging modality. EEG performed between seizures is neither a sensitive nor specific test for diagnosing epilepsy in the elderly.[62] Older age is associated with generalised slowing and a higher prevalence of focal abnormalities making test results harder to interpret.[64] It is only appropriate for use by specialists. A lumbar puncture can be helpful when rare causes of seizures are suspected (e.g. subarachnoid haemorrhage, encephalitis or meningitis).

TABLE 5.4 Clinical features to help distinguish between syncope and epilepsy

Clinical feature	Syncope	Epilepsy
Onset	Events often related to posture (typically when standing) or exercise (cardiac arrhythmias)	Events may occur in any situation
Prodromal symptoms	Nausea, sweating, light-headedness or palpitations	Aura (e.g. taste or smell) if temporal lobe origin (but less common in old age)
Limb movements	Brief myoclonic jerks	Rhythmical and prolonged
Urinary incontinence	Possible	Possible
Tongue biting	May bite tip of tongue	Deep bites to lateral tongue suggests epilepsy
Colour during event	Pale or grey	Cyanosis
After event	Rapidly back to normal	Prolonged confusion (>1 hour)

Treatment

Appropriate driving advice should be given to those who still drive.[46] Where possible, underlying provocative factors (e.g. drugs and metabolic imbalances) should be corrected. It is not clear whether drug treatment should be started after a single seizure. It probably makes sense when recurrence is likely due to persisting underlying pathology. In other cases the decision may be guided by patient preference, bearing in mind the patient is likely to be on lifelong treatment. Data to aid comparison between treatment options in the elderly are limited. One study has compared carbamazepine with lamotrigine and gabapentin in older patients (mean age, 72 years) with a new diagnosis of epilepsy (most commonly secondary to stroke).[65] Seizure control was similar with all three drugs. Discontinuation because of side effects was most common with carbamazepine (31%) than for either lamotrigine (12%) or gabapentin (22%). However, the side effects of carbamazepine may be diminished by using a controlled-release preparation.[62]

Medication choice is often guided by potential side effects. Drugs should be started at low doses and gradually titrated upwards until seizures are controlled or unacceptable side effects occur. All anti-epileptic drugs may cause sedation in older patients, and a sensation of imbalance or dizziness is also frequently reported.[66] Sodium valproate and lamotrigine are currently recommended as first-line drugs in the UK for the management of both focal and generalised epilepsy.[67,68] In elderly patients sodium valproate is associated with tremor severe enough to necessitate drug dose change or discontinuation in around 11% of cases, and significant confusion is seen in 5%–10% of people on lamotrigine.[66] Occasionally sodium valproate can induce a state of reduced consciousness associated with a raised serum ammonia level (termed 'valproate-induced hyperammonaemic encephalopathy').[69] Levetiracetam has also been effectively used in the elderly but currently mainly as an add-on therapy in those who are not controlled on a single agent.[70] Potential side effects include confusion and changes in personality (e.g. excessive irritability).

Carbamazepine can cause a rash and hyponatraemia (secondary to the syndrome of inappropriate antidiuretic hormone secretion – *see* p. 75). It also induces some hepatic enzymes, which can lead to drug interactions (*see* p. 300). Gabapentin may precipitate cognitive impairment.[66] Because of toxicity, especially sedation and cognitive impairment, phenobarbital is best avoided in the elderly. Phenytoin has zero order kinetics, which increases its risk of toxicity with small dose changes, which may lead to ataxia. It can also cause bone loss (anti-vitamin D effects) and megaloblastic anaemia (anti-folate effects). For these reasons, phenytoin is no longer a drug of first choice.

Currently, there is insufficient evidence to determine if anti-epileptic drugs can be safely withdrawn from the elderly after a period of seizure freedom (e.g. 2 years).[60] As a result, most patients remain on treatment for life.

Status epilepticus

Status epilepticus is traditionally defined as continuous seizures or two or more seizures with incomplete recovery of consciousness in between lasting more than 30 minutes.[71] However, recent studies have shown that among patients with prolonged seizures (more than 10 minutes), 57% will progress to true status epilepticus without medication and the mortality increases for seizures lasting more than 30 minutes to 19% compared with 3% for those lasting 10–29 minutes.[72] For these reasons, a more practical definition of status epilepticus is seizures lasting more than 10 minutes.

Seizures can be either convulsive or non-convulsive. Non-convulsive status may present as delirium,[73] but it is less harmful than convulsive status, which

TABLE 5.5 The assessment and management of status epilepticus

Recognition	Most normal seizures last less than 2 minutes
	Generalised seizure activity for greater than 10 minutes is a medical emergency
History	Previous diagnosis of epilepsy
	Previous history of status epilepticus
	Recent withdrawal or change in medication
	Recent infection/vomiting
Investigations	Venous glucose
	Urea and electrolytes, calcium, magnesium, creatine kinase
	Anti-epileptic drug levels
	Chest X-ray
	Blood gases
	Blood cultures
	Head CT scan
	Urine for toxicology
Immediate treatment	Initial emergency treatment – airway, breathing, circulation
	Pulse oximetry, high flow oxygen, consider nasopharyngeal airway
	Check capillary blood glucose
	Obtain iv access and give iv lorazepam 2–4 mg (slowly)
	If evidence of poor nutrition or alcoholism then give iv B vitamins (e.g. Pabrinex high potency two pairs of ampules) and iv glucose (e.g. 50 mL of 20%)
	If seizures continue after 10 minutes give phenytoin (15–18 mg/kg) diluted in normal saline over 30 minutes with ECG monitoring
	If seizures stop, continue with maintenance phenytoin, iv or oral
	Continue with patient's usual anti-epileptic treatment
	If no improvement, contact intensive treatment unit for ventilation and general anaesthesia with thiopentone, propofol or midazolam
Failure to respond	Consider:
	• inadequate doses of phenytoin (check levels)
	• failure to continue maintenance therapy
	• medical complications – e.g. acidosis or electrolyte imbalance
	• possible pseudostatus (but rare in older people)

Abbreviation: iv = intravenous

can lead to severe cognitive impairment, multisystem failure and death. Once status becomes established it becomes self-perpetuating and more resistant to drug treatment. The efficacy of benzodiazepines drops twentyfold during the first 30 minutes of continuous seizures.[74] The mortality is higher in older people who also may have less cognitive reserve. For this reason, status epilepticus is a medical emergency, especially in older people, and prompt treatment saves brain function as well as lives.[75] Non-convulsive status requires a high level of suspicion for diagnosis, which is made by EEG testing.[62]

Common causes include anti-epileptic drug non-adherence or discontinuation, withdrawal syndromes following discontinuation of alcohol, baclofen, barbiturates or benzodiazepines, acute structural injury (such as a stroke or brain tumour), infection (encephalitis or meningitis), metabolic abnormalities (e.g. hypoglycaemia, hyponatraemia, hypocalcaemia) or the use/overdose of drugs that lower the seizure threshold (e.g. theophyllines, tricyclic antidepressants, phenothiazines). Initial treatment is intravenous lorazepam (Table 5.5), which is preferred to diazepam because it has a longer duration of action.[76,77] If this is not effective then the next step is intravenous phenytoin. Phenytoin has the advantage that it is not very sedating, but it can cause arrhythmias and hypotension and so cardiac monitoring is necessary. It is important to continue the patient's usual maintenance therapy using a nasogastric tube if necessary. The underlying cause for the status should also be looked for and treated (Table 5.3). Prompt treatment of status epilepticus is particularly important in older people to protect the more vulnerable brain. Prolonged seizures can also lead to rhabdomyolysis (*see* p. 73).

KEY POINTS

- Syncope and epilepsy are usually distinguished by the history of events (including a witness account) and clinical signs.
- Epilepsy in the old is usually secondary to underlying pathology – look for reversible causes.
- Careful consideration is needed when prescribing anti-epileptic drugs – they are likely to cause side effects and are usually continued for life.
- Patients who still drive need to be given appropriate advice.
- Status epileptics is a medical emergency and should be considered present when there has been a seizure lasting for more than 10 minutes or more than one seizure with incomplete recovery between events.
- Status epilepticus can sometimes present in a non-convulsive form with clinical features of delirium.

REFERENCES

1. Kenny RA, Traynor G. Carotid sinus syndrome: clinical characteristics in elderly patients. *Age Ageing.* 1991; **20**(6): 449–54.
2. Scuffham P, Chaplin S, Legood R. Incidence and costs of unintentional falls in older people in the United Kingdom. *J Epidemiol Community Health.* 2003; **57**(9): 740–4.

3. Gillespie LD, Robertson MC, Gillespie WJ, *et al.* Interventions for preventing falls in older people living in the community. Cochrane Database Syst Rev. 2012; 9: CD007146.
4. Davies AJ, Kenny RA. Falls presenting to the accident and emergency department: types of presentation and risk factor profile. *Age Ageing.* 1996; **25**(5): 362–6.
5. Close J, Ellis M, Hooper R, *et al.* Prevention of falls in the elderly trial (PROFET): a randomised controlled trial. *Lancet.* 1999; **353**(9147): 93–7.
6. Baraff LJ, Lee TJ, Kader S, *et al.* Effects of a practice guideline for emergency department care of falls in elder patients on subsequent falls and hospitalizations for injuries. *Acad Emerg Med.* 1999; **6**(12): 1224–31.
7. Bell AJ, Talbot-Stern JK, Hennessy A. Characteristics and outcomes of older patients presenting to the emergency department after a fall: a retrospective analysis. *Med J Aust.* 2000; **173**(4): 179–92.
8. Russell MA, Hill KD, Blackberry I, *et al.* Falls risk and functional decline in older fallers discharged directly from emergency departments. *J Gerontol.* 2006; **61**(10): 1090–5.
9. Tinetti ME, Williams CS. The effect of falls and fall injuries on functioning in community-dwelling older persons. *J Gerontol.* 1998; **53**(2): M112–19.
10. Close JCT, Halter M, Elrick A, *et al.* Falls in the older population: a pilot study to assess those attended by London Ambulance Service but not taken to A&E. *Age Ageing.* 2002; **31**(6): 488–9.
11. Donaldson MG, Khan KM, Davis JC, *et al.* Emergency department fall-related presentations do not trigger fall risk assessment: a gap in care of high-risk outpatient fallers. *Arch Gerontol Geriatr.* 2005; **41**(3): 311–17.
12. Covinsky KE, Kahana E, Kahana B, *et al.* History and mobility exam index to identify community-dwelling elderly persons at risk of falling. *J Gerontol.* 2001; **56**(4): M253–9.
13. Close JCT, Hooper R, Glucksman E, *et al.* Predictors of falls in a high risk population: results from the prevention of falls in the elderly trial (PROFET). *Emerg Med J.* 2003; **20**(5): 421–5.
14. Cummings SR, Nevitt MC, Kidd S. Forgetting falls: the limited accuracy of recall of falls in the elderly. *J Am Geriatr Soc.* 1988; **36**(7): 613–16.
15. Davison J, Bond J, Dawson P, *et al.* Patients with recurrent falls attending Accident & Emergency benefit from multifactorial intervention: a randomised controlled trial. *Age Ageing.* 2005; **34**(2): 162–8.
16. Teno J, Kiel DP, Mor V. Multiple stumbles: a risk factor for falls in community-dwelling elderly, a prospective study. *J Am Geriatr Soc.* 1990; **38**(12): 1321–5.
17. Vellas BJ, Wayne SJ, Romero L, *et al.* One-leg balance is an important predictor of injurious falls in older persons. *J Am Geriatr Soc.* 1997; **45**(6): 735–8.
18. Carpenter CR, Scheatzle MD, D'Antonio JA, *et al.* Identification of fall risk factors in older adult emergency department patients. *Acad Emerg Med.* 2009; **16**(3): 211–19.
19. Richardson JK, Hurvitz EA. Peripheral neuropathy: a true risk factor for falls. *J Gerontol.* 1995; **50**(4): M211–15.
20. Moreland JD, Richardson JA, Goldsmith CH, *et al.* Muscle weakness and falls in older adults: a systematic review and meta-analysis. *J Am Geriatr Soc.* 2004; **52**(7): 1121–9.
21. Menz HB, Morris ME, Lord SR. Foot and ankle risk factors for falls in older people: a prospective study. *J Gerontol.* 2006; **61**(8): 866–70.
22. Lord SR, Dayhew J, Howland A. Multifocal glasses impair edge-contrast sensitivity and depth perception and increase the risk of falls in older people. *J Am Geriatr Soc.* 2002; **50**(11): 1760–6.
23. Hirani V, Primatesta P. Vitamin D concentrations among people aged 65 years and over

living in private households and institutions in England: population survey. *Age Ageing.* 2005; **34**(5): 485–91.

24. Anderson F. Vitamin D for older people: how much, for whom and – above all – why? *Age Ageing.* 2005; **34**(5): 425–6.

25. Venning G. Recent developments in vitamin D deficiency and muscle weakness among elderly people. *BMJ.* 2005; **330**(7490): 524–6.

26. Flicker L, MacInnis RJ, Stein MS, *et al.* Should older people in residential care receive vitamin D to prevent falls? Results of a randomized trial. *J Am Geriatr Soc.* 2005; **53**(11): 1881–8.

27. Leipzig RM, Cumming RG, Tinetti ME. Drugs and falls in older people: a systematic review and meta-analysis: I. Psychotropic drugs. *J Am Geriatr Soc.* 1999; **47**(1): 30–9.

28. Landi F, Onder G, Cesari M, *et al.* Psychotropic medications and risk for falls among community-dwelling frail older people: an observational study. *J Gerontol.* 2005; **60**(5): 622–6.

29. Leipzig RM, Cumming RG, Tinetti ME. Drugs and falls in older people: a systematic review and meta-analysis: II. Cardiac and analgesic drugs. *J Am Geriatr Soc.* 1999; **47**(1): 40–50.

30. Carter SE, Campbell EM, Sanson-Fisher RW, *et al.* Environmental hazards in the homes of older people. *Age Ageing.* 1997; **26**(3): 195–202.

31. Davison J, Brady S, Kenny RA. 24-hour ambulatory electrocardiographic monitoring is unhelpful in the investigation of older persons with recurrent falls. *Age Ageing.* 2005; **34**(4): 382–6.

32. Gangavati AS, Kiely DK, Kulchycki LK, *et al.* Prevalence and characteristics of traumatic intracranial hemorrhage in elderly fallers presenting to the emergency department without focal findings. *J Am Geriatr Soc.* 2009; **57**(8): 1470–4.

33. Baraff LJ, Lee TJ, Kader S, *et al.* Effects of a practice guideline for emergency department care of falls in elder patients on subsequent falls and hospitalizations for injuries. *Acad Emerg Med.* 1999; **6**(12): 1224–31.

34. Salter AE, Khan KM, Donaldson MG, *et al.* Community-dwelling seniors who present to the emergency department with a fall do not receive guideline care and their fall risk profile worsens significantly: a 6-month prospective study. *Osteoporos Int.* 2006; **17**(5): 672–83.

35. Gates S, Fisher JD, Cooke MW, *et al.* Multifactorial assessment and targeted intervention for preventing falls and injuries among older people in community and emergency care settings: a systematic review and meta-analysis. *BMJ.* 2008; **336**(7636): 130–3.

36. Cameron ID, Murray GR, Gillespie LD, *et al.* Interventions for preventing falls in older people in nursing care facilities and hospitals. Cochrane Database Syst Rev. 2010; 1: CD005465.

37. Shaw FE, Bond J, Richardson DA, *et al.* Multifactorial intervention after a fall in older people with cognitive impairment and dementia presenting to the accident and emergency department: randomised controlled trial. *BMJ.* 2003; **326**(7380): 73–8.

38. Van der Velde N, van der Meiraker AH, Pols H, *et al.* Withdrawal of fall-risk-increasing drugs in older persons: effect on tilt-table test outcomes. *J Am Geriatr Soc.* 2007; **55**(5): 734–9.

39. Lord SR, Menz HB, Sherrington C. Home environment risk factors for falls in older people and the efficacy of home modifications. *Age Ageing.* 2006; **35**(Suppl. 2): ii55–9.

40. Patient Safety First Campaign. *The 'How To' Guide for Reducing Harm from Falls.* London: Patient Safety First; 2009. Available at: www.patientsafetyfirst.nhs.uk/ashx/ Asset.ashx?path=/Intervention-support/FALLSHow-to%20Guide%20v4.pdf (accessed 24 January 2013).

41. Sarasin FP, Louis-Simonet M, Carballo D, *et al.* Prospective evaluation of patients with syncope: a population-based study. *Am J Med.* 2001; **111**(3): 177–84.
42. Reed MJ, Gray A. Collapse query cause: the management of adult syncope in the emergency department. *Emerg Med J.* 2006; **23**(8): 589–94.
43. Linzer M, Yang EH, Estes M, *et al.* Diagnosing syncope: part 1: value of history, physical examination, and electrocardiography. *Ann Intern Med.* 1997; **126**(12): 989–96.
44. Del Rosso A, Ungar A, Maggi R, *et al.* Clinical predictors of cardiac syncope at initial evaluation in patients referred urgently to a general hospital: the EGSYS score. *Heart.* 2008; **94**(12): 1620–6.
45. Galizia G, Abete P, Mussi C, *et al.* Role of early symptoms in assessment of syncope in elderly people: results from the Italian group for the study of syncope in the elderly. *J Am Geriatr Soc.* 2009; **57**(1): 18–23.
46. Driver and Vehicle Licensing Agency (DVLA). *DVLA at a Glance Guide to the Current Medical Standards of Fitness to Drive.* Swansea: DVLA; 2012. Available at: www.dft.gov.uk/dvla/medical/ataglance.aspx (accessed 24 January 2013).
47. Kapoor WN. Syncope in older persons. *J Am Geriatr Soc.* 1994; **42**(4): 426–36.
48. Sagrista-Sauleda J, Romero-Ferrer B, Moya A, *et al.* Variations in diagnostic yield of head-up tilt test and electrophysiology in groups of patients with syncope of unknown origin. *Eur Heart J.* 2001; **22**(10): 857–65.
49. Saccilotto RT, Nickel CH, Bucher HC, *et al.* San Francisco Syncope Rule to predict short-term serious outcomes: a systematic review. *CMAJ.* 2011; **183**(15): E1116–26.
50. Armstrong VL, Lawson J, Kamper AM, *et al.* The use of an implantable loop recorder in the investigation of unexplained syncope in older people. *Age Ageing.* 2003; **32**(2): 185–8.
51. Sarasin FP, Junod A, Carballo D, *et al.* Role of echocardiography in the evaluation of syncope: a prospective study. *Heart.* 2002; **88**(4): 363–7.
52. European Society of Cardiology. Guidelines for the diagnosis and management of syncope. *Eur Heart J.* 2009; **30**(21): 2631–71.
53. Lipsitz LA, Nyquist RP, Wei JY, *et al.* Postprandial reduction in blood pressure in the elderly. *N Engl J Med.* 1983; **309**(2): 81–3.
54. Mussi C, Ungar A, Salvioli G, *et al.* Orthostatic hypotension as a cause of syncope in patients older than 65 years admitted to emergency departments for transient loss of consciousness. *J Gerontol.* 2009; **64**(7): 801–6.
55. Freeman R, Wieling W, Axelrod FB, *et al.* Consensus statement on the definition of orthostatic hypotension, neurally mediated syncope and the postural tachycardia syndrome. *Clin Auton Res.* 2011; **21**(2): 69–72.
56. Allcock LM, Ullyart K, Kenny RA, *et al.* Frequency of orthostatic hypotension in a community based cohort of patients with Parkinson's disease. *J Neurol Neurosurg Psychiatry.* 2004; **75**(10): 1470–1.
57. Fan CW, Walsh C, Cunningham CJ. The effect of sleeping with the head of the bed elevated six inches on elderly patients with orthostatic hypotension: an open randomised controlled trial. *Age Ageing.* 2011; **40**(2): 187–92.
58. Gaeta TJ, Fiorini M, Ender K, *et al.* Potential drug-drug interactions in elderly patients presenting with syncope. *J Emerg Med.* 2002; **22**(2): 159–62.
59. Wallace H, Shorvon S, Tallis R. Age-specific incidence and prevalence rates of treated epilepsy in an unselected population of 2,052,922 and age-specific fertility rates of women with epilepsy. *Lancet.* 1998; **352**(9145): 1970–3.
60. Brodie MJ, Kwan P. Epilepsy in elderly people. *BMJ.* 2005; **331**(7528): 1317–22.

61. Mendez MF, Lim GTH. Seizures in elderly patients with dementia: epidemiology and management. *Drugs Aging*. 2003; **20**(11): 791–803.

62. Brodie MJ, Elder AT, Kwan P. Epilepsy in later life. *Lancet Neurol*. 2009; **8**(11): 1019–30.

63. Cloyd J, Hauser W, Towne A, *et al*. Epidemiological and medical aspects of epilepsy in the elderly. *Epilepsy Res*. 2006; **68**(Suppl. 1): S39–48.

64. Thomas RJ. Seizures and epilepsy in the elderly. *Arch Intern Med*. 1997; **157**(6): 605–17.

65. Rowan AJ, Ramsay RE, Collins JF, *et al*. New onset geriatric epilepsy: a randomized study of gabapentin, lamotrigine, and carbamazepine. *Neurology*. 2005; **64**(11): 1868–73.

66. Arif H, Buchsbaum R, Pierro J, *et al*. Comparative effectiveness of 10 antieplileptic drugs in older adults with epilepsy. *Arch Neurol*. 2010; **67**(4): 408–15.

67. Scottish Intercollegiate Guidelines Network. *Diagnosis and Management of Epilepsy in Adults: Clinical guideline 70*. Edinburgh: Scottish Intercollegiate Guidelines Network; 2003. Available at: www.sign.ac.uk/pdf/sign70.pdf (accessed 20 February 2013).

68. National Institute for Health and Clinical Excellence. *The Diagnosis and Management of the Epilepsies in Adults and Children in Primary and Secondary Care*: NICE guideline 20. London: NIHCE; 2004. Available at: www.nice.org.uk/nicemedia/pdf/CG020NICEguideline.pdf (accessed 20 February 2013).

69. Segura-Bruna N, Rodriguez-Campello A, Puente V, *et al*. Valproate-induced hyperammonemic encephalopathy. *Acta Neurol Scand*. 2006; **114**(1): 1–7.

70. Werhahn KJ, Klimpe S, Balkaya S, *et al*. The safety and efficacy of add-on levetiracetam in elderly patients with focal epilepsy: a one-year observational study. *Seizure*. 2011; **20**(4): 305–11.

71. Working Group on Status Epilepticus. Treatment of convulsive status epilepticus. Recommendations of the Epilepsy Foundation of America's working group on status epilepticus. *JAMA*. 1993; **270**(7): 854–9.

72. Hunter G, Young B. Status epilepticus: a review, with emphasis on refractory causes. *Can J Neurol Sci*. 2012; **39**(2): 157–69.

73. Beyenburg S, Elger CE, Reuber M. Acute confusion or altered mental state: consider nonconvulsive status epilepticus. *Gerontology*. 2007; **53**(6): 388–96.

74. Mazarati AM, Baldwin RA, Sankar R, *et al*. Time-dependent decrease in the effectiveness of anti-epileptic drugs during the course of self-sustaining status epilepticus. *Brain Res*. 1998; **814**(1–2): 179–85.

75. Rossetti AO, Hurwitz S, Logroscino G, *et al*. Prognosis of status epilepticus: role of aetiology, age and consciousness impairment at presentation. *J Neurol Neurosurg Psychiatry*. 2006; **77**(5): 611–15.

76. Leppik IE, Derivan AT, Homan RW, *et al*. Double blind study of lorazepam and diazepam in status epilepticus. *JAMA*. 1983; **249**(11): 1452–4.

77. Alldredge BK, Gelb AM, Isaacs SM, *et al*. A comparison of lorazepam, diazepam and placebo for the treatment of out of hospital status epilepticus. *N Engl J Med*. 2001; **345**(9): 631–7.

CHAPTER 6

Surgical care

Presentations of surgical conditions in older patients are frequently vague, sometimes resulting in patients erroneously being admitted initially to medical wards.[1] This can delay effective treatment. Physiological changes make older individuals more susceptible to the stress of surgical intervention. In addition, changes in the skin increase the risk of post-operative infections and can impair wound healing.[2] Patients with poorer functional status are more likely to develop multidrug-resistant surgical wound infections.[3] The frail elderly have a higher risk of adverse post-operative events such as falls and delirium. A confidential enquiry into deaths in patients aged over 80 years within 30 days of surgery in the UK recommended that daily input from geriatricians should be available to elderly people undergoing surgery.[4] Older frail patients often survive major operations only to die from a complication that could have been prevented by high-quality shared post-operative care. It makes sense that frail older patients in acute surgical settings, just as in acute medical settings, would benefit from comprehensive geriatric assessment. Traditionally a divide existed between surgery and geriatrics, but this gap is narrowing because of both integrated working patterns and, hopefully, improved education for all regarding high-quality care for elderly patients.

This is not a book about surgical management, but we provide some discussion about presentations of common surgical disease in the elderly. We have chosen to focus on abdominal pain and trauma. A specialist surgical opinion is recommended to aid the management of these conditions.

PERIOPERATIVE CARE

In non-emergency surgery it is possible to detect and optimise the management of co-morbid conditions prior to the operation to reduce the risk of complications. In the frail elderly this should include many of the components of comprehensive geriatric assessment. It is vital that preoperative cognitive assessment is performed to be able to detect changes following the procedure. Echocardiography is usually recommended if clinical examination reveals a murmur suggestive of aortic stenosis.[5] The high prevalence of diabetes and more frequent prescription of warfarin in the elderly can complicate perioperative care. These should be managed in accordance with local protocols. Careful consideration also needs to be given to medication intake around the time of surgery for those with Parkinson's disease (*see* p. 258).

Excessive administration of fluids leading to water, sodium and chloride overload is a recognised cause of increased post-operative morbidity and mortality.[6] However, the prescription of fluids is often delegated to the most junior member of the medical team. Post-operative oliguria is a common phenomenon and should not alone be used to judge fluid status, which is best assessed by a combination of factors including trends in pulse and blood pressure, capillary refill and jugular venous pressure.[6] It is recommended that physiologically balanced solutions (e.g. Hartmann's or Ringer's) should be used in preference to normal saline in most situations (*see* p. 71). The exception to this is where excess chloride loss is anticipated (e.g. vomiting or gastric drainage).[6] Dextrose saline or 5% dextrose pose a risk of hyponatraemia in the elderly.[7] The aim is to return to normal oral food and fluid intake as soon as possible following the surgery.

Preoperative beta-blockade has been suggested as potentially beneficial to those at risk of cardiovascular events. The use of metoprolol compared with placebo in patients with vascular risk factors (e.g. previous vascular disease or diabetes) having non-cardiac surgery did reduce the incidence of perioperative myocardial infarct (4.2% vs 5.7%), but the overall mortality rate was higher (3.1% vs 2.3%).[8] The use of statin drugs is associated with lower complication rates around the time of non-cardiac vascular surgery.[9]

Outcomes

Surgery has a higher risk for those with co-morbidities (especially cardiac disease) and those requiring emergency procedures. The post-operative mortality rate for non-cardiac surgery in patients aged over 80 years is around 5%, with a morbidity rate around 25%.[10] High-risk patients are typically the elderly with severe co-morbidities and having major surgery. This group has a mortality rate around 12% and they account for 84% of all surgical deaths.[11] Predictors of post-operative complications other than older age include high body mass index (>25), chronic obstructive pulmonary disease and longer operation times.[12] Frailty is also a risk factor for post-operative complications, longer length of stay and discharge to a care home.[13]

The use of laparoscopic procedures may lower the risk of complications. A review of 129 patients aged 71 and over (mean age, 76 years) found lower morbidity rates with laparoscopic than open surgery (24% vs 51%), but 6% of laparoscopic patients required conversion to open procedures.[14] Laparoscopic operations may take longer and this has to be balanced against the possible shorter recovery time.

Post-operative delirium has been detected in 13% of those aged over 65 years undergoing surgery (emergency or elective), but this study excluded those with pre-existing dementia, so the true incidence may have been higher.[15] Another group have reported that around 55% of patients aged over 65 undergoing non-cardiac surgery develop delirium in the first 2 days after their operation.[16] Older age (>75 years), multiple co-morbidities, cognitive impairment, depression and abnormal gylcaemic control are linked with greater risk. It is associated with longer lengths of stay and increased mortality rates. Higher rates of delirium have been detected in those following surgery for fractured neck of femur (*see* p. 165). The route of anaesthesia does not seem to be an important factor.[17] Avoiding hypoxia, correcting fluid and electrolyte imbalances, controlling pain, rationalising medications and the early restoration of nutritional intake and mobility can reduce the incidence of post-operative delirium.[18] The diagnosis and management of delirium is discussed on page 107.

Post-operative cognitive decline is a reported subacute to chronic hazard of surgery that differs from delirium, possibly induced by perioperative cerebral hypoxia. Cognitive decline following coronary artery bypass graft surgery of one standard deviation or more in any cognitive domain has been detected in 53% of patients at discharge, and 24% at 6 months.[19] A study had estimated it to have a prevalence of around 10% at 3 months after major non-cardiac surgery in people aged over 60 years.[20] However, more recent data that assessed preoperative cognitive function and compared with controls did not find a significant association.[21] So uncertainty surrounds the phenomenon of post-operative cognitive decline at the current time.[22]

The systematic approach term 'Enhanced Recovery After Surgery' may improve outcomes. It has four key elements: (1) comprehensive preoperative evaluation, (2) optimal anaesthesia and minimally invasive techniques, (3) post-operative care (pain control and early mobilisation), and (4) rapid resumption of normal diet. This is very intensive and requires significant nursing and therapy input and it typically also involves the regular input of geriatricians on surgical units.

- Frail elderly patients are at greater risk of adverse outcomes following surgery – comprehensive assessment with appropriate intervention is vital to reduce this risk.
- High-quality perioperative fluid management is an important component of care.
- Mortality rates are higher for emergency procedures and in those with background co-morbidities.
- Post-operative delirium is common – clinicians should take steps to reduce the risk, be vigilant to allow an early diagnosis and when detected take appropriate actions.
- Surgical outcomes are likely to be improved when there is a comprehensive preoperative evaluation, optimal anaesthesia and surgical technique, high-quality post-operative care (including pain control) and the early resumption of mobility and normal diet.

ABDOMINAL PAIN

Abdominal pain accounts for approximately 3%–6% of emergency department (ED) visits in patients aged over 65 years.[23,24] Around 10%–37% of these patients require acute surgical intervention.[24–28] Older patients have higher rates of surgery and mortality than younger cases.[29] They represent a challenging group to the ED physician.[30] It should be remembered that abdominal pain can occasionally be the presenting complaint of patients with non-abdominal disorders (e.g. myocardial infarction).

Diagnosis

The initial diagnostic accuracy is lower in older adults than in younger adults, falling from around 45%–55% in young adults, to 29%–44% in those aged 80 and over.[31,32] Inaccurate initial diagnosis puts patients at greater risk of morbidity.[33] Serious problems that are frequently initially misdiagnosed include ischaemic bowel, malignancy and pancreatitis.[34] Urinary retention should be considered, especially in elderly men.

Table 6.1 shows the frequency of the most common diagnoses in patients presenting acutely with non-traumatic abdominal pain at different ages.[25,27,32,34] Table 6.2 shows the most common reasons for emergency surgery for abdominal pain in the elderly.[26,35,36]

Presenting temperature and serum white blood cell counts have been found to be poor markers to detect the patients that required surgical intervention.[26] In a group of patients aged 80 and over (mean age 85 years) with acute abdominal pain requiring operation, 30% had a temperature <37.5°C and a serum white cell count (WCC) <10.5 × 10⁹/L.[35] Compared with those aged 64 and under, patients aged 80 and above who required surgical intervention were less likely to be found to have rebound tenderness (29% vs 62%), rectal tenderness (18% vs 32%) or abdominal rigidity (34% vs 43%).[32] Guarding and rebound tenderness sometimes only present late in the disease and may herald perforation or gangrene.[37] The reduced association with muscular guarding could also be explained by reduced muscle size and strength secondary to sarcopenia.

TABLE 6.1 Common causes of abdominal pain in patients assessed in hospital aged over 65 and over 80 years

Diagnosis (%)	Age (years)	
	65+	80+
Non-specific abdominal pain	14–26	22
Gall bladder disease	8–23	14
Small bowel obstruction	11–12	–
Diverticulitis	5–12	4
Peptic ulcer disease	4–11	–
Constipation	2–9	9
Hernia	1–6	–
Pancreatitis	2–4	4
Appendicitis	1–4	3
Renal colic	4	1

Note: Data obtained from Bugliosi et al.,[25] Kizer and Vassar,[27] Laurell et al.,[32] and Abi-Hanna and Gleckman[34]

TABLE 6.2 The commonest reasons for emergency surgery for abdominal pain in patients aged over 65 and over 80 years

Surgical diagnosis (%)	Age (years)	
	65+	80+
Gall bladder disease	26–43	25
Bowel obstruction	16–25	17
Hernia	5–20	21
Perforation	9–12	9
Ischaemic bowel	8–11	9
Appendicitis	7	3

Note: Data obtained from Parker et al.,[26] Potts and Vukov,[35] and Ozkan et al.[36]

Investigations

Abdominal X-rays are good for detecting bowel obstruction and can demonstrate constipation (*see* Figure 6.1). Ultrasound scans are good for imaging the biliary tree and bladder scans can demonstrate urinary retention. CT scanning is useful for poorly differentiated abdominal pain, or those with suspected obstruction, pancreatitis, appendicitis or abdominal aortic aneurysm in the absence of shock.[38] A study of 337 patients aged over 60 (mean age, 73 years) presenting with acute non-traumatic abdominal pain to an ED found that 37% had an abdominal CT performed.[29] These scans were diagnostic in 57% of this patient group. The commonest abnormalities detected were diverticulitis (18%), bowel obstruction (18%), nephrolithiasis (10%), gall bladder disease (10%), mass/neoplasm (8%), pyelonephritis (7%) and pancreatitis (6%). A study that performed abdominal CT scans in 104 consecutive cases of patients aged over 65 (mean age, 75 years) presenting to the ED with acute non-traumatic abdominal pain found that CT scanning altered the suspected diagnosis in 45% of cases and the decision to admit or discharge in 26% of cases.[39] As would be expected, physicians tend to order CT scans when the diagnosis is unclear.[40]

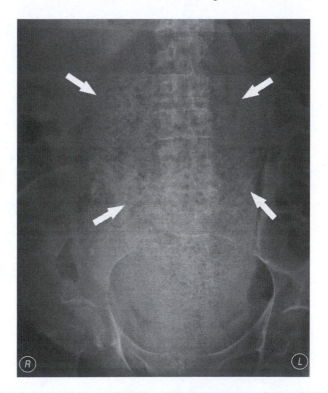

FIGURE 6.1 An abdominal X-ray showing an extreme case of constipation – the large central area of mottled shadowing (outlined by white arrows) is caused by faeces

Prognosis

Mortality rates for patients admitted with acute abdominal pain are higher in older than younger patients, reaching 5%–7% in those aged 80 and over.[31,32] The prognosis is worse in those who require surgery.

Around 10%–20% of gastrointestinal surgery is performed on patients over the age of 75.[41] Mortality rates are higher (4%–5% vs <1%) and complications are more frequent (including pulmonary emboli, pneumonia, acute kidney injury, myocardial infarction and stroke) than for patients aged 55 or younger. This is particularly true for patients requiring emergency rather than elective surgery. The reasons for this include a lack of time for thorough evaluation and to correct physiological abnormalities (e.g. shock, electrolyte disorders and acidosis).

In a group of patients aged over 80 (n = 215; mean age, 84 years) having surgery, morbidity and mortality rates of 49% and 14% were described overall.[42] Mortality was 19% in those having emergency procedures, compared with 8% in the elective group. Another study found a mortality rate after emergency abdominal surgery in patients aged 65 and over (n = 92; mean age, 73 years) of 15%.[36] One series of patients aged 80 and over (n = 132; mean age, 85 years) who were admitted to hospital with acute abdominal disorders found a perioperative mortality rate of 34%.[33] However, another series of patients aged 85 and over (n = 179; mean age, 89 years) having abdominal surgery (64% emergency procedures) found a mortality rate of 17%.[43] A review of 32 patients aged 90 and over who underwent surgery found an overall mortality rate of 9% (elective cases 0%, emergency 14%).[44] These data show quite wide variation, suggesting that appropriate patient selection is of key importance.

Those with impaired cardiac or respiratory function are more likely to develop complications.[45] A low albumin level is also associated with a worse prognosis.[42] However, regarding emergency surgery in the elderly, no preoperative risk assessment score is sufficiently accurate to be a surrogate for clinical judgement.[46]

Specific conditions

The common causes of acute non-traumatic abdominal pain in the elderly are outlined below. Table 6.3 shows a simple overview of clinical features to aid differentiation.

Biliary tract disease

Gallstones are present in around 30% of men and 40% of women over the age of 80 years, but just 30% of these cause symptoms.[47] Around 80% of those aged over 90 years who live in a care home have evidence of gallstones or have previously had a cholecystectomy.[48] The commonest presentations are obstructive

TABLE 6.3 A simple overview of the clinical features of common causes of acute non-traumatic abdominal pain in the elderly

Condition	Location of pain	Nature of pain	Comments
Cholecystitis	Right UQ	Colicky/constant	Murphy's sign may be present LFT likely to be abnormal
Obstruction	Diffuse	Colicky	Abnormal abdominal X-ray Check for hernias if small bowel obstructed
Perforation	Diffuse	Sudden onset, worse on movement	May see gas under diaphragm on erect chest X-ray
Appendicitis	Central then moving to right IF	Constant	May have a tender local mass
Diverticulitis	Left IF	Constant, may reduce after passing flatus	May have a tender local mass Can cause lower GI bleeding
Aortic aneurysm	Diffuse/back	Severe	May have a pulsatile mass with or without shock
Ischaemic bowel	Diffuse	Severe, worse on movement	Few physical signs in early stages Likely to have vascular risk factors/AF
Pancreatitis	Epigastric	Worse on movement, may radiate to back	Serum amylase very high

Abbreviations: UQ = upper quadrant, LFT = liver function test, IF = iliac fossa, GI = gastrointestinal, AF = atrial fibrillation

jaundice (30%), biliary colic (30%), pancreatitis (15%) and acute cholecystitis (14%).[47] Patients presenting with right upper quadrant pain are most likely to have a disorder of the biliary tract.[34] The pain may be constant rather than colicky in nature.[37] Endoscopic retrograde cholangiopancreatography is typically appropriate for stones within the common bile duct of patients unsuitable for surgery. However, a magnetic resonance cholangiopancreatography may be required first to definitely identify stones before subjecting a frail elderly person to the significant risks of an endoscopic retrograde cholangiopancreatography. Early elective cholecystectomy, where possible, appears to be a better option than a non-surgical approach in this age group.[47]

Acute cholecystitis is a common reason for emergency surgery in the elderly. A review reported the presenting clinical features of 168 patients aged over 65 (mean age, 74 years) who required urgent cholecystectomy.[49] Overall, 65% had right upper quadrant pain, 5% had no pain, 56% were apyrexial (<37.0°C) and 41% had normal serum WCCs. Nausea and vomiting are also less commonly reported by older patients.[50] Murphy's sign has a lower sensitivity in older people.[38] There may be mild jaundice. Ultrasound scanning is reliable for detecting gallstones, but less reliable at detecting cholecystitis (which may be acalculous in the old).[37] Complications include gangrenous cholecystitis, empyema formation and perforation, which are more common in the elderly.[38] These may be more reliably detected by CT scanning.

Bowel obstruction

Bowel obstruction typically causes diffuse colicky pain with nausea and vomiting. Diarrhoea may be present in the early stages due to hyperperistalsis distal to the lesion. A change in nature of the pain to severe and constant might indicate the development of strangulation or perforation; this may be accompanied by fever and shock.[38] Vomiting, distension, tenderness and abnormal bowel sounds may not be detected at initial presentation.[37] The diagnosis is typically made by plain abdominal X-ray (*see* Figure 6.2), but these can appear normal in cases of small bowel obstruction.[51] CT scanning is more sensitive and is more likely to identify the underlying cause or show signs of strangulated bowel.[38] The presence of strangulated bowel is likely to necessitate immediate surgical intervention.

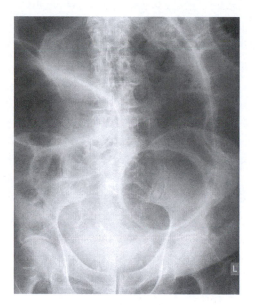

FIGURE 6.2 An abdominal X-ray showing very dilated large bowel caused by a sigmoid volvulus

Small bowel obstruction is most commonly due to adhesions (secondary to prior surgery) (50%–70%) or hernias (15%–30%) and less commonly due to gallstone ileus or neoplasia.[37,50,51] The finding of a tender mass in the inguinal-femoral triangle or abdominal midline suggests a hernia as the cause.[38]

Large bowel obstruction is most commonly due to malignancy, diverticulitis or volvulus.[37,50,51] In the frail elderly it may also be caused by faecal impaction. The onset can be gradual over several days with non-specific initial symptoms. Colorectal cancer is suggested by a history of changed bowel habit, weight loss, abdominal pain and/or rectal bleeding.[37] Volvulae cause around 15% of large bowel obstructions in older patients, with 80% of these due to sigmoid volvulae (the remainer involving the caecum). Sigmoid volvulae tend to be associated with a more gradual onset of pain, compared with a more acute presentation with those affecting the caecum.[50] They are more likely to occur in patients taking laxatives, sedatives, anticholinergics or anti-Parkinsonian medications. On abdominal X-ray, sigmoid volvulae produce a pattern of dilated colon arising from the left lower quadrant and projected towards the right (caecal volvulae arise from the right lower quadrant).

Acute pseudo-obstruction of the colon

Acute pseudo-obstruction of the colon (also known as Ogilvies' syndrome) is characterised by massive dilatation of the large bowel in the absence of a true blockage. It is probably caused by an impairment of the autonomic nervous system. Overall it is a rare condition, but more common in the elderly.[6] It is associated with neurodegenerative conditions (e.g. Parkinson's disease and Alzheimer's dementia), electrolyte disturbances (e.g. hypokalaemia and hypomagnesaemia), post-operative patients and some medications (e.g. anticholinergics and opiates).[52]

Patients tend to present with painless abdominal distension plus constipation, nausea and vomiting. When pain is present it is usually mild. Bowel sounds are usually present. Very dilated large bowel (>12 cm) may perforate – this is suggested by peritonism, fever and a rising serum WCC. Abdominal X-rays show dilatation of the right colon (>9 cm) without air-fluid levels, and usually with gaseous distension of the rectum (which is not seen in genuine obstruction). Either water-soluble contrast enema or CT scanning can differentiate it from bowel obstruction.[52] Also it should not be confused with toxic megacolon secondary to *Clostridium difficile* infection (*see* p. 189).

Initial treatment is to correct any fluid and electrolyte abnormalities and to discontinue any potentially causative drugs, particularly those with anticholinergic properties (*see* p. 306). Intestinal decompression with a nasogastric tube and rectal cannula may be tried. The cholinesterase inhibitor neostigmine has been successfully used in this condition.[6] More severe and unresponsive cases can be decompressed endoscopically. Occasionally surgery is required to form a caecal stoma or in cases of perforation.

Perforated bowel

Visceral perforations are most commonly due to peptic ulcers (50%), but large bowel causes include diverticula and tumours.[38] The typical pain is of sudden onset and severe in nature causing the patient to lie motionless. There is associated tachycardia and tachypnoea. The classic rigid abdomen may not be present in elderly patients. Pneumoperitoneum is seen on erect chest X-ray in around 55%–70% of cases but can be detected more frequently by CT scanning.[1,38]

The age-specific incidence of perforation due to peptic ulcers has fallen following the widespread use of medications such as proton pump inhibitors. Compared to people aged below 65 years, those 65 and over are less likely to have classic epigastric pain (59% vs 85%), less likely to have a history of peptic ulcer disease (55% vs 68%), less likely to have epigastric tenderness and guarding (24% vs 70%), but more likely to be shocked (blood pressure <90 mmHg) (21% vs 2%).[1] Mortality rates for those requiring emergency surgery following perforated peptic ulcers is around 27% for those aged 70–79 and around 45% for those aged 80 and over.[53]

Appendicitis

The classic presentation of appendicitis is a combination of right lower abdominal pain, fever (>37.6°C), raised serum WCC (>10 × 10⁹/L), nausea and vomiting. Among elderly patients this occurs in around 15%–30% of cases.[54,55] Right lower quadrant pain is present in 70%–75%, fever (>37.6°C) in 23%–37%, and a raised WCC ($>10 \times 10^9$/L) in 74%–78%. The initial presentation may mimic bowel obstruction in the old.[38] In a series of 113 patients aged over 60 (mean age, 72 years), 51% were perforated (incidence in younger people around 20%), and the mortality rate was 4% (compared with <1% in younger cases).[54] However, more recent data suggests that improvements in care (including better preoperative diagnosis rates because of CT scanning and greater use of laparoscopic surgery) have resulted in lower perforation (27%) and mortality rates (1%) in older patients.[55]

Diverticular disease

In Western countries the prevalence of bowel diverticula (diverticulosis) is associated with age, being rare before the age of 40 but present in more than half of people over the age of 80.[56] Around 1%–2% will require hospitalisation for complications and more than half of those admitted are aged over 70 years.

Painful (or symptomatic) diverticular disease causes episodes of localised abdominal pain (most commonly left lower quadrant) in the absence of signs of systemic inflammation. The pain may be made worse by eating and reduced by passing flatus or stools.[57] Diverticula are also a common cause of large lower gastrointestinal bleeds, typically without pain (*see* p. 252).[37]

Diverticulitis is the combination of painful diverticular disease plus signs of systemic inflammation. Features include low-grade fever, leukocytosis, nausea/vomiting, diarrhoea and mild abdominal distension.[37,38] Bowel sounds may be increased or reduced, and there may be a palpable abdominal mass.[57] There may be micro-perforation of one or more diverticula.[51] This can develop into peritonitis, abscess formation, fistulae (e.g. colovesical or colovaginal) or bowel obstruction. Diverticulitis is usually a clinical diagnosis, but if in doubt CT scanning may help (colonoscopy and barium enema should be avoided due to risk of enlarging any perforation).[51]

Abdominal aortic aneurysm

Abdominal aortic aneurysms (AAAs) occur more commonly in men with a history of peripheral vascular disease or vascular risk factors (especially smoking), and are typically infrarenal in location.[51] They are estimated to be present in 4%–8% of people over the age of 65.[58] They are often asymptomatic, but may cause abdominal pain, back pain or claudication. In the event of a rupture, the classic presentation is with severe abdominal pain, hypotension and a palpable pulsatile mass. This carries a high mortality rate, at around 50%.[59] Hypotension is sometimes absent because of tamponade in the retroperitoneal space.[50] A study found that 30% of patients (n = 152; mean age, 70 years) presenting with a ruptured AAA were initially misdiagnosed.[59] Only 9% of this group of patients had all three of abdominal pain, back pain and a pulsatile mass. This latter sign was detected in 26% of patients, compared with 72% of those with an initial correct diagnosis. A ruptured AAA may be confused with renal colic, as the pain may radiate to the groin, and there may be associated haematuria due to irritation of the ureters.[50] Alternatively, it can be wrongly labelled as musculoskeletal back pain. Dissection typically causes pain in the back or abdomen, which can vary in intensity (*see* p. 233).[37] This can be diagnosed by CT scanning.

Ischaemic bowel

Acute mesenteric ischaemia presents with abdominal pain (typically severe, poorly localised and with few physical findings), vomiting, diarrhoea, reduced bowel sounds and shock.[37] Peritonism and bloody stools are late features suggesting bowel infarction.[50] It can be caused by emboli (e.g. from the heart), non-occlusive (e.g. reduced cardiac output), local arterial thrombus formation (often preceded by chronic symptoms including post-prandial pain and weight loss) or venous thrombus. The superior mesenteric artery is most commonly involved. There may be risk factors for vascular disease including atrial fibrillation (present in 50%).[50] It is suggested by a raised serum WCC (mean value around 20 000 cells/mm³), but metabolic acidosis may only be a late feature (i.e. bowel infarction).[38] Initial X-rays are often normal. Angiography is the best diagnostic test. The mortality rate is high: 60%–90%.[36,38] A high index of suspicion is required to make a timely diagnosis.

Pancreatitis

Acute pancreatitis in the old usually has a similar presentation to that seen in the young (epigastric pain, nausea, vomiting, low-grade fever and dehydration),[37] but it may present atypically. Blood tests show a high serum amylase and lipase, but more minor elevations in amylase can be seen with other conditions, including mesenteric ischaemia.[50] Gallstones are the commonest cause in the old. Other causes include alcohol excess, adverse drug reactions (e.g. azathioprine, diuretics, non-steroidal anti-inflammatory drugs and erythromycin), hypercalcaemia and hypothermia. An increased mortality rate is seen in older patients (around 20%–40% in those aged over 70 years).[38,50] Abdominal CT scanning may be useful to differentiate causes in the scenario of mild increases in serum amylase levels. CT scanning can also detect pancreatic necrosis.

KEY POINTS

- Consider non-abdominal causes of abdominal pain – such as myocardial infarction.
- Urinary retention may present as abdominal pain.
- Typical features of significant intra-abdominal disease (e.g. fever, raised serum WCC, abdominal rigidity or rebound tenderness) are often absent at initial presentation in the frail elderly.
- The mortality rate in patients aged over 80 admitted with acute non-traumatic abdominal pain is around 5%–7%, and in those requiring emergency surgery it rises to around 14%–34%.
- Gallstones are common in older patients and acute cholecystitis is a common reason for emergency surgery – suspect in cases of right upper quadrant pain.
- Acute mesenteric ischaemia typically presents with severe abdominal pain that is poorly localised and with few physical findings.

- CT scanning is the best investigation for older patients with unexplained abdominal pain.

TRAUMA

Around 12% of people aged over 65 and 20% of people aged over 85 present to an ED following an injury each year.[60] Among patients presenting to an ED with injuries, 48%–62% in the over-65s, and 66%–81% in the over-85s are because of falls.[60,61] Fractures account for about 22% of injuries. Overall 20% of patients are admitted, but this figure rises to 30% in the over-85s.

Falls account for 71%–84% of injuries to older adults admitted because of trauma.[62,63] Injury rates following falls are high in the elderly because of the high prevalence of osteoporosis and reduced self-protecting reflexes (e.g. putting out arms to protect the head). The majority of older patients (65 years and over) admitted with trauma secondary to falls have sustained fractures (89%),[62] with 48% of these due to hip fracture (mortality rate 6%). Intracranial injuries are present in around 4%, and this group have a high mortality rate (24%). The second-commonest cause of injury is road traffic accidents.[63] These include injuries to those driving or passengers in a car, and to pedestrians hit by vehicles. In addition, the incidence of sternal fractures from seat belts is increased in the elderly.[2]

Mortality rates following trauma seem to increase after the age of 70 years, irrespective of injury severity.[64] The in-hospital mortality for patients aged over 65 is around 5%–10%.[61,63] Trauma scores used for predicting prognosis may be less accurate in the frail elderly sustaining low energy injuries.[65] Elderly patients who do survive trauma are likely to lose independence and to have a reduced quality of life.[66,67] Those who are discharged from the ED without hospitalisation are likely to need additional short-term support (which is often provided by family members).[68]

Factors associated with a poor prognosis include hypotension (systolic blood pressure <90 mmHg), hypoventilation (respiratory rate <10 breaths per minute) and low Glasgow Coma Scale (GCS) score.[69] Older adults may not demonstrate a compensatory tachycardia in response to hypovolaemia and shock (e.g. beta-blocker use).[2] A high level of suspicion of serious injury is required. Serum lactate or arterial blood gas sampling may demonstrate tissue hypoperfusion. Persisting high lactate or low pH levels despite initial resuscitation suggest inadequate treatment, ongoing haemorrhage, or the development of complications.[2]

Fractures

Osteoporosis is highly prevalent in the frail elderly. Fractures typically occur after falling from the patient's own height or less, which is termed a 'fragility fracture'. Around 90% of women aged over 65 years who have had a previous fracture at any site have either osteoporosis or osteopenia, with 69% of those aged over 75 having osteoporosis.[70] Mortality following all fragility fractures is increased in older men and women compared with age-matched controls.[71-73] After a fragility fracture, the risk of future fracture is doubled in both men and women.[74] This emphasises the need for preventive strategies – to reduce the risk of falls and treat osteoporosis. Osteoporotic vertebral fractures are discussed on page 277. Pathological fractures are also possible because of underlying Paget's disease, metastatic cancer (e.g. bronchus, breast, kidney or prostate) or myeloma.

Hip fracture

The mean age of presentation following hip fracture is currently around 79–82 years with about 80% being women.[75,76] Hip fracture is diagnosed in around 20% of patients aged over 70 who attend an ED because of a fall.[77] It is associated with dementia. In patients aged 85 years, a prevalence of prior hip fracture of 28% has been found in those with dementia, compared to 12% in those without ($p < 0.01$).[78] This difference may be partly explained by a higher use of psychotropic drugs in demented patients, which are associated with an increased risk of falls. There did not appear to be significant differences in bone mineral density between the groups. Acute confusional states are also common in elderly patients with hip fractures and they are associated with worse outcomes,[79] yet clinicians are often poor at routinely assessing cognition and diagnosing impairment.[80]

Assessment

In a patient presenting following a fall, or with hip pain, the presence of hip fracture is usually obvious when displaced as the leg is shortened and externally rotated. This is then confirmed on X-ray (*see* Figure 6.3). If not, then try doing straight leg raising, internal and external rotation at the hip and palpate over the pelvic bones. If the patient experiences pain then an undisplaced fracture (*see* Figure 6.4) should be suspected. Evaluation in the ED should include assessment for pain, nutrition and hydration, pressure ulcer risk, mental state and functional status.[5]

A diagnosis is delayed for more than 24 hours in around 14% of patients.[81] This is most frequently because of a failure of the patient to see a doctor or the doctor not requesting a hip X-ray, but hip X-rays do not always demonstrate a

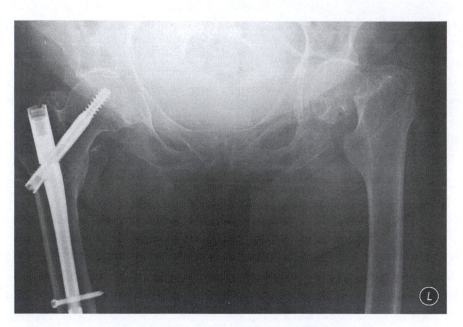

FIGURE 6.3 This patient has an acute fracture of the left hip (note that they have previously had surgery to repair a broken right hip)

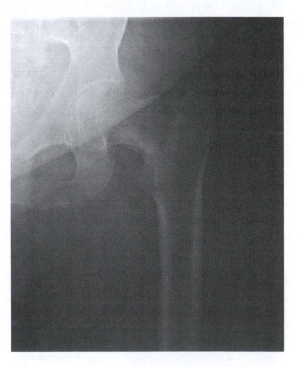

FIGURE 6.4 An X-ray showing a minimally displaced fracture of the left hip

fracture, especially if it is undisplaced. Around 1% of initial X-rays will fail to show a fracture that later becomes apparent (most often by becoming displaced).[81] Other imaging modalities may increase the early detection rate. A prevalence of hip or pelvic fracture of 4.4% was identified by MRI of patients who attended an ED with hip pain but had no fracture seen on initial X-ray.[82] The use of MRI in patients aged 70 and over with negative X-rays but a high clinical suspicion of fracture (persisting pain, unable to weight bear and pain on straight leg raising or hip rotation) seems particularly beneficial. A study detected a proximal femoral fracture in 21 of 25 (84%) such patients, with a further three having pelvic fractures.[83] CT or bone scans are alternative but less sensitive imaging techniques. Another option is to simply repeat the hip X-ray after 24–48 hours.[5]

Analgesia

There is evidence that a large proportion of people attending an ED with painful conditions do not receive adequate analgesia.[84] It is important to assess and treat pain following an injury. This should include documentation of both the presence of pain and a measure of its intensity (e.g. on a 0–10 scale), with reassessment after giving analgesia. The risk of delirium is not a valid reason to avoid opioids as pain itself could also be a trigger. One should consider co-prescribing laxatives with opiates given the increased risk of constipation in the elderly.[85]

There is evidence of under treatment of pain in older patients following hip fracture, including seldom use of opioid drugs.[86] One study found that 81% of elderly patients (mean age, 83 years) with hip fracture in an ED complained of pain, yet 36% of these people received no analgesia.[87] Of those who did receive analgesia, there was a mean time of 141 minutes from presentation to receipt of medication. Compared with younger people with fractures, patients aged over 70 are less likely to receive analgesia in the ED (66% vs 80%) and they receive, on average, lower doses.[88]

A study comparing cognitively impaired adults presenting with hip fracture to those without cognitive impairment found that similar proportions reported pain (60%–65%) and the intensity rating was also similar.[89] However, the cognitively impaired patients received significantly less opioid analgesia (first 48 hours post-operatively daily equivalent of morphine 13.2 vs 21.0 mg). Fear of worsening cognitive impairment should not be a barrier to providing adequate pain relief and pain itself may worsen cognition.

Management

Guidelines have described the key elements of good care.[5,90] Clinicians should aim to perform a hip X-ray, administer intravenous (iv) fluids and analgesia (usually opiates), and move onto a pressure-relieving mattress within 2 hours of arrival in the ED. There should be prompt admission to orthopaedic care (within four hours). Comprehensive assessment by medical, surgical and anaesthetic teams should be rapid. Good communication and collaboration between these specialities is essential. The current recommended model is for orthogeriatric input on an orthopaedic ward. Secondary prevention including bone protection and a falls assessment is essential (*see* Chapter 5).

Surgical fixation

Surgical fixation is almost always appropriate as conservative management is associated with chronic pain and immobility. Surgery should be performed as soon as possible because delays are associated with increased mortality rates (which may be explained by the presence of co-morbidities) and more complications including pressure ulcers.[91] The aim is to operate within 48 hours of admission, providing the patient is fit enough. Those on warfarin with an international normalised ratio >1.5 should have their warfarin withheld and be given iv vitamin K. The use of antiplatelet drugs should not postpone surgery.

The best method for surgical fixation is unclear.[91] The technique used is influenced by the location of the fracture – typically, intra- or extracapsular (*see* Figure 6.5). The most commonly used techniques are to join the broken bones back together with a dynamic hip screw (for extracapsular fractures), or to replace the broken section of bone with a hemi-arthroplasty or total hip replacement (for intracapsular fractures). Osteoporotic bone can be a challenge for the surgeon to effectively repair, and the bone tends to heal more slowly.[90] Regional anaesthesia appears to be associated with lower perioperative mortality rates.[91]

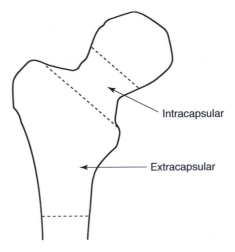

Intracapsular

Extracapsular

FIGURE 6.5 The common locations of hip fracture

Complications

Around 20% of patients develop post-operative complications.[76] Pressure-relieving mattresses should be used to reduce the incidence of pressure ulcers.[91] Patients admitted with hip fracture are at high risk of underlying malnutrition, which could delay post-operative healing. Overall, there is only weak evidence of a benefit from nutritional supplementation,[92] but screening to detect malnutrition (*see* p. 58) and giving oral supplements when found would be reasonable. Post-operative delirium is found in around 28%–40% of elderly patients with fractured neck of femur (*see* Chapter 4).[93,94] Symptomatic deep vein thrombosis develops in around 3% and pulmonary embolus in around 1%.[90] Low-molecular-weight heparins, factor X inhibitors (e.g. fondaparinux) or mechanical compression devices can reduce the risk of deep vein thrombosis, but they can increase the risk of other complications, and there is a lack of widespread consensus on their optimal use.[5,90,91] Early mobilisation is also important. Antibiotic prophylaxis (single dose) reduces the risk of deep wound infections.[95]

Osteoporosis

Dual-energy X-ray absorptiometry scanning is used to evaluate bone density. A T-score of 2.5 standard deviations or more below the normal value for a person of the same sex aged 25 years is used to define osteoporosis. Patients aged over 75 who have sustained a fragility fracture are very likely to have osteoporosis and this is a reasonable assumption when dual-energy X-ray absorptiometry scanning is unavailable or inappropriate.[96]

Inadequate vitamin D levels are highly prevalent in the UK, with insufficiency affecting around 50% and severe deficiency 16% in the winter and spring.[97] This is especially true for patients who have limited sunlight exposure, which includes the frail elderly with reduced mobility or residing in care homes. Vitamin D deficiency can also be provoked by some medications (e.g. phenytoin, sodium valproate and carbamazepine) or malabsorption (e.g. coeliac disease). Clinical features of vitamin D deficiency in adults include proximal muscle weakness and pain in the ribs, hips, pelvis or feet.[97] Blood tests may show an elevated alkaline phosphatase, low calcium and low phosphate levels, but these are not always present. When clinically suspected, the best way to assess vitamin D status is to measure serum 25-hydroxyvitamin D levels. Vitamin D deficiency leads to osteomalacia that worsens osteoporosis. Calcium and vitamin D supplements are usually appropriate for the frail elderly following a fragility fracture (also *see* p. 129).

Other possible secondary causes or contributory factors to osteoporosis include steroid use, Cushing's syndrome, hyperparathyroidism, hypothyroidism, pan-hypopituitarism, alcohol excess and smoking. These should also be considered as part of a comprehensive evaluation.

The bisphosphonate alendronate is the current recommended first-line drug to treat osteoporosis (risedronate or etidronate can be considered if alendronate is not tolerated).[96] Second-line options include strontium ranelate and raloxifene. Teriparatide (a recombinant form of parathyroid hormone) and denosumab (a monoclonal antibody that inhibits osteoclasts) are other possible therapeutic options. There is evidence that secondary prevention is suboptimal. In a review of prescriptions between 1995 and 2004 for patients who had a previous hip fracture and now resided in nursing homes, just 12% were prescribed medications to treat osteoporosis.[98]

Rehabilitation

Various models of post-operative rehabilitation have been proposed. These include rehabilitation on the orthopaedic ward, within a specialised orthogeriatric unit, or at the patient's own home with a supported discharge service. Prompt mobilisation ideally from the first post-operative day, usually allowing full weight bearing, is recommended. A multidisciplinary rehabilitation approach should be adopted. Early supported discharge and ongoing community rehabilitation is often appropriate. There is some evidence that early geriatric multidisciplinary intervention can reduce complications and mortality rates.[99]

Prognosis

Mortality is around 5%–10% after 1 month, being higher in the oldest, most frail and those with co-morbidities.[76,100] An overall 90-day mortality rate of 18% was found in one study.[101] The rate was 15% for those with intracapsular and 22% for extracapsular fractures. The 1-year mortality rate is around 33%–38%.[75,76] Patients with three or more co-morbidities or those who develop either post-operative heart failure or chest infection are at greatest risk of death. In those who survive, there is often significant associated functional impairment. In a cohort of elderly patients (mean age 80 years) who had sustained a hip fracture, only 54% were independently mobile at 1 year, compared with 87% pre-admission.[102] A significant number of patients will require placement within a care home.[75]

Head trauma

Head trauma in the elderly is most commonly caused by falls (51%–59%), with road traffic accidents (as passenger or pedestrian) being next most common (9%–33%).[103,104] This differs from younger patients (43% due to motor accidents,

28% following an assault, 23% after a fall). The initial assessment should include calculation of the GCS score and a full neurological examination.

CT scans

CT head scanning is performed on most patients with significant head trauma. In a review of cases that had a head CT scan following presenting to an ED after blunt head trauma, 20% of patients over the age of 60 (compared with 13% of younger cases) had a traumatic brain injury and 17% of these patients required neurosurgical intervention.[103] But it is unknown which patients with minor head trauma should be scanned. Various clinical decision aids have been developed to guide the use of head CT scans in mild closed head trauma. None offers ideal sensitivity and specificity to detect significant intracranial lesions.[105] Current National Institute for Health and Clinical Excellence guidance recommends CT head scans for patients aged 65 and over with a GCS score of 15 if on warfarin, or if any amnesia for loss of consciousness has occurred since the injury.[106]

A study that recruited 133 patients over the age of 65 with minor head trauma (GCS score of 13–15 on admission) (mean age, 84 years; 85% had GCS score of 15, 95% presented following a fall or syncope) who underwent CT head scanning, found an intracranial injury in 14% of cases.[107] No symptoms were reported by 26% of these patients, and 21% required neurosurgical intervention. No significant association with either alcohol or anticoagulant use was detected. A different review of 89 cases of patients on anticoagulants who had a CT scan following head trauma found evidence of intracranial bleeding in 7 (8%).[108] All patients with bleeds had a GCS score below 15 and/or a focal neurological deficit.

Occult head injury (GCS score of 15, no focal neurological deficit or evidence of skull fracture) may be more common in the elderly. This could be explained by brain atrophy allowing mass lesions not to compress other structures. Low-impact injuries (e.g. falls from own height) may not lead to significant external evidence of injury. A study of CT scans performed for all blunt head trauma in those aged 65 years and over detected an intracranial injury in 12.5% (compared with 7.9% of younger adults) and a clinically significant injury (requiring intervention or associated with long-term disability) in 9.2% (compared with 6.1% of younger adults).[109] In the overall population, a clinically significant head injury presented in an occult way in 2.2% (compared with 0.8% of younger adults). The findings from these studies suggest that emergency physicians should have a low threshold for head CT scanning of older patients presenting with minor head trauma.

Subdural haematoma

Subdural haematoma (SDH) can result from trivial head trauma in the elderly and present weeks to months after the event.[110] The elderly appear more susceptible to SDH, in part due to brain atrophy (approximately a 200 g reduction in mass) and subsequent stretching of the bridging veins.[2] Other risks factors include alcoholism and anticoagulant use. SDH most commonly presents with altered mental status or conscious level, focal neurological symptoms (which may be progressive, fluctuating or transient), recurrent falls (possibly as a cause or effect), seizures and/or headache. A diagnosis is made by CT head scan. Acute bleeding appears white, and this slowly darkens over time. After around 7–10 days the blood will become isodense with normal brain tissue and then hypodense (i.e dark grey or black). There may be evidence of acute bleeding into a more chronic SDH (*see* Figure 6.6). Cases should be discussed with a neurosurgical team. Corticosteroids have been suggested as a therapeutic option in SDH, but their role is currently unclear.[111]

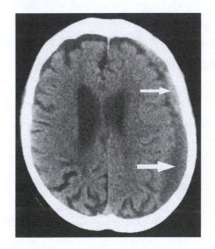

FIGURE 6.6 An acute on chronic subdural haematoma – the acute bleed is white (thin arrow) and the older haematoma is dark grey (fat arrow)

KEY POINTS

- Falls are the commonest cause of traumatic injuries in the frail elderly.
- Following trauma all patients should be assessed for pain relief. Cognitive impairment should not be a barrier to prescribing appropriate levels of analgesia.
- The management of fragility fractures includes looking for underlying risk factors for falls and osteoporosis and formulating an appropriate plan of action.

- Undisplaced hip fractures may have few clinical signs and may not be evident on initial X-ray images.
- With suspected hip fracture the aim is to perform a hip X-ray, administer iv fluids and analgesia, and move the patient onto a pressure-relieving mattress within 2 hours of arrival in the ED.
- Surgical repair of fractured hips should be within 48 hours of admission.
- Delirium following hip fixation is very common.
- The 30-day mortality rate following hip fracture is around 5%–10%, and many of the survivors will have a persisting functional deficit.
- Frail elderly patients are at risk of significant brain injury even following minor trauma and clinicians should have a low threshold for head CT scanning.
- SDH can occur secondary to trivial head trauma and the onset of symptoms may be delayed. Presentations include altered mental status or conscious level, focal neurological symptoms, recurrent falls, seizures or headache.

REFERENCES

1. Kum CK, Chong YS, Koo CC, *et al.* Elderly patients with perforated peptic ulcers: factors affecting morbidity and mortality. *J R Coll Surg Edinb.* 1993; **38**(6): 344–7.
2. Aschkenasy MT, Rothenhaus TC. Trauma and falls in the elderly. *Emerg Med Clin North Am.* 2006; **24**(2): 413–32.
3. Chen T, Anderson DJ, Chopra T, *et al.* Poor functional status is an independent predictor of surgical site infections due to Methicillin-Resistant *Staphylococcus aureus* in older adults. *J Am Geriatr Soc.* 2010; **58**(3): 527–32.
4. Wilkinson K, Martin IC, Gough MJ, *et al. An Age Old Problem: a review of the care received by elderly patients undergoing surgery.* London: NCEPOD; 2010. Available at: www.ncepod.org.uk/2010report3/downloads/EESE_fullReport.pdf (accessed 24 January 2013).
5. Scottish Intercollegiate Guidelines Network. *Management of Hip Fracture in Older People: SIGN guideline 111.* Edinburgh: SIGN; 2009. Available at: www.sign.ac.uk/pdf/sign111.pdf (accessed 24 January 2013).
6. Tack J. Acute colonic pseudo-obstruction (Ogilvie's syndrome). *Curr Treat Options Gastroenterol.* 2006; **9**(4): 361–8.
7. Lane N, Allen K. Hyponatraemia after orthopaedic surgery. *BMJ.* 1999; **318**(7195): 1363–4.
8. POISE Study Group. Effects of extended-release metoprolol succinate in patients undergoing non-cardiac surgery (POISE trial): a randomised-controlled trial. *Lancet.* 2008; **371**(9627): 1839–47.
9. Desai H, Aronow WS, Ahn C, *et al.* Incidence of perioperative myocardial infarction and of 2-year mortality in 577 elderly patients undergoing noncardiac vascular surgery treated with and without statins. *Arch Gerontol Geriatr.* 2010; **51**(2): 149–51.
10. Liu LL, Leung JM. Predicting adverse postoperative outcomes in patients aged 80 years or older. *J Am Geriatr Soc.* 2000; **48**(4): 405–12.
11. Pearse RM, Harrison DA, James P, *et al.* Identification and characterisation of the high-risk surgical population in the United Kingdom. *Crit Care.* 2006; **10**(3): R81.

12. Kennedy GD, Rajamanickam V, O'Connor ES, *et al.* Optimizing surgical care of colon cancer in the older adult population. *Ann Surg.* 2011; **253**(3): 508–14.

13. Makary MA, Segev DL, Pronovost PJ, *et al.* Frailty as a predictor of surgical outcomes in older patients. *J Am Coll Surg.* 2010; **210**(6): 901–8.

14. Tei M, Ikeda M, Haraguchi N, *et al.* Postoperative complications in elderly patients with colorectal cancer: comparison of open and laparoscopic surgical procedures. *Surg Laparosc Endosc Percutan Tech.* 2009; **19**(6): 488–92.

15. Ansaloni L, Catena F, Chattat R, *et al.* Risk factors and incidence of postoperative delirium in elderly patients after elective and emergency surgery. *Br J Surg.* 2010; **97**(2): 273–80.

16. Leung JM, Sands LP, Paul S, *et al.* Does postoperative delirium limit the use of patient-controlled analgesia in older surgical patients? *Anesthesiology.* 2009; **111**(3): 625–31.

17. Marcantonio ER, Goldman L, Orav EJ, *et al.* The association of intraoperative factors with the development of postoperative delirium. *Am J Med.* 1998; **105**(5): 380–4.

18. Marcantonio ER, Flacker JM, Wright RJ, *et al.* Reducing delirium after hip fracture: a randomized trial. *J Am Geriatr Soc.* 2001; **49**(5): 516–22.

19. Newman MF, Kirchner JL, Phillips-Bute B, *et al.* Longitudinal assessment of neurocognitive function after coronary-artery bypass surgery. *N Engl J Med.* 2001; **344**(6): 395–402.

20. Moller JT, Cluitmans P, Rasmussen LS, *et al.* Long-term postoperative cognitive dysfunction in the elderly: ISPOCD1 study. *Lancet.* 1998; **351**(9106): 857–61.

21. Avidan MS, Searleman AC, Storandt M, *et al.* Long-term cognitive decline in older subjects was not attributable to noncardiac surgery or major illness. *Anesthesiology.* 2009; **111**(5): 964–70.

22. Avidan MS, Evers AS. Review of clinical evidence for persistent cognitive decline or incident dementia attributable to surgery or general anesthesia. *J Alzheimers Dis.* 2011; **24**(2): 201–16.

23. Wofford JL, Schwartz E, Timerding BL, *et al.* Emergency department utilization by the elderly: analysis of the National Hospital Ambulatory Medical Care Survey. *Acad Emerg Med.* 1996; **3**(7): 694–9.

24. Marco CA, Schoenfeld CN, Keyl PM, *et al.* Abdominal pain in geriatric emergency patients: variables associated with adverse outcomes. *Acad Emerg Med.* 1998; **5**(12): 1163–8.

25. Bugliosi TF, Meloy TD, Vukov LF. Acute abdominal pain in the elderly. *Ann Emerg Med.* 1990; **19**(12): 1383–6.

26. Parker JS, Vukov LF, Wollan PC. Abdominal pain in the elderly: use of temperature and laboratory testing to screen for surgical disease. *Fam Med.* 1996; **28**(3): 193–7.

27. Kizer KW, Vassar MJ. Emergency department diagnosis of abdominal disorders in the elderly. *Am J Emerg Med.* 1998; **16**(4): 357–62.

28. Lewis LM, Banet GA, Blanda M, *et al.* Etiology and clinical course of abdominal pain in senior patients: a prospective, multicenter study. *J Gerontol A Biol Sci Med Sci.* 2005; **60**(8): 1071–6.

29. Hustey FM, Meldon SW, Banet GA, *et al.* The use of abdominal computed tomography in older ED patients with acute abdominal pain. *Am J Emerg Med.* 2005; **23**(3): 259–65.

30. Kamin RA, Nowicki TA, Courtney DS, *et al.* Pearls and pitfalls in the emergency department evaluation of abdominal pain. *Emerg Med Clin North Am.* 2003; **21**(1): 61–72.

31. De Dombal FT. Acute abdominal pain in the elderly. *J Clin Gastroenterol.* 1994; **19**(4): 331–5.

32. Laurell H, Hansson LE, Gunnarsson U. Acute abdominal pain among elderly patients. *Gerontology.* 2006; **52**(6): 339–44.

33. Van Geloven AAW, Biesheuvel TH, Luitse JSK, *et al.* Hospital admissions of patients aged over 80 with acute abdominal complaints. *Eur J Surg.* 2000; **166**(11): 866–71.

34. Abi-Hanna P, Gleckman R. Acute abdominal pain: a medical emergency in older patients. *Geriatrics.* 1997; **52**(7): 72–4.

35. Potts FE, Vukov LF. Utility of fever and leukocytosis in acute surgical abdomens in octogenarians and beyond. *J Gerontol A Biol Sci Med Sci.* 1999; **54**(2): M55–8.

36. Ozkan E, Fersahoglu MM, Dulundu E, *et al.* Factors affecting mortality and morbidity in emergency abdominal surgery in geriatric patients. *Ulus Travma Acil Cerrahi Derg.* 2010; **16**(5): 439–44.

37. Sanson TG, O'Keefe KP. Evaluation of abdominal pain in the elderly. *Emerg Med Clin North Am.* 1996; **14**(3): 615–27.

38. Hendrickson M, Naparst TR. Abdominal emergencies in the elderly. *Emerg Med Clin North Am.* 2003; **21**(4): 937–69.

39. Esses D, Birnbaum A, Bijur P, *et al.* Ability of CT to alter decision making in elderly patients with acute abdominal pain. *Am J Emerg Med.* 2004; **22**(4): 270–2.

40. Lewis LM, Klippel AP, Bavolek RA, *et al.* Quantifying the usefulness of CT in evaluating seniors with abdominal pain. *Eur J Radiol.* 2007; **61**(2): 290–6.

41. Bentrem DJ, Cohen ME, Hynes DM, *et al.* Identification of specific quality improvement opportunities for the elderly undergoing gastrointestinal surgery. *Arch Surg.* 2009; **144**(11): 1013–20.

42. Huang T, Hu F, Fan C, *et al.* A simple novel model to predict hospital mortality, surgical site infection, and pneumonia in elderly patients undergoing operation. *Dig Surg.* 2010; **27**(3): 224–31.

43. Mirbagheri N, Dark JG, Watters DAK. How do patients aged 85 and older fare with abdominal surgery? *J Am Geriatr Soc.* 2010; **58**(1): 104–8.

44. Rigberg D, Cole M, Hiyama D, *et al.* Surgery in the nineties. *Am Surg.* 2000; **66**(9): 813–16.

45. Gerson MC, Hurst JM, Hertzberg VS, *et al.* Prediction of cardiac and pulmonary complications related to elective abdominal and noncardiac thoracic surgery in geriatric patients. *Am J Med.* 1990; **88**(2): 101–7.

46. Rix TE, Bates TE. Pre-operative risk scores for the prediction of outcome in elderly people who require emergency surgery. *World J Emerg Surg.* 2006; **2**: 16.

47. Arthur JDR, Edwards PR, Chagla LS. Management of gallstone disease in the elderly. *Ann R Coll Surg Engl.* 2003; **85**(2): 91–6.

48. Ratner J, Lisbona A, Rosenbloom M, *et al.* The prevalence of gallstone disease in very old institutionalized persons. *JAMA.* 1991; **265**(7): 902–3.

49. Parker LJ, Vukov LF, Wollan PC. Emergency department evaluation of geriatric patients with acute cholecystitis. *Acad Emerg Med.* 1997; **4**(1): 51–5.

50. Martinez JP, Mattu A. Abdominal pain in the elderly. *Emerg Med Clin North Am.* 2006; **24**(2): 371–88.

51. Lyon C, Clark DC. Diagnosis of acute abdominal pain in older patients. *Am Fam Physician.* 2006; **74**(9): 1537–44.

52. De Giorgio R, Knowles CH. Acute colonic pseudo-obstruction. *Br J Surg.* 2009; **96**(3): 229–39.

53. Su Y, Yeh C, Lee C, *et al.* Acute surgical treatment of perforated peptic ulcer in the elderly patients. *Hepato-gastroenterology.* 2010; **57**(104): 1608–13.

54. Storm-Dickerson TL, Horattas MC. What have we learned over the past 20 years about appendicitis in the elderly? *Am J Surg.* 2003; **185**(3): 198–201.

55. Paranjape C, Dalia S, Pan J, *et al.* Appendicitis in the elderly: a change in the laparoscopic era. *Surg Endosc.* 2007; **21**(5): 777–81.

56. Jeyarajah S, Faiz O, Bottle A, *et al.* Diverticular disease hospital admissions are increasing, with poor outcomes in the elderly and emergency admissions. *Aliment Pharmacol Ther.* 2009; **30**(11–12): 1171–82.

57. Farrell RJ, Farrell JJ, Morrin MM. Diverticular disease in the elderly. *Gastroenterol Clin North Am.* 2001; **30**(2): 475–96.

58. Winters ME, Kluetz P, Zilberstein J. Back pain emergencies. *Med Clin North Am.* 2006; **90**(3): 505–23.

59. Marston WA, Ahlquist R, Johnson G, *et al.* Misdiagnosis of ruptured abdominal aortic aneurysms. *J Vasc Surg.* 1992; **16**(1): 17–22.

60. Carter MW, Gupta S. Characteristics and outcomes of injury-related ED visits among older adults. *Am J Emerg Med.* 2008; **26**(3): 296–303.

61. Richmond TS, Kauder D, Strumpf N, *et al.* Characteristics and outcomes of serious traumatic injury in older adults. *J Am Geriatr Soc.* 2002; **50**(2): 215–22.

62. Peel NM, Kassulke DJ, McClure RJ. Population based study of hospitalised fall related injuries in older people. *Inj Prev.* 2002; **8**(4): 280–3.

63. Aitken LM, Burmeister E, Lang J, *et al.* Characteristics and outcomes of injured older adults after hospital admission. *J Am Geriatr Soc.* 2010; **58**(3): 442–9.

64. Caterino JM, Valasek T, Werman HA. Identification of an age cutoff for increased mortality in patients with elderly trauma. *Am J Emerg Med.* 2010; **28**(2): 151–8.

65. Pickering SAW, Esberger D, Moran CG. The outcome following major trauma in the elderly: predictors of survival. *Injury.* 1999; **30**(10): 703–6.

66. Inaba K, Goecke M, Sharkey P, *et al.* Long-term outcomes after injury in the elderly. *J Trauma.* 2003; **54**(3): 486–91.

67. Grossman M, Scaff DW, Miller D, *et al.* Functional outcomes in octogenarian trauma. *J Trauma.* 2003; **55**(1): 26–32.

68. Wilber ST, Blanda M, Gerson LW, *et al.* Short-term functional decline and service use in older emergency department patients with blunt injuries. *Acad Emerg Med.* 2010; **17**(7): 679–86.

69. Knudson MM, Lieberman J, Morris JA, *et al.* Mortality factors in geriatric blunt trauma patients. *Arch Surg.* 1994; **129**(4): 448–53.

70. Brankin E, Mitchell C, Munro R. Closing the osteoporosis management gap in primary care: a secondary prevention of fracture programme. *Curr Med Res Opin.* 2005; **21**(4): 475–82.

71. Cauley JA, Thompson DE, Ensrud KC, *et al.* Risk of mortality following clinical fractures. *Osteoporos Int.* 2000; **11**(7): 556–61.

72. O'Brien DP, Luchette FA, Pereira SJ, *et al.* Pelvic fracture in the elderly is associated with increased mortality. *Surgery.* 2002; **132**(4): 710–15.

73. Bliuc D, Nguyen ND, Milch VE, *et al.* Mortality risk associated with low-trauma osteoporotic fracture and subsequent fracture in men and women. *JAMA.* 2009; **301**(5): 513–21.

74. Center JR, Bliuc D, Nguyen TV, *et al.* Risk of subsequent fracture after low-trauma fracture in men and women. *JAMA.* 2007; **297**(4): 387–94.

75. Keene GS, Parker MJ, Pryor GA. Mortality and morbidity after hip fractures. *BMJ.* 1993; **307**(6914): 1248–50.

76. Roche JJW, Wenn RT, Sahota O, *et al.* Effect of comorbidities and postoperative complications on mortality after hip fracture in elderly people: prospective observational cohort study. *BMJ.* 2005; **331**(7529): 1374.

77. Donaldson MG, Khan KM, Davis JC, *et al.* Emergency department fall-related presentations

do not trigger fall risk assessment: a gap in care of high-risk outpatient fallers. *Arch Gerontol Geriatr.* 2005; **41**(3): 311–17.

78. Johansson C, Skoog I. A population-based study on the association between dementia and hip fractures in 85-year olds. *Aging (Milano).* 1996; **8**(3): 189–96.

79. Dolan MM, Hawkes WG, Zimmerman SI, *et al.* Delirium on hospital admission in aged hip fracture patients: prediction of mortality and 2-year functional outcomes. *J Gerontol A Biol Sci Med Sci.* 2000; **55**(9): M527–34.

80. Gustafson Y, Brannstrom B, Norberg A, *et al.* Underdiagnosis and poor documentation of acute confusional states in elderly hip fracture patients. *J Am Geriatr Soc.* 1991; **39**(8): 760–5.

81. Pathak G, Parker MJ, Pryor GA. Delayed diagnosis of femoral neck fractures. *Injury.* 1997; **28**(4): 299–301.

82. Dominguez S, Liu P, Roberts C, *et al.* Prevalence of traumatic hip and pelvic fractures in patients with suspected hip fracture and negative initial standard radiographs: a study of emergency department patients. *Acad Emerg Med.* 2005; **12**(4): 366–9.

83. Chana R, Noorani A, Ashwood N, *et al.* The role of MRI in the diagnosis of proximal femoral fractures in the elderly. *Injury.* 2006; **37**(2): 185–9.

84. Selbst SM, Clark M. Analgesic use in the emergency department. *Ann Emerg Med.* 1990; **19**(9): 1010–13.

85. Terrell KM, Hustey FM, Hwang U, *et al.* Quality indicators for geriatric emergency care. *Acad Emerg Med.* 2009; **16**(5): 441–9.

86. Ardery G, Herr K, Hannon BJ, *et al.* Lack of opioid administration in older hip fracture patients. *Geriatr Nurs.* 2003; **24**(6): 353–60.

87. Hwang U, Richardson LD, Sonuyi TO, *et al.* The effect of emergency department crowding on the management of pain in older adults with hip fracture. *J Am Geriatr Soc.* 2006; **54**(2): 270–5.

88. Jones JS, Johnson K, McNinch M. Age as a risk factor for inadequate emergency department analgesia. *Am J Emerg Med.* 1996; **14**(2): 157–60.

89. Felt KS, Ryden MB, Miles S. Treatment of pain in cognitively impaired compared with cognitively intact older patients with hip fracture. *J Am Geriatr Soc.* 1998; **46**(9): 1079–85.

90. British Orthopaedic Society. *The Care of Patients with Fragility Fracture.* London: British Orthopaedic Society; 2007.

91. Beaupre LA, Jones CA, Saunders LD, *et al.* Best practices for elderly hip fracture patients: a systematic overview of the evidence. *J Gen Intern Med.* 2005; **20**(11): 1019–25.

92. Avenell A, Handoll HHG. Nutritional supplementation for hip fracture aftercare in older people. Cochrane Database Syst Rev. 2010; 1: CD001880.

93. Edland A, Lundstrom M, Lundstrom G, *et al.* Clinical profile of delirium in patients treated for femoral neck fractures. *Dement Geriatr Cogn Disord.* 1999; **10**(5): 325–9.

94. Marcantonio E, Ta T, Duthie E, *et al.* Delirium severity and psychomotor types: their relationship with outcomes after hip fracture repair. *J Am Geriatr Soc.* 2002; **50**(5): 850–7.

95. Gillespie WJ, Walenkamp GHIM. Antibiotic prophylaxis for surgery for proximal femoral and other closed long bone fractures. Cochrane Database Syst Rev. 2010; 3: CD000244.

96. National Institute for Health and Clinical Excellence. Alendronate, Etidronate, Risedronate, Raloxifene, Strontium Ranelate and Teriparatide for the Secondary Prevention of Osteoporotic Fragility Fractures in Postmenopausal Women (Amended). London: NIHCE; 2011. Available at: www.nice.org.uk/guidance/TA161 (accessed 24 January 2013).

97. Pearce SHS, Cheetham TD. Diagnosis and management of vitamin D deficiency. *BMJ.* 2010; **340**: 142–6.

98. Parikh S, Mogun H, Avorn J, *et al*. Osteoporosis medication use in nursing home patients with fractures in 1 US state. *Arch Intern Med*. 2008; **168**(10): 1111–15.

99. Vidan M, Serra JA, Moreno C, *et al*. Efficacy of a comprehensive geriatric intervention in older patients hospitalized for hip fracture: a randomized, controlled trial. *J Am Geriatr Soc*. 2005; **53**(9): 1476–82.

100. Parker M, Johansen A. Hip fracture. *BMJ*. 2006; **333**(7557): 27–30.

101. Todd CJ, Freeman CJ, Camilleri-Ferrante C, *et al*. Differences in mortality after fracture of hip: the east Anglian audit. *BMJ*. 1995; **310**(6984): 904–8.

102. Magaziner J, Simonsick EM, Kashner TM, *et al*. Predictors of functional recovery one year following hospital discharge for hip fracture: a prospective study. *J Gerontol*. 1990; **45**(3): M101–7.

103. Nagurney JT, Borczuk P, Thomas SH. Elder patients with closed head trauma: a comparison with nonelder patients. *Acad Emerg Med*. 1998; **5**(7): 678–84.

104. Thompson HJ, McCormick WC, Kagan SH. Traumatic brain injury in older adults: epidemiology, outcomes, and future implications. *J Am Geriatr Soc*. 2006; **54**(10): 1590–5.

105. Stein SC, Fabbri A, Servadei F, *et al*. A critical comparison of clinical decision instruments for computed tomographic scanning in mild closed traumatic brain injury in adolescents and adults. *Ann Emerg Med*. 2009; **53**(2): 180–8.

106. National Institute for Health and Clinical Excellence. Head Injury: triage, assessment, investigation and early management of head injury in infants, children and adults; NICE guideline 56. London: NIHCE; 2007. Available at: www.nice.org.uk/nicemedia/live/11836/36259/36259.pdf (accessed 20 February 2013).

107. Mack LR, Chan SB, Silva JC, *et al*. The use of head computed tomography in elderly patients sustaining minor head trauma. *J Emerg Med*. 2003; **24**(2): 157–62.

108. Gittleman AM, Ortiz O, Keating DP, *et al*. Indications for CT in patients receiving anticoagulation after head trauma. *AJNR Am J Neuroradiol*. 2005; **26**(3): 603–6.

109. Rathlev NK, Medzon R, Lowery D, *et al*. Intracranial pathology in elders with blunt head trauma. *Acad Emerg Med*. 2006; **13**(3): 302–7.

110. Adhiyaman V, Asghar M, Ganeshram KN, *et al*. Chronic subdural haematoma in the elderly. *Postgrad Med J*. 2002; **78**(916): 71–5.

111. Berghauser Pont LM, Dirven CM, Dippel DW, *et al*. The role of corticosteroids in the management of chronic subdural hematoma: a systematic review. *Eur J Neurol*. 2012; **19**(11): 1397–403.

CHAPTER 7

Infection

Older people are more susceptible to infections, with higher mortality rates than younger people. Explanations for this include the physiological changes of frailty, co-morbidities (including malnutrition), reduced immune system activity, pharmacological factors (e.g. polypharmacy, adverse drug reactions and changed pharmacokinetics) and delayed diagnosis due to atypical disease presentations. This latter factor can postpone the receipt of antibiotics, increasing the risk of death.[1]

A frequent feature in the frail elderly is the absence of significant pyrexia despite serious systemic bacterial infection. Occasionally, patients may even demonstrate hypothermia due to tissue hypo-perfusion. There is some evidence that older people, on average, have lower baseline body temperatures than younger people (*see* Table 7.1).[2] However, differences are small and are unlikely to explain the absence of pyrexia seen with some infections.

TABLE 7.1 Average baseline temperatures for men and women at different ages

Age (years)	Women	Men
20–29	36.5°C	36.3°C
80+	36.3°C	36.1°C

PROGNOSTIC MARKERS

In older patients presenting with fever, serious illness (e.g. bacteraemia, death, or prolonged admission) has been associated with the presence of a high maximum temperature (>39.4°C), leukocytosis, respiratory rate of 30 breaths per minute or higher, heart rate of 120 bpm or higher, or an infiltrate seen on chest X-ray.[3] However, half of patients with a serious illness have none of these clinical features. In patients aged 65 and over with suspected infection, a number of clinical characteristics have been associated with an increased risk of death – *see* Table 7.2.[4]

TABLE 7.2 Clinical features in elderly people with suspected infection that are associated with a worse outcome

Clinical features	28-day mortality rate depending on number of features present	
	Features (n)	Mortality rate (%)
Respiratory rate >20 breaths per minute	0	0.5%
Hypoxia (oxygen saturation <90%)	1	3%
Tachycardia (≥120 bpm)	2	14%
Systolic blood pressure <90 mmHg	3+	47%
Serum lactate ≥4.0 mmol/L		
Platelet count <150 × 10^9/L		
Pre-existing terminal illness		

BACTERAEMIA

Bacteraemia is the presence of bacteria within the blood stream. It has no clinical signs or symptoms that are pathognomonic. Infectious organisms within the bloodstream result in the release of inflammatory mediators and activation of the coagulation cascade.[5] This leads to microvascular injury that causes tissue hypoxia and organ dysfunction. Younger people are more likely to show the classic signs of sepsis than older people with bacteraemia.[6] Older patients are more likely to develop septic shock and renal failure than the young.[7]

In studies of patients aged over 65 with community-acquired bacteraemia presenting to an emergency department (ED), the commonest sources have been found to be urinary tract (32%–44%) and chest infections (17%–26%), but the site of origin was often not identified (11%–26%).[6,8–10] The commonest organism was *Escherichia coli*, which accounted for 29%–48% of bacteraemias. An overall mortality rate of 38% has been found, but this appears to be lower in those with *E. coli* infections (15%).[8] A presenting temperature of <37°C was present in 21%–24% of cases.[8,9] The absence of fever is associated with higher mortality rates.[10,11] Other predictors of adverse outcome include the presence of shock and functional dependence prior to admission.[10] Confusion was the only presenting symptom in 19% in one series.[8] A normal serum white cell count (WCC) has been found in 24%–26% of cases.[6,9] Hypothermia is a possible but uncommon (<4%) presenting feature of bacteraemia.[7]

Bacteraemia in patients in long-term care facilities is also most commonly of urinary tract origin (56%) and carries a similar mortality rate (35%).[12] In a study of patients admitted from a nursing home (NH) to an ED, where 90% of patients had blood cultures collected, a prevalence of bacteraemia of 10% (when false positives due to contamination were excluded) was found.[13] No symptoms or signs were useful in predicting those patients with bacteraemia, and 30% did not have a fever.

Blood cultures

Given the lack of pathognomonic signs of bacteraemia, it can only reliably be diagnosed by blood cultures. When these were ordered in an adult population presenting to an ED, they were positive in 13%, with 7% being suspected contaminants and just 6% being true positives.[14] Overall, 3% of results altered patient management. However, the group of patients with positive cultures had a higher mean age (68 vs 57 years). Around 18% of patients aged over 65 presenting to an ED with fever will have a positive blood culture.[3] These data suggest that clinicians assessing frail elderly patients with unexplained functional or cognitive decline, even in the absence of pyrexia, should have a low threshold for performing blood cultures (i.e. if any of the clinical features of sepsis are found – *see* next section).

SEPSIS

Sepsis is defined as an infection accompanied by signs of systemic involvement (*see* bullet list in the following paragraph).[15] The term systemic inflammatory response syndrome is used to describe the clinical features of sepsis when not caused by infection (e.g. pancreatitis, organ ischaemia or immune-mediated disorders).[16] Severe sepsis is defined as sepsis plus evidence of organ dysfunction or tissue hypoperfusion, and septic shock is sepsis resulting in hypotension (i.e. systolic blood pressure <90 mmHg despite fluid resuscitation).[15] Tissue hypoperfusion is defined as septic shock or elevated serum lactate (4.0 mmol/L or more) or oliguria (<0.5 mL/kg/hour). Severe sepsis and septic shock have overall mortality rates around 50%.[5] This figure is likely to be much higher in the frail elderly.

The clinical features of sepsis are one or more of the following:[16]

➤ temperature >38°C or <36°C
➤ pulse >90 bpm
➤ respiratory rate >20 breaths per minute (or reduced partial pressure of arterial carbon dioxide because of hyperventilation)
➤ serum WCC >12 or $<4 \times 10^9$/L.

Patients aged 65 and over account for around two-thirds of hospitalised patients with sepsis in developed countries (relative risk is 13 times greater than for younger adults).[17] The commonest sources of infection are respiratory (37%), genitourinary tract (28%), gastrointestinal (11%) and skin, soft tissue or bone (4%). A number of patients (around 20%) presenting to the ED with sepsis but without initial features of shock develop shock within the next 72 hours.[18] Older patients are at an increased risk of this.

The key steps in the initial treatment of severe sepsis are:[15]

➤ resuscitation starts immediately (intravenous (iv) fluids)
➤ consider a urinary catheter in this situation to monitor urine output
➤ obtain blood cultures before starting antibiotics (plus any other relevant cultures when possible)
➤ begin iv antibiotics as soon as possible (always <1 hour of recognition)
➤ use broad-spectrum empirical antibiotics initially
➤ the site of infection should be identified as soon as possible (within 6 hours from presentation).

A fluid challenge of up to 1 L of crystalloid or 500 mL of colloid over 30 minutes may be appropriate.[15] Caution is required in those with co-existent heart failure, where an initial 250 mL challenge may be tried first.

ANTIBIOTICS

Antibiotics can cause harm to the frail elderly. This can be because of direct effects of the medication (e.g. a rash caused by penicillin) or through the development of antibiotic-associated infections (e.g. *Clostridium difficile*-associated diarrhoea – *see* p. 189). Multidrug-resistant organisms are classified as those that are resistant to one or more classes of antimicrobial agent. These include methicillin-resistant *Staphylococcus aureus* (MRSA), vancomycin-resistant enterococci and some Gram-negative bacilli (including those producing extended-spectrum beta-lactamases). These pathogens commonly affect the frail elderly, particularly those in longer-term care settings.[19] Their emergence is linked to the inappropriate use of antibiotics in some patients and is potentially a major threat to world health.

Choosing the right agent can be difficult. Patients with renal impairment may be unable to secrete nitrofurantoin in therapeutic concentrations into their urine, and gentamicin can be nephrotoxic. Quinolones are linked with MRSA (*see* p. 192) and may cause confusion. *C. difficile* infection (CDI) is associated with many antibiotics. As a general principle it is best to start with an empiric broad-spectrum agent in cases of severe infections. Once the causative organism has been identified it may be possible to switch to a narrower-spectrum drug. In cases of milder infections it may be possible to obtain relevant culture results

before prescribing treatment. The choice of drug should be guided by local antibiotic policies that reflect patterns of resistance in your area.

PNEUMONIA

Pneumonia is a term for a chest infection causing inflammation of the lungs.
It can be classified as 'lobar pneumonia' (consolidation seen in a specific lung
region) or 'bronchopneumonia' (more widespread lung shadowing). It can also
be classified by location of onset into 'community-acquired pneumonia' (CAP),
'hospital-acquired pneumonia' ('nosocomial') or 'nursing home-acquired pneumonia' (NHAP). The higher prevalence of chronic chest disease (e.g. chronic
obstructive pulmonary disease (COPD)) may hamper diagnosis in the elderly.

Patients aged 75 and over account for around 41% of CAP in the UK.[20] It is
more common in those with underlying COPD, heart disease or dementia.[21] The
development of pneumonia is more likely in people taking antipsychotic medications (odds ratio, 1.6; 95% confidence interval, 1.3–2.1), particularly atypical
agents (odds ratio, 3.1; 95% confidence interval, 1.9–5.1), with the highest risk
occurring in the first week after their commencement.[22] This may be explained
by higher rates of aspiration (*see* p. 181).

Presenting features

Older patients with pneumonia are less likely than younger people to report
cough, shortness of breath or pleuritic chest pain,[23] yet an elevated respiratory

rate is more commonly seen in the elderly (65% of those aged 75 and over vs 44% aged 45–64). A review of 48 veterans aged over 65 (mean age, 78 years) with acute pneumonia on chest X-ray found that 10% of patients did not report any of fever, cough or shortness of breath.[24] The peak temperature recorded was below 37.7°C in 40% of patients, and 31% had a serum WCC $<10 \times 10^9/L$. A different study compared 81 patients aged 65 and over (mean age, 77 years) with pneumonia with 57 patients aged below 65 (mean age, 46 years).[25] The older patients were more likely to be afebrile (temperature 37.0°C or less) at the time of admission (57% vs 26%; $p < 0.01$). Another study found that just 23% of patients aged 70 and over (mean age, 83 years) had a temperature >37.8°C, 69% had cough, 68% had shortness of breath, and 41% had acute confusion.[26] Over 90% had relevant signs on chest examination. In an evaluation of elderly patients (mean age, 72 years) admitted with CAP, the absence of fever (<37.8°C) and raised serum WCC ($<10 \times 10^9/L$) was associated with an increased mortality rate (29% vs 4%).[27]

Causative organism

The most common organism causing pneumonia is *Streptococcus pneumoniae*, underlying 23%–48% of cases in the old.[21,28] Other isolated pathogens include *Chlamydia*, *Mycoplasma pneumoniae* and *Haemophilus influenzae*, but these atypical agents may be less common in older than younger people.[21] Around 12% of cases are associated with viral infections.[28] This may explain the higher incidence in winter months. Evaluation of the causative organism is often difficult because of colonisation of upper airways by enteric Gram-negative bacilli and *S. aureus*, particularly in NH residents. It is typically difficult to obtain reliable, uncontaminated sputum samples. In many cases the underlying causative agent remains unknown.

Nursing home-acquired pneumonia

NHAP accounts for around 9% of all patients admitted to hospital from the community with pneumonia in the UK, and for 14% of those aged 65 or over.[29] Compared with patients aged 65 and over with CAP, those with NHAP (associated with acute radiographic changes) were less likely to present with productive cough (30%–35% vs 53%–61%) or pleuritic chest pain (3%–14% vs 17%–32%) but were more likely to have confusion (30%–70% vs 12%–37%).[29,30] Similar rates of shortness of breath and fever have been seen between these groups. Mortality rates for NHAP are higher than those seen in CAP in older adults (19%–53% vs 8%–21%).[29-31]

Current evidence suggests that, similar to CAP, the commonest causative organisms are *S. pneumoniae*, *Chlamydophila pneumoniae*, *H. influenzae* and *M. pneumoniae*, and it may also be due to viral infections.[29,32] Suitable sputum cultures may only be obtainable in 5%–10% of NH residents with suspected pneumonia.[32] Oropharyngeal aspiration may be an aetiological mechanism in some particularly severe cases. The provision of oral care to NH residents may reduce the incidence of pneumonia.[33] Risk factors include witnessed aspiration and the use of sedative medications.[34]

Aspiration pneumonia

Gastric contents are typically considered sterile due to the high acidity. However, this is unlikely to be the case in older adults on acid-suppressing medications or those with atrophic gastritis. There is also a risk of secondary bacterial infection to an area of inflamed lung tissue. Aspiration may initially go unnoticed by the patient or carers (termed 'silent aspiration'). Silent aspiration may be a more common cause of CAP than traditionally thought. One study found evidence of aspiration in 71% of patients with CAP (mean age, 77 years) compared with 10% of controls (mean age, 73 years).[35] Perhaps as many as half of normal healthy individuals aspirate small amounts of matter during sleep.[36] Aspiration is more common in the old and is believed to be the cause of 5%–15% of cases of CAP.[21,36] It is likely to be a factor in many more cases of NHAP.

Pneumonia is more likely to develop in those with dental decay who harbour potentially causative organisms within their mouths.[37] Other risk factors include dysphagia, dementia, diabetes, malnutrition, reduced saliva production (e.g. anticholinergic drugs), impaired cough reflex and antipsychotic drugs.[38,39]

The organisms causing aspiration pneumonia are likely to be similar to those causing other pneumonias, but there may be a higher incidence of Gram-negative organisms and anaerobes.[36,40] These latter groups seem to be more likely in those from NH and with poor dentition. Broad-spectrum antibiotics such as piperacillin-tazobactam, possibly with anaerobic cover (e.g. metronidazole), are typically recommended.[36] Angiotensin-converting enzyme inhibitors may have a protective benefit.[41] Improving dental hygiene may reduce the risk of future events.

Assessing severity

Clinical features can help define the severity of CAP. Patients with bilateral chest X-ray changes, tachycardia (>100 bpm) or absence of pyrexia (<37°C) have been found to be at a higher risk of death.[20]

Simple scales have also been developed. One such tool is the CURB-65 score. Here one point for each of **C**onfusion, a raised serum **U**rea (>7 mmol/L), a **R**espiratory rate of 30 breaths per minute or greater, a low **B**lood pressure (systolic <90 mmHg or diastolic <60 mmHg), and age **65** or above. The CRB-65 is a simpler version that omits blood urea so that it can be used in the initial assessment of patients in the community. A study using the CRB-65 found 30-day mortality rates in older people (mean age, 77 years) of <1% for a score of 0 or 1, 8% for a score of 2, and 17% for a score of 3.[42] Hospitalisation is typically recommended for those with a score of 2 or more.

The CURB-65 and CRB-65 seem to have better predictive value than either the standardised early warning score or systemic inflammatory response syndrome criteria,[43] but the CURB-65 score seems to be a little less accurate than the more lengthy Pneumonia Severity Index in identifying low-risk patients.[44] Unfortunately, both sets of criteria appear less predictive in older patients than in younger patients.[45]

Investigations

Blood tests should include serum WCC and C-reactive protein (CRP) as markers of an infective process. Hyponatraemia can be caused by syndrome of inappropriate antidiuretic hormone (*see* p. 75). Urea is a marker of illness severity. The collection of blood cultures within 24 hours of admission is associated with improved survival rates.[46] Sputum culture may be helpful but it is not always obtainable, the patient may have already received antibiotics, and the culture can be contaminated with bacteria or fungi that colonise the upper airways.[25] Chest X-rays should be performed but these can be difficult to interpret in the frail elderly (*see* Figure 2.2). Arterial blood gases should be considered when hypoxia is present or in cases of severe sepsis.

Treatment

Basic initial treatment should address hypoxia and hypovolaemia. Once pneumonia has been diagnosed, it is important to start appropriate antibiotic therapy rapidly. The administration of antibiotics within 4 hours of hospital admission for older adults with CAP is associated with reduced mortality rates and shorter lengths of stay.[47] The significant proportion due to atypical organisms has led to it being common practice to cover these organisms with empirical antibiotic therapy.[48]

Prognosis

Patients aged 65 and over admitted to hospital with CAP have been found to have a 6% 30-day mortality rate and 24% mortality rate at 18 months.[49] Those with worse functional status were most likely to die. Another study found an in-hospital mortality rate for CAP in the over-65s of 11% and a 12-month mortality rate of 41%.[50] These figures rose from 8% and 31% (in-hospital mortality rate and 12-month mortality rate, respectively) in those aged 65–69, up to 16% and 57% (in-hospital mortality rate and 12-month mortality rate, respectively) in those aged over 90. The mortality rates for CAP exceeded the averages for non-pneumonia hospitalised elderly in this study, which is consistent with CAP being a marker of poorer prognosis.

Acute respiratory distress syndrome is a severe complication of pneumonia that is associated with mortality in younger patients. Following CAP, patients aged over 85 years or those with aspiration pneumonia are less likely to develop acute respiratory distress syndrome than younger patients without aspiration pneumonia.[51]

KEY POINTS

- Older patients with pneumonia are less likely to report cough, shortness of breath or pleuritic chest pain – particularly those from NHs.
- Frail patients with pneumonia who lack pyrexia and a raised serum WCC have a worse prognosis.
- *S. pneumoniae* is the commonest bacterial cause, but a proportion will be due to viruses.
- Aspiration is a significant cause of pneumonia and it may be 'silent'.
- Antipsychotic drug use increases the risk of pneumonia.
- Simple risk scores such as the CURB-65 can be used to guide which patients require hospital admission.
- Around 6%–11% of elderly patients will not survive an acute hospital admission because of pneumonia.

INFLUENZA

Influenza types A and B can cause serious illnesses in frail older adults. The typical presentation of cough and fever occurs after a 2-day incubation period. Outbreaks are more common in the winter (November to April in the northern hemisphere) and spread rapidly in care homes. It is estimated to affect 5%–20% of the population each year. The virus is limited to the respiratory tract. Deaths are most often due to superimposed bacterial pneumonia. This is likely to occur between 5 and 7 days after initial symptoms and it is most often due to *S. pneumoniae*.

A number of viral subtypes have been identified according to variations in haemagglutinin (H) and neuraminidase (N) surface proteins. The H1N1, H2N2 and H3N2 subtypes most commonly infect humans. There is also seasonal variation in virus strains. Minor changes are termed 'antigenic drift' and cause annual epidemics, due to avoiding memory T-cells and circulating antibodies. Pandemics are caused by major virus changes such as recombination of RNA, which is termed 'antigenic shift'. Rapid serological tests are usually used for diagnosis.

Treatment

To be effective, antiviral medications need to be commenced within 48 hours of symptom onset. Neuraminidase inhibitors have been found to reduce the duration of symptoms by one to two days. Oseltamivir is taken orally and can cause nausea and vomiting. Zanamivir is an inhaled medication that may cause bronchospasm and should be avoided in people with COPD or asthma. Barrier nursing can reduce the spread of infection around hospitals or care homes.

Vaccination

Influenza vaccination can prevent infection. However, it may take 4–6 weeks from administration to achieving sufficient antibody response. The protection lasts a few months and so it is usually given in October–November to cover the annual winter peak in incidence. Ageing of the immune system tends to make vaccines less effective in the frail elderly. Estimation of the true efficacy of the vaccines is difficult due to potential bias in study populations. Some studies have found a significant benefit for older people.[52] A Cochrane review suggested only modest benefits for the elderly living in care homes and no benefit for those living in the community.[53] Another review was unclear on the benefit of vaccinating healthcare workers to try and reduce influenza outbreaks among NH residents.[54] Vaccination may reduce the risk of developing secondary bacterial pneumonia. Studies to date have also been inconclusive.[55,56]

URINARY TRACT INFECTION

Urinary tract infections (UTIs) are more common in older adults. This is partly because of reduced immune system activity related to frailty. In addition, older adults are more prone to incomplete bladder emptying (typically related to prostatic enlargement in men) and higher rates of urinary catheter insertion (sometimes inappropriately – *see* p. 90).

However, the tendency among physicians is for overdiagnosis. UTIs are frequently blamed for non-specific declines in physical and/or cognitive function in older people, but this practice is not evidence based.[57] The diagnosis of UTI in hospitalised patients aged 75 and over is probably incorrect around 40% of the time.[58] This results in inappropriate exposure to antibiotics and delays in establishing the correct diagnosis.

Asymptomatic bacteriuria

A major challenge in diagnosing UTIs in the frail elderly is the high prevalence of asymptomatic bacteriuria (ASB), which is defined as the presence of bacteria in the urine of people without attributable symptoms. This is rare in younger people but it becomes common in old age. Over 75 years it is detected in 7%–10% of men and 17%–20% of women who live in the community and up to 40%–50% of non-catheterised people in care homes.[59–61] All long-term catheter users have bacteriuria, whether symptomatic or not.

White blood cells are found in the urine (termed 'pyuria') in over 90% of people with ASB.[60] Some patients presenting with symptoms unrelated to the urinary tract are coincidentally found to have ASB, and this can wrongly reinforce the concept that most non-specific presentations in older people are due to UTIs. Giving antibiotics to eradicate ASB does not reduce mortality or morbidity but does increase the risk of antibiotic-related adverse events and colonisation of the urinary tract with resistant organisms.[62,63]

Symptomatic urinary tract infection

Symptomatic UTI is defined as bacteriuria causing urinary tract symptoms. This can be classified as upper (i.e. pyelonephritis) or lower (i.e. cystitis), the former classically causing flank pain and renal angle tenderness, the latter causing dysuria, frequency and urgency of micturition. UTIs can further be divided into complicated and uncomplicated forms. A complicated UTI is one that occurs in a person with an abnormal urinary tract or an increased susceptibility to infection. This definition typically includes people with urinary catheters or diabetes, and all men (as usually associated with prostatic enlargement). Bacteraemic UTI is defined as simultaneously identifying the same organisms on both urine and blood cultures. Guidelines designed for diagnosing UTIs in younger people typically rely on the presence of relevant urinary tract symptoms.[61]

Diagnostic problems in the frail elderly

One diagnostic difficulty in the frail elderly is that many presenting with a genuine UTI do not have urinary tract symptoms.[58,64] Even in cases of bacteraemic UTI, they are reported by just 18%–51% of the elderly.[65,66] Patients can present in non-specific ways such as functional or cognitive decline (*see* p. 67). In addition, those with urinary catheters would not be expected to get typical symptoms such as urgency and dysuria, and those with cognitive impairment (including delirium) may not reliably report such symptoms. In addition, chronic urinary symptoms unrelated to acute infections, such as urinary incontinence or nocturia, are more common. Only symptoms that have started in the last few days should be considered relevant to a diagnosis of UTI.

These problems lead to a diagnostic grey area between ASB and symptomatic UTI. In this situation, a UTI should only be considered if there is evidence of a septic illness (e.g. pyrexia, raised serum WCC, or elevated inflammatory markers) and in the absence of signs of a more likely source (e.g. chest infection).

Urine testing

There are two key limitations with urine testing in the frail elderly. First, the high prevalence of ASB means that false-positive results are likely. Second, a reliable sample for testing may be hard to collect. Problems include cognitive impairment, urinary incontinence, sample contamination and the prior receipt of antibiotics.

If a urine culture that is collected before the patient gets antibiotic therapy is negative for growth, then a UTI is effectively excluded. Although of limited diagnostic value, urine cultures are useful to guide the appropriate choice of antibiotic once a clinical diagnosis of UTI has been made.

Regarding UTIs, urine dipsticks typically test for both leukocyte esterase (a marker for pyuria) and urinary nitrites (coliform bacteria reduce nitrates to nitrites). Coliform bacteria (Gram-negative organisms found in the intestine, e.g. *E. coli*, klebsiella, proteus and enterobacter) are the commonest cause of UTI overall. However, Gram-positive (e.g. enterococci) and atypical organisms (e.g. pseudomonas) cause a larger proportion of UTIs in the elderly.[67] These organisms do not reduce urinary nitrates to nitrites. Urine dipsticks negative for both leukocytes and nitrites makes a diagnosis of UTI less likely, but the high rate of positive tests leads to only a small number of tested patients being excluded and it has a false-negative rate of 10%–20%.[68] So urinary dipsticks have only a very limited role in diagnosing UTIs in the elderly.

Blood tests

A raised serum WCC or CRP level is consistent with an infective illness. A blood culture positive for a known uropathogen in the absence of an alternative, more likely source suggests UTI, especially if urine culture is simultaneously positive for the same organism.

Making a diagnosis

Patients who report an acute onset of classical urinary symptoms such as dysuria and urgency are likely to have a UTI. Frail patients with an acute decline in functional or cognitive status don't always report such symptoms, especially if there is cognitive impairment or an indwelling urinary catheter. The following questions should be considered:

➤ Does the patient have evidence of a septic illness? For example, pyrexia, raised serum WCC and/or CRP.

➤ If so, is the source of the sepsis most likely to be the urinary tract? For example, there is no alternative more likely explanation (e.g. no clinical features of pneumonia or cellulitis).

Only if the response to both questions is positive is a UTI likely. Figure 7.1 shows a suggested diagnostic approach for UTI in the frail elderly – note that urine dipstick results are not considered.

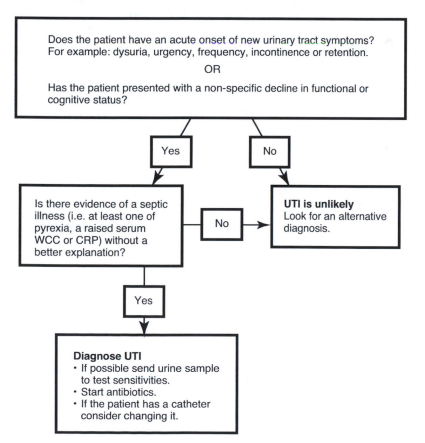

FIGURE 7.1 A suggested diagnostic approach for UTI in the frail elderly

Treatment

As stated earlier, it is appropriate to aim for a narrow-spectrum antibiotic whenever possible to reduce the risk of hospital-acquired infections. Unfortunately, resistance to commonly used antibiotics, especially amoxicillin and trimethoprim, is increasing. Infections with resistant organisms are more common in older adults, especially those with catheters or residing in care homes.[69]

Uncomplicated UTIs are typically caused by less resistant organisms, and initial treatment with a narrow-spectrum drug is appropriate (e.g. trimethoprim). Complicated UTIs should initially be treated with a broad-spectrum antibiotic (e.g. co-amoxiclav). This could be changed later to a narrower-spectrum agent if sensitivities obtained from cultures suggest this would be effective.

Evidence supports just 3-day courses of antibiotics for patients with uncomplicated UTIs,[70] but courses of 7 days or more are recommended for complicated UTIs.[61] Patients with urinary catheters should have them changed prior to antibiotic treatment as this leads to more rapid improvement and lower risk of treatment failure.[71] It can also provide a chance to obtain a urine sample from the bladder, which is less likely to be contaminated.

Preventing urinary tract infection

A key step in preventing unnecessary UTIs in hospitalised patients is through limiting the use of urinary catheters. There is evidence that they are frequently used inappropriately in the elderly and are associated with longer lengths of hospital stay and higher mortality rates (*see* p. 90).[72] Sometimes patients with recurrent UTIs are commenced on long-term prophylactic antibiotics. There is no convincing evidence for efficacy in the frail elderly and there are concerns that this can lead to colonisation with resistant organisms. In addition, there may be complications related to prolonged drug exposure (e.g. pulmonary fibrosis and peripheral neuropathy with nitrofurantoin).

KEY POINTS

- Older people are frequently diagnosed as having a UTI, but 40% of cases may be wrongly labelled.
- UTIs often present with non-specific illnesses without urinary tract symptoms, which makes distinguishing a UTI from ASB difficult.
- Diagnosis depends on comprehensive assessment rather than a specific test in isolation.
- Antibiotic use should be limited to the shortest effective duration with the narrowest-spectrum agent.

- Urinary catheters should be inserted only when absolutely necessary and removed as soon as possible.

CLOSTRIDIUM DIFFICILE INFECTION

C. difficile-associated diarrhoea is the leading cause of infectious diarrhoea in hospitals and has a high morbidity and mortality. It is a particular problem in older people as its prevalence and recurrence rates increase with age. The mortality rate may be up to 25% in the elderly.[73] C. difficile is an anaerobic spore-forming organism that produces illness by releasing toxins (type A and B) that act on the colon. It is responsible for a spectrum of illnesses ranging from mild diarrhoea to pseudo-membranous colitis and toxic megacolon. CDI increases the length of hospital stay and costs the National Health Service at least an extra £4000 per case.[74]

Transmission and pathogenesis

C. difficile spores are excreted from patients with diarrhoea and contaminate the environment and can survive for months or years. Spore ingestion can lead to asymptomatic colonisation. Up to 50% of patients in long-term facilities have been found to be asymptomatic carriers of C. difficile.[75] In elderly people, the normal gut flora is less dense and contains fewer bacterial species. Also, gut immunity declines with increasing age.[76] In susceptible people colonised with C. difficile, exposure to antibiotics leads to disruption of the normal flora and the release of toxins, with subsequent diarrhoea. Key risk factors for developing CDI are shown in Table 7.3. Virtually all antibiotics have been associated with CDI, but particular high-risk antibiotics are listed in Table 7.4 and should be avoided in older people as far as possible. Fluoroquinolones are associated with the particularly virulent 027 strain.

TABLE 7.3 Major risk factors for *Clostridium difficile* infection

Risk factor
Current or recent use of antimicrobial agents
Increasing age
Prolonged hospital stay
Serious underlying diseases
Surgical procedures (especially bowel procedures)
Immunocompromising conditions
Use of proton pump inhibitors

TABLE 7.4 High-risk antibiotics

Antibiotic
Third-generation cephalosporins (e.g. ceftriaxone or cefotaxime)
Broad-spectrum penicillins (e.g. co-amoxiclav)
Clindamycin
Fluoroquinolones (e.g. ciprofloxacin)

Prevention

The basis of prevention is to stop colonisation and reduce disease in patients already colonised. This can be achieved by prudent antimicrobial prescribing, hand hygiene, environmental cleaning, isolation nursing and use of personal protective equipment (i.e. gloves and aprons).[74] Avoiding the use of third generation cephalosporins has been successful in reducing the incidence of CDI.[77] These factors are summarised in Figure 7.2.

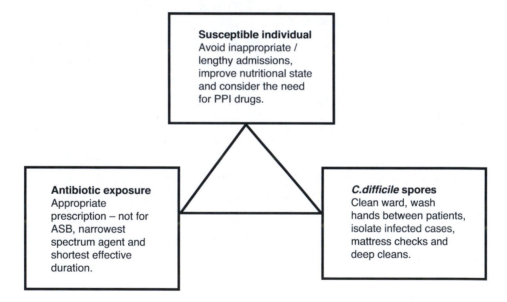

FIGURE 7.2 Factors that can be targeted to reduce the risk of CDI

Clinical presentation

CDI should always be considered as a differential diagnosis in patients who present with diarrhoea. The diagnosis is confirmed by the identification of *C. difficile* toxin in the stool of a patient who has had diarrhoea in the last 48 hours, not attributable to any other cause. Patients' stools can be classified with numerical assessments tools such as the Bristol Stool Scale (*see* p. 91). A thorough assessment is mandatory to exclude colitis, bowel perforation and other diagnoses.

Blood samples from patients with severe or relapsing CDI tend to show low albumin, low potassium and a very high WCC.

Treatment

The precipitating antibiotic(s) should be stopped if possible. Patients with CDI should be barrier nursed in a side room. Supportive care should be given, including attention to hydration, electrolytes and nutrition. Patients with mild or moderate CDI should be treated with oral metronidazole (iv route also possible), but patients with markers for severe CDI (*see* Table 7.5) should be treated with a 10-day course of oral vancomycin.[78] Iv vancomycin is ineffective in CDI but it can be given via a nasogastric tube in those with an impaired swallow. Patients with severe disease should be assessed daily for hypotension, fluid balance, bowel movement frequency, urea and electrolytes, WCC and signs of toxic megacolon, ileus or perforation with CT scanning if necessary. Colectomy is required in some patients with toxic megacolon (dilatation more than 10 cm), perforation or septic shock. This should occur before the blood lactate rises above 5 mmol/L.[79] A Cochrane review evaluated the effect of probiotic preparations on the treatment of CDI and concluded that, on current evidence, their use could not be recommended.[80]

TABLE 7.5 Severity indicators of *Clostridium difficile* infection

Severity indicator
Temperature >38.5°C
Major risk factors (e.g. immunosuppression, ITU admission)
Suspicion of:
• pseudo-membranous colitis
• toxic megacolon
• ileus
Colonic dilatation on abdominal X-ray or CT scan (>6 cm)
Serum WCC >15 × 10^9/L
Creatinine >1.5 × baseline value

Abbreviations: ITU = intensive therapy unit, WCC = white cell count

Relapse and recurrence

Relapse and recurrence occur in 15%–25% of treated patients with CDI.[73] Older age and frailty are predictors for recurrent disease. First line treatment for recurrent disease is oral vancomycin for 10 days, which can be followed by pulsed doses.[73] In a recent systematic review there was little difference between metronidazole and vancomycin in effectiveness in treatment of CDI, but the recurrence rate was significantly less with fidaxomicin compared to vancomycin (15% vs 25%).[81]

METHICILLIN-RESISTANT *STAPHYLOCOCCUS AUREUS*

MRSA produces an enzyme that provides resistance to beta-lactam antibiotics such as penicillins and cephalosporins. It is spread by direct person-to-person contact or through contaminated environments. It can survive for months on inanimate objects such as stethoscopes.[82] Older adults are at an increased risk of colonisation, partly due to higher rates of hospital admission and higher prevalence within care homes. Asymptomatic carriage has been found in 22% of UK care home residents.[83] This is usually detected by culturing swabs of the nose and throat. Invasive infections are associated with high mortality rates.[84,85] These occur most often in patients with indwelling lines or following surgical procedures.

Treatment

Patient isolation and effective barrier nursing are important ways to prevent cross-contamination. The injudicious use of broad-spectrum antibiotics promotes the spread of MRSA. Fluoroquinolones have particularly been implicated.[86,87] Topical colonisation can be treated with nasal mupirocin and antiseptic body washes. Iv vancomycin is the most commonly used antibiotic for invasive infections. Sodium fusidate or rifampicin may be used together or in combination with vancomycin for soft tissue infections. Tetracycline or clindamycin can also be used for some soft tissue infections and bronchiectasis. MRSA UTI is sometimes sensitive to tetracycline, trimethoprim or nitrofurantoin. Newer agents that can be effective include teicoplanin, linezolid, daptomycin and tigecycline.

KEY POINTS

- CDI occurs when susceptible people (e.g. the frail elderly) are exposed to certain antibiotics and spores of the organism.
- It should be suspected in all diarrhoea of recent onset in frail elderly patients.
- Key steps in prevention are rationalising the use of high-risk antibiotics and limiting the spread of spores through containment measures and deep cleaning.
- Signs of severe illness include high temperature (>38.5°C), serum WCC >15 × 10^9/L, creatinine >1.5 × baseline value and evidence of colonic dilatation (e.g. on abdominal X-ray).
- It is usually managed with oral metronidazole or vancomycin plus careful maintenance of fluid and electrolyte balance.

- MRSA colonisation is common among elderly residents of care homes.
- Some broad-spectrum antibiotics, especially fluoroquinolones, can promote the spread of MRSA.
- Invasive MRSA infections are typically treated with iv vancomycin.

INFECTIVE ENDOCARDITIS

The incidence of infective endocarditis (IE) increases with age and is currently at an all-time high.[88] Reasons for the increased rate in older people include a higher prevalence of degenerative valve disease and higher rates of invasive procedures and implanted devices compared with younger patients. Furthermore, older age is associated with a higher mortality rate.[89] The onset is usually insidious, sometimes the presenting symptoms are less severe resulting in delayed diagnosis and more aggressive pathogens can cause the infection. Older people are less likely to have surgery for endocarditis than younger patients (36% aged over 65 compared with 51% aged below 65).[90]

Causes

The commonest cause of IE in the elderly is *S. aureus*, but IE is more likely to be due to gastrointestinal sources in older patients, compared with younger people, especially *Streptococcus bovis*, which is associated with colonic pathology – in particular, neoplasia – as well as the involvement of multiple valves and embolic complications.[89,90] Enterococcus infections are also more common in the elderly. Pathogens from the urinary tract are a more frequent cause of endocarditis in older people and this is thought to be because of the higher proportion of urethral and prostatic procedures carried out in the old.[91] It is thought that valve vegetations are generally smaller in the elderly with reduced embolic risk.[89] IE due to pacemaker implantation increases with age and has a poorer prognosis, often because of delays in diagnosis.[92]

Diagnosis

The clinical diagnosis of IE is based on the Duke criteria, which include positive blood cultures, suggestive features on echocardiography, predisposing heart disease, fever and vascular and immunological phenomena.[90] However, in the elderly the onset of IE can be insidious and the classic signs are often absent.[91] IE should always be considered in the elderly in the presence of sepsis with no obvious source. Table 7.6 lists the common presentations in the elderly. Fever is less often associated, but anaemia is seen more frequently and delirium is often a prominent feature in older people. New or changing murmurs are heard less frequently in the elderly. At least three sets of blood cultures should be taken before administration of any antibiotics. Transthoracic and transoesophageal echocardiography are helpful in diagnosis with transoesophageal echocardiography being more sensitive for detecting valve abnormalities and vegetations.[93]

TABLE 7.6 Typical presentations of infectious endocarditis (IE) in the elderly

Typical presentation
Sepsis of unknown origin
Fever associated with:
• intracardiac prosthetic material, including pacemakers
• congestive cardiac failure
• recent cardiac interventions
• positive blood cultures with possible IE causative organism
• previous history of IE
• non-specific neurological symptoms or signs

Management

When IE is suspected and after three sets of blood cultures, broad-spectrum antibiotics (according to the local hospital policy) should be administered intravenously. When the results of blood cultures and sensitivities are known, then a more targeted antibiotic should be commenced. Prosthetic valve and pacemaker endocarditis, which is more common in the elderly, requires 4–6 weeks of iv antibiotics.[93] Treatment involves close liaison with microbiology and the local cardiology service. Surgery can be life-saving in IE, even in very elderly patients. Indications for surgery include heart failure, uncontrolled infection and prevention of embolic events.[94] In a Spanish study, the outcomes of 365 patients over 65 years were compared with 605 younger patients.[90] Surgery showed a lower percentage mortality compared with medical treatment (23% vs 31%) in the younger group, but a higher mortality was observed with both options in the elderly (48% vs 40%).

MENINGITIS

Meningitis can occur at any age, but the largest spikes in incidence occur in infants and in people older than 60 years.[95] Mortality increases with age and this may be due to delay in diagnosis, other co-morbidities or related to the specific pathogens. Pathogens associated with community-acquired meningitis include *S. pneumoniae*, *Neisseria meningitidis* and *Listeria monocytogenes*. In a Dutch meningitis cohort study, 257 (37%) cases of community-acquired meningitis in patients over 60 years were compared with 439 (63%) cases in patients

17–59 years old.[96] In older adults meningitis was most often due to *S. pneumoniae* (68%) and they more often developed complications (75% vs 57%; $p < 0.001$) which resulted in a higher mortality rate (34% vs 13%; $p < 0.001$).

Clinical features

Elderly people often present with the classical triad of symptoms: fever, neck stiffness and altered mental status, including delirium.[96] Headache is also likely to be present. However, neck stiffness is less common than in younger people and older people are more likely to present with focal neurological features. Neck stiffness can be a difficult sign to reliably elicit in the old as it may be due to other co-morbidities.[97] Older patients with meningitis commonly have other predisposing conditions such as otitis, sinusitis or pneumonia.[96] The elderly patient with meningitis may not have a high fever and the mental status changes are frequently incorrectly ascribed to other conditions such as psychosis, a transient ischaemic attack or stroke. Fever, when present, may be mistakenly attributed to pneumonia or UTI.[98] Tuberculous meningitis is particularly insidious in both young and old with sometimes days or weeks of non-specific symptoms.[99] A delay in diagnosis and treatment of meningitis may have devastating consequences. Therefore, it is important to have a low index of suspicion for both meningitis and encephalitis in older people and to start treatment early in suspected cases.

Management

As soon as meningitis is suspected, treatment should be started with a third generation cephalosporin (e.g. cefotaxime or ceftriaxone) and amoxicillin (to cover listeria) plus dexamethasone 8 mg iv (repeated 6-hourly) given immediately before antibiotics. Corticosteroids have been shown to reduce hearing loss and short-term neurological sequelae in acute bacterial meningitis and reduce mortality in *S. pneumoniae* meningitis.[100] Blood cultures should be taken immediately, but lumbar puncture (LP) should wait until after an urgent CT head scan. A normal CT does not exclude raised intracranial pressure and the LP should be deferred if there is a suspicion of this (e.g. presence of seizures or reduced level of consciousness). The recommended list of cerebrospinal fluid (CSF) tests in suspected meningitis and/or encephalitis is given in Table 7.7.[101] Subsequent antibiotics should be guided by the results of the LP and local microbiological advice (Table 7.8). Tuberculous meningitis should be suspected if there is a CSF leucocytosis (predominantly lymphocytes), the CSF protein is raised and the CSF to plasma glucose ratio is less than 50%.[99] Diagnostic yield is greater if large volumes of CSF (i.e. more than 6 mL) are submitted for examination. A CSF lactate level <2 mmol/L is said to rule out bacterial disease.[102]

TABLE 7.7 Recommended laboratory tests for suspected meningitis/encephalitis in older people

Cerebrospinal fluid	Blood
Protein	Glucose
Total WCC	Cultures
Differential WCC	
Microscopy and Gram stain	
Bacterial culture	
Glucose	
Lactate	
PCR for viruses (HSV, VSV and enteroviruses)	
Specific tests as indicated: • ZN stain and culture for TB • Cryptococcal antigen and India ink preparation • Nucleic acid amplification tests (e.g. multiplex PCR) • Cytology and flow cytometry (if malignancy suspected)	Serological tests (e.g. VDRL)

Abbreviations: WCC = white cell count, PCR = polymerase chain reaction, HSV = herpes simplex virus, VSV = varicella zoster virus, ZN = Ziehl–Neelsen, TB = tuberculosis, VDRL = venereal disease research laboratory test

TABLE 7.8 Typical changes in the cerebrospinal fluid (CSF) in different types of meningitis

Change	Normal	Viral	Bacterial	Tuberculosis
Appearance	Crystal clear	Clear	Turbid or purulent	Turbid or viscous
Mononuclear cells (per cubic millimetre)	<5	10–100	<50	100–300
Polymorph cells (per cubic millimetre)	Nil	Nil*	>200	0–200
Protein (g/L)	0.2–0.4	0.4–0.8	0.5–2.0	0.5–3.0
CSF glucose (proportion of blood value)	2/3 to 1/2	>1/2	<1/2	<1/3

Note: *Some polymorph cells may be seen in the early stages of viral meningitis or encephalitis.

ENCEPHALITIS

Encephalitis is a diffuse infection of the brain most often caused by viruses, particularly enteroviruses. The brain damage caused by encephalitis is the result of intracellular viral replication and the host's inflammatory response. The presence or absence of normal brain function is the important distinguishing feature between encephalitis and meningitis. Classically, patients with meningitis are uncomfortable, lethargic and distracted by their headache, but cerebral function is normal. In encephalitis, however, there is altered mental status (delirium or coma), motor or sensory deficits, altered behaviour and personality change, speech or movement disorders. The distinction between the two is blurred, especially in older patients who may have both a meningeal process and a parenchymal process and clinical features of both. Encephalitis, like meningitis, affects people at the two extremes of age – young and old. In older people encephalitis is frequently missed as the change in cerebral function is attributed to a stroke and the underlying infective process is missed.[103]

Although relatively rare, it is important not to miss treatable causes for viral encephalitis such as herpes simplex. Herpes simplex encephalitis is the most common form of sporadic necrotising encephalitis and has a second peak of incidence in the older age group with a high mortality.[104] Typically, herpes simplex encephalitis presents with a flu-like illness with headache and fever followed by seizures, cognitive impairment, behavioural changes and focal neurological signs. It usually affects the temporal and frontal lobes, often causing behavioural symptoms, disorientation and dysphasia. CT scanning has a low sensitivity for the brain changes and so treatment with aciclovir should be started as soon as the diagnosis is suspected until both polymerase chain reaction testing of the CSF and MRI brain scanning are negative.[104] The CSF typically shows a raised lymphocyte count, sometimes with red blood cells, indicating the haemorrhagic nature of the encephalitis, mildly raised protein and normal or mildly decreased glucose.[105] However, initial LP can be normal and should be repeated after 24–48 hours and treatment started in the interim if clinical suspicion is high.

Aciclovir reduces the overall mortality from 70% to 19%, but neurological sequelae are common, including dysphasia, seizures and memory problems.[104] It should be given for at least 14 days because of the risk of relapse.[105] Although it is relatively safe, it can cause a reversible nephropathy after four days of iv therapy and the risk of this should be minimised by ensuring adequate hydration, monitoring renal function and stopping iv aciclovir promptly when shown not to be indicated.[105]

SKIN AND SOFT TISSUE INFECTIONS

Cellulitis is an acute spreading pyogenic inflammation of the lower dermis and associated subcutaneous tissue. It accounts for roughly 1.6% of emergency hospital admissions in England and Wales.[106] Older people are particularly susceptible to cellulitis and other skin and soft tissue infections because of increased risk factors (e.g. diabetes, peripheral vascular disease, venous insufficiency, ulcers and trauma). Ageing of the skin also leads to decreased epidermal renewal and thinning of the epidermis resulting in the skin being a less effective barrier, delayed wound healing and greater opportunities for microorganisms to invade.[107]

Cellulitis ranges from mild localised infection to serious, life-threatening infections such as necrotising fasciitis. *S. aureus* accounts for 56% and *Streptococcus pyogenes* accounts for around 21% of cases of cellulitis.[106] Other soft tissue infections – e.g. diabetic foot ulcers, infected pressure ulcers and surgical site infections – are also common in the elderly and can lead to urgent admission to hospital. Skin and soft tissue infections account for around 5% of cases of sepsis in patients over 65 years of age.[17]

Diagnosis

Cellulitis most commonly affects the legs and presents as an acute tender, erythematous and swollen area of skin. In severe cases there may be blisters, oedema, ulcers, lymphangitis and lymphadenopathy associated with fever. Features of sepsis may occur with hypotension and tachycardia. The differential diagnosis includes other causes of a red, swollen limb – for example, a deep venous thrombosis, pyoderma gangrenosum, hypersensitivity, stasis dermatitis or a local drug reaction. Bilateral cellulitis is rare and bilateral red, swollen legs are more likely due to dermatitis due to hypersensitivity or venous stasis. There may be evidence of a portal of infection – for example, eczema, tinea pedis, pressure ulcers, trauma, insect bites or venous/arterial ulcers. Necrotising fasciitis is a rare, severe form of cellulitis that causes rapidly spreading necrosis of fascia and subcutaneous tissues, including muscles, and is characterised by severe pain, skin necrosis, crepitus and a severe systemic illness with a markedly raised WCC, CRP and creatinine.[108] Blood cultures are not particularly useful in the diagnosis of cellulitis, only being positive in around 2% of cases.[109] Similarly, wound swabs may be of limited benefit because of the presence of colonising bacteria. Ultrasound may guide management of cellulitis by detection of occult abscesses and MRI may help in diagnosing necrotising fasciitis.[106]

Treatment

General measures in treatment of cellulitis include rest, elevation and analgesia. If there is severe oedema, short-term diuretics may speed up recovery. The area of redness should be marked and reviewed daily for evidence of response to antibiotics. Patients who are systemically unwell, or who have significant co-morbidities (e.g. diabetes, obesity, venous insufficiency) are usually managed in hospital with iv antibiotics, at least initially.[110] Suggested antibiotics are included in Table 7.9, but it is always wise to discuss options with your local microbiologists as empiric antibiotic treatment is based on local epidemiology of antimicrobial resistance. A review of clinical studies failed to come to a conclusion as to the best antibiotic treatment of cellulitis.[111] If there is a poor response to treatment then it is necessary to reconsider the diagnosis (e.g. underlying deep vein thrombosis, severe dermatitis or lymphoedema) and consider an alternative second-line antibiotic (e.g. clindamycin).

TABLE 7.9 Skin and soft tissue infections in the elderly

Clinical presentation	Likely infecting organism	Suggested antibiotic(s)	Comments
Cellulitis	*Staphylococcus aureus, Streptococcus pyogenes*	Flucloxacillin	Blood cultures unlikely to be helpful Use intravenous antibiotics if systemic features or co-morbidities
Cellulitis plus penicillin allergy	*S. aureus, S. pyogenes*	Clarithromycin or clindamycin	High risk of *Clostridium difficile* infection with clindamycin
Necrotising fasciitis	Group A streptococcus or poly-microbial (Gram-negative and anaerobic organisms)	Benzylpenicillin or clindamycin	Urgent intravenous antibiotics Surgical debridement Mortality 20%–40%
Infected diabetic foot ulcers	*S. aureus*, Group B streptococci	Flucloxacillin – may need to be a broad-spectrum agent, depending on wound cultures	Good diabetic control and liaison with the diabetic team and vascular surgeons (possible revascularisation) Alleviation of mechanical load
Infected pressure ulcers	Multiple infectious organisms – Gram-positive, Gram-negative and anaerobics	Dependent on sensitivities (e.g. from blood cultures) – may need to be broad-spectrum	Systemic antibiotics usually only if bacteraemia or osteomyelitis Debride necrotic tissue Relieve pressure

Patients with necrotising fasciitis are severely ill and need immediate iv antibiotics and often urgent surgical debridement. Diabetic foot ulcers are a common cause for older diabetic patients to be admitted to hospital (*see* p. 266). Diabetic foot ulcers need specialised management in conjunction with the diabetic multidisciplinary team and vascular surgeons with optimal control of the diabetes, offloading of the affected area, surgical debridement and antibiotics, especially when underlying bone involvement is suspected. Diabetic foot ulcers are the most important risk factors for lower extremity amputation.[112] Routine systemic antibiotics are not recommended in pressure ulcers or chronic leg ulcers unless there are local or systemic signs of infection, bacteraemia or osteomyelitis[107] – local cleansing, debridement and relief of pressure are more important.

- IE can present more insidiously in older people and can lead to a delay in diagnosis and worse outcomes.
- IE should be suspected in cases of sepsis without an obvious cause, especially when there is a history of cardiac disease or interventions.
- A delay in the diagnosis of meningitis and encephalitis increases the risk of adverse outcomes – it is important to have a low index of suspicion for these conditions in older people and to start treatment early.
- When considering sources of infection in older people do not forget the skin and soft tissue as a possible source (e.g. pressure ulcers).

REFERENCES

1. Waterer GW, Kessler LA, Wunderink RG. Delayed administration of antibiotics and atypical presentation in community-acquired pneumonia. *Chest*. 2006; **130**(1): 11–15.
2. Waalen J, Buxbaum JN. Is older colder or colder older? The association of age with body temperature in 18,630 individuals. *J Gerontol A Biol Sci Med Sci*. 2011; **66**(5): 487–92.
3. Marco CA, Schoenfeld CN, Hansen KN, *et al*. Fever in geriatric emergency patients: clinical features associated with serious illness. *Ann Emerg Med*. 1995; **26**(1): 18–24.
4. Caterino JM, Kulchycki LK, Fischer CM, *et al*. Risk factors for death in elderly emergency department patients with suspected infection. *J Am Geriatr Soc*. 2009; **57**(7): 1184–90.
5. Nguyen HB, Rivers EP, Abrahamian FM, *et al*. Severe sepsis and septic shock: review of the literature and emergency department guidelines. *Ann Emerg Med*. 2006; **48**(1): 28–54.
6. Chassagne P, Perol M, Doucet J, *et al*. Is presentation of bacteremia in the elderly the same as in younger patients? *Am J Med*. 1996; **100**(1): 65–70.
7. Lee C, Chen S, Chang I, *et al*. Comparison of clinical manifestations and outcome of community-acquired bloodstream infections among the oldest old, elderly, and adult patients. *Medicine (Baltimore)*. 2007; **86**(3): 138–44.
8. Whitelaw DA, Rayner BL, Willcox PA. Community-acquired bacteremia in the elderly: a prospective study of 121 cases. *J Am Geriatr Soc*. 1992; **40**(10): 996–1000.
9. Fontanarosa PB, Kaeberlein FJ, Gerson LW, *et al*. Difficulty in predicting bacteremia in elderly emergency patients. *Ann Emerg Med*. 1992; **21**(7): 842–8.
10. Deulofeu F, Cervello B, Capell S, *et al*. Predictors of mortality in patients with bacteremia: the importance of functional status. *J Am Geriatr Soc*. 1998; **46**(1): 14–18.
11. Caterino JM, Jalbuena T, Bogucki B. Predictors of acute decompensation after admission in ED patients with sepsis. *Am J Emerg Med*. 2010; **28**(5): 631–6.
12. Setia U, Serventi I, Lorenz P. Bacteremia in a long-term care facility: spectrum and mortality. *Arch Intern Med*. 1984; **144**(8): 1633–5.
13. Sinclair D, Svendsen A, Marrie T. Bacteremia in nursing home patients: prevalence among patients presenting to an emergency department. *Can Fam Physician*. 1998; **44**: 317–22.
14. Mountain D, Bailey PM, O'Brien D, *et al*. Blood cultures ordered in the adult emergency department are rarely useful. *Eur J Emerg Med*. 2006; **13**(2): 76–9.
15. Dellinger RP, Levy MM, Carlet JM, *et al*. Surviving sepsis campaign: international guidelines for management of severe sepsis and septic shock: 2008. *Intensive Care Med*. 2008; **34**(1): 17–60.

16. Bone RC, Balk RA, Cerra FB, *et al*. Definitions for sepsis and organ failure and guidelines for the use of innovative therapies in sepsis. ACCP/SCCM Consensus Conference Committee. *Chest*. 1992; **101**(6): 1644–55.

17. Martin GS, Mannino GM, Moss M. The effect of age on the development and outcome of adult sepsis. *Crit Care Med*. 2006; **34**(1): 15–21.

18. Glickman SW, Cairns CB, Otero RM, *et al*. Disease progression in hemodynamically stable patients presenting to the emergency department with sepsis. *Acad Emerg Med*. 2010; **17**(4): 383–90.

19. O'Fallon E, Pop-Vicas A, D'Agata E. The emerging threat of multidrug-resistant Gram-negative organisms in long-term care facilities. *J Gerontol A Biol Sci Med Sci*. 2009; **64**(1): 138–41.

20. Lim WS, Macfarlane JT. Defining prognostic factors in the elderly with community acquired pneumonia: a case controlled study of patients aged ≥75 yrs. *Eur Respir J*. 2001; **17**(2): 200–5.

21. Fernandez-Sabe N, Carratala J, Roson B, *et al*. Community-acquired pneumonia in very elderly patients: causative organisms, clinical characteristics, and outcomes. *Medicine (Baltimore)*. 2003; **82**(3): 159–69.

22. Knol W, van Marum RJ, Jansen PAF, *et al*. Antipsychotic drug use and risk of pneumonia in elderly people. *J Am Geriatr Soc*. 2008; **56**(4): 661–6.

23. Metlay JP, Schulz R, Li Y, *et al*. Influence of age on symptoms at presentation in patients with community-acquired pneumonia. *Arch Intern Med*. 1997; **157**(13): 1453–9.

24. Harper C, Newton P. Clinical aspects of pneumonia in the elderly veteran. *J Am Geriatr Soc*. 1989; **37**(9): 867–72.

25. Marrie TJ, Haldane EV, Faulkner RS, *et al*. Community-acquired pneumonia requiring hospitalisation: is it different in the elderly? *J Am Geriatr Soc*. 1985; **33**(10): 671–80.

26. Starczewski AR, Allen SC, Vargas E, *et al*. Clinical prognostic indices of fatality in elderly patients admitted to hospital with acute pneumonia. *Age Ageing*. 1988; **17**(3): 181–6.

27. Ahkee S, Srinath L, Ramirez J. Community-acquired pneumonia in the elderly: association of mortality with lack of fever and leukocytosis. *South Med J*. 1997; **90**(3): 296–8.

28. Jokinen C, Heiskanen L, Juvonen H, *et al*. Microbial etiology of community-acquired pneumonia in the adult population of 4 municipalities in eastern Finland. *Clin Infect Dis*. 2001; **32**(8): 1141–54.

29. Lim WS, Macfarlane JT. A prospective comparison of nursing home acquired pneumonia with community acquired pneumonia. *Eur Respir J*. 2001; **18**(2): 362–8.

30. Marrie TJ, Blanchard W. A comparison of nursing home-acquired pneumonia patients with patients with community-acquired pneumonia and nursing home patients without pneumonia. *J Am Geriatr Soc*. 1997; **45**(1): 50–5.

31. Meehan TP, Chua-Reyes JM, Tate J, *et al*. Process of care performance, patient characteristics, and outcomes in elderly patients hospitalized with community-acquired or nursing home-acquired pneumonia. *Chest*. 2000; **117**(5): 1378–85.

32. Mylotte JM. Nursing home-acquired pneumonia: update on treatment options. *Drugs Aging*. 2006; **23**(5): 377–90.

33. Yoneyama T, Yoshida M, Ohrui T, *et al*. Oral care reduces pneumonia in older patients in nursing homes. *J Am Geriatr Soc*. 2002; **50**(3): 430–3.

34. Vergis EN, Brennen C, Wagener M, *et al*. Pneumonia in long-term care: a prospective case-control study of risk factors and impact on survival. *Arch Intern Med*. 2001; **161**(19): 2378–81.

35. Kikuchi R, Watabe N, Konno T, *et al.* High incidence of silent aspiration in elderly patients with community-acquired pneumonia. *Am J Resp Crit Care Med.* 1994; **150**(1): 251–3.
36. Marik PE. Aspiration pneumonitis and aspiration pneumonia. *N Engl J Med.* 2001; **344**(9): 665–71.
37. Terpenning MS, Taylor GW, Lopatin DE, *et al.* Aspiration pneumonia: dental and oral risk factors in an older veteran population. *J Am Geriatr Soc.* 2001; **49**(5): 557–63.
38. Marik PE, Kaplan D. Aspiration pneumonia and dysphagia in the elderly. *Chest.* 2003; **124**(1): 328–36.
39. Van der Maarel-Wierink CD, Vanobbergen JNO, Bronkhorst EM, *et al.* Risk factors for aspiration pneumonia in frail older people: a systematic literature review. *J Am Med Dir Assoc.* 2011; **12**(5): 344–54.
40. El-Solh AA, Pietrantoni C, Bhat A, *et al.* Microbiology of severe aspiration pneumonia in institutionalized elderly. *Am J Respir Crit Care Med.* 2003; **167**(12): 1650–4.
41. Arai T, Sekizawa K, Ohrui T, *et al.* ACE inhibitors and protection against pneumonia in elderly patients with stroke. *Neurology.* 2005; **64**(3): 573–4.
42. Bont J, Hak E, Hoes AW, *et al.* Predicting death in elderly patients with community-acquired pneumonia: a prospective validation study reevaluating the CRB-65 severity assessment tool. *Arch Intern Med.* 2008; **168**(13): 1465–8.
43. Barlow G, Nathwani D, Davey P. The CURB65 pneumonia severity score outperforms generic sepsis and early warning scores in predicting mortality in community-acquired pneumonia. *Thorax.* 2007; **62**(3): 253–9.
44. Aujesky D, Auble TE, Yealy DM, *et al.* Prospective comparison of three validated prediction rules for prognosis in community-acquired pneumonia. *Am J Med.* 2005; **118**(4): 384–92.
45. Chen J, Chang S, Liu JJ, *et al.* Comparison of clinical characteristics and performance of pneumonia severity score and CURB-65 among younger adults, elderly and very old subjects. *Thorax.* 2010; **65**(11): 971–7.
46. Meehan TP, Fine MJ, Krumholz HM, *et al.* Quality of care, process, and outcomes in elderly patients with pneumonia. *JAMA.* 1997; **278**(23): 2080–4.
47. Houck PM, Bratzler DW, Nsa W, *et al.* Timing of antibiotic administration and outcomes for Medicare patients hospitalized with community-acquired pneumonia. *Arch Intern Med.* 2004; **164**(6): 637–44.
48. Arnold FW, Summersgill JT, Lajoie AS, *et al.* A worldwide perspective of atypical pathogens in community-acquired pneumonia. *Am J Respir Crit Care Med.* 2007; **175**(10): 1086–93.
49. Torres OH, Munoz J, Ruiz D, *et al.* Outcome predictors of pneumonia in elderly patients: importance of functional assessment. *J Am Geriatr Soc.* 2004; **52**(10): 1603–9.
50. Kaplan V, Clermont G, Griffin MF, *et al.* Pneumonia: still the old man's friend? *Arch Intern Med.* 2003; **163**(3): 317–23.
51. Toba A, Yamazaki M, Mochizuki H, *et al.* Lower incidence of acute respiratory distress syndrome in community-acquired pneumonia patients aged 85 years or older. *Respirology.* 2010; **15**(2): 319–25.
52. Groenwold RHH, Hoes AW, Hak E. Impact of influenza vaccination on mortality risk among the elderly. *Eur Respir J.* 2009; **34**(1): 56–62.
53. Jefferson T, Di Pietrantonj C, Al-Ansary LA, *et al.* Vaccines for preventing influenza in the elderly. Cochrane Database Syst Rev. 2010; 2: CD004876.
54. Thomas RE, Jefferson T, Demicheli V, *et al.* Influenza vaccination for healthcare workers who work with the elderly. Cochrane Database Syst Rev. 2006; 3: CD005187.
55. Nichol KL, Nordin JD, Nelson DB, *et al.* Effectiveness of influenza vaccine in the community-dwelling elderly. *N Engl J Med.* 2007; **357**(14): 1373–81.

56. Jackson ML, Nelson JC, Weiss NS, *et al.* Influenza vaccination and risk of community-acquired pneumonia in immunocompetent elderly people: a population-based, nested case-control study. *Lancet.* 2008; **372**(9636): 398–405.

57. Ducharme J, Neilson S, Ginn JL. Can urine cultures and reagent test strips be used to diagnose urinary tract infection in elderly emergency department patients without focal urinary symptoms? *CJEM.* 2007; **9**(2): 87–92.

58. Woodford HJ, George J. Diagnosis and management of urinary tract infection in hospitalized older people. *J Am Geriatr Soc.* 2009; **57**(1): 107–14.

59. Baldassarre JS, Kaye D. Special problems of urinary tract infection in the elderly. *Med Clin North Am.* 1991; **75**(2): 375–90.

60. Nicolle LE. Urinary infections in the elderly: symptomatic or asymptomatic? *Int J Antimicrob Agents.* 1999; **11**(3–4): 265–8.

61. Scottish Intercollegiate Guideline Network. *Management of Suspected Bacterial Urinary Tract Infection in Adults: Guideline 88.* Edinburgh: SIGN; 2006. Available at: www.sign.ac.uk/pdf/sign88.pdf (accessed 25 January 2013).

62. Nicolle LE, Mayhew WJ, Bryan L. Prospective randomized comparison of therapy and no therapy for asymptomatic bacteriuria in institutionalized elderly women. *Am J Med.* 1987; **83**(1): 27–33.

63. Abrutyn E, Berlin J, Mossey J, *et al.* Does treatment of asymptomatic bacteriuria in older ambulatory women reduce subsequent symptoms of urinary tract infection? *J Am Geriatr Soc.* 1996; **44**(3): 293–5.

64. Barkham TM, Martin FC, Eykyn SJ. Delay in the diagnosis of bacteraemic urinary tract infection in elderly patients. *Age Ageing.* 1996; **25**(2): 130–2.

65. Esposito AL, Gleckman RA, Cram S, *et al.* Community-acquired bacteraemia in the elderly: analysis of one hundred consecutive episodes. *J Am Geriatr Soc.* 1980; **28**(7): 315–19.

66. Woodford HJ, Graham C, Meda M, *et al.* Bacteremic urinary tract infection in hospitalized older patients: are any currently available diagnostic criteria sensitive enough? *J Am Geriatr Soc.* 2011; **59**(3): 567–8.

67. Ronald A. The etiology of urinary tract infection: traditional and emerging pathogens. *Am J Med.* 2002; **113**(Suppl. 1A): 14–19S.

68. Ouslander JG, Schapira M, Fingold S, *et al.* Accuracy of rapid urine screening tests among incontinent nursing home residents with asymptomatic bacteriuria. *J Am Geriatr Soc.* 1995; **43**(7): 772–5.

69. Wright SW, Wrenn KD, Haynes M, *et al.* Prevalence and risk factors for multidrug resistant uropathogens in ED patients. *Am J Emerg Med.* 2000; **18**(2): 143–6.

70. Vogel T, Verreault R, Gourdeau M, *et al.* Optimal duration of antibiotic therapy for uncomplicated urinary tract infection in older women: a double-blind randomized controlled trial. *CMAJ.* 2004; **170**(4): 469–73.

71. Raz R, Schiller D, Nicolle LE. Chronic indwelling catheter replacement before antimicrobial therapy for symptomatic urinary tract infection. *J Urol.* 2000; **164**(4): 1254–8.

72. Holroyd-Leduc JM, Sen S, Bertenthal D, *et al.* The relationship of indwelling urinary catheters to death, length of hospital stay, functional decline, and nursing home admission in hospitalized older medical patients. *J Am Geriatr Soc.* 2007; **55**(2): 227–33.

73. Ewan V, Newton JL. Management of *Clostridium difficile* infection. *J R Coll Physicians Edinb.* 2008; **38**: 144–7.

74. Department of Health. *Saving Lives: reducing infection, delivering clean and safe care.* High impact intervention No. 7. London: Department of Health; 2007. Available at: www.

dh.gov.uk/en/Publicationsandstatistics/Publications/PublicationsPolicyAndGuidance/DH_124265 (accessed 25 January 2013).

75. Riggs MM, Sethi AK, Zabarsky TF, *et al*. Asymptomatic carriers are a potential source for transmission of epidemic and non epidemic *Clostridium difficile* strains among long-term care facility residents. *Clin Infect Dis*. 2007; **45**(8): 992–8.

76. Hebuterne X. Gut changes attributed to ageing effects on intestinal microflora. *Curr Opin Clin Nutr Metab Care*. 2003; **6**(1): 49–54.

77. Gouliouris T, Brown NM, Aliyu SH. Prevention and treatment of *Clostridium difficile* infection. *Clin Med*. 2011; **11**(1): 75–9.

78. Department of Health and Health Protection Agency. Clostridium difficile *Infection: how to deal with the problem*. London: Department of Health and Health Protection Agency; 2008.

79. Lamontagne F, Labbe AC, Haeck O, *et al*. Impact of emergency colectomy on survival of patients with fulminant *Clostridium difficile* colitis during an epidemic caused by a hyper-virulent strain. *Ann Surg*. 2009; **245**(2): 267–72.

80. Pillai A, Nelson R. Probiotics for the treatment of *Clostridium difficile*-associated colitis in adults. Cochrane Database Syst Rev. 2008; 1: CD004611.

81. Drekonja DM, Butler M, McDonald R, *et al*. Comparative effectiveness of *Clostridium difficile* treatments: a systematic review. *Ann Intern Med*. 2011; **155**(12): 839–47.

82. Kluytmans J, Stuelens M. Meticillin resistant *Staphylococcus aureus* in the hospital. *BMJ*. 2009; **338**: 532–7.

83. Barr B, Wilcox MH, Brady A, *et al*. Prevalence of methicillin-resistant *Staphylococcus aureus* colonization among older residents of care homes in the United Kingdom. *Infect Control Hosp Epidemiol*. 2007; **28**(7): 853–9.

84. Wyllie DH, Crook DW, Peto TEA. Mortality after *Staphylococcus aureus* bacteraemia in two hospitals in Oxfordshire, 1997–2003: cohort study. *BMJ*. 2006; **333**(7562): 281–6.

85. Laupland KB, Ross T, Gregson DB. *Staphylococcus aureus* bloodstream infections: risk factors, outcomes, and the influence of methicillin resistance in Calgary, Canada, 2000–2006. *J Infect Dis*. 2008; **198**(3): 336–43.

86. Weber SG, Gold HS, Hooper DC, *et al*. Fluoroquinolones and the risk for methicillin-resistant *Staphylococcus aureus* in hospitalized patients. *Emerg Infect Dis*. 2003; **9**(11): 1415–22.

87. Charbonneau P, Parienti JJ, Thibon P, *et al*. Fluoroquinolone use and methicillin-resistant *Staphylococcus aureus* isolation rates in hospitalized patients: a quasi experimental study. *Clin Infect Dis*. 2006; **42**(6): 778–84.

88. Dhawan VK. Infective endocarditis in elderly patients. *Clin Infect Dis*. 2002; **34**(6): 806–12.

89. Durante-Mangoni E, Bradley S, Selton-Suty C, *et al*. Current features of infective endocarditis in elderly patients. *Arch Intern Med*. 2008; **168**(19): 2095–103.

90. Ramirez-Duque E, Garcia-Cabrera R, Ivanova-Georgieva R, *et al*. Surgical treatment of infective endocarditis in elderly patients. *J Infect*. 2011; **63**(2): 131–8.

91. Vahanian A. The growing burden of infective endocarditis in the elderly. *Eur Heart J*. 2003; **24**(17): 1539–40.

92. Remadi JP, Nadji G, Goissen T, *et al*. Infective endocarditis in elderly patients: clinical characteristics and outcome. *Eur J Cardiothorac Surg*. 2009; **35**(1): 123–9.

93. Prendergast BD. The changing face of infective endocarditis. *Heart*. 2006; **92**(7): 879–85.

94. European Society of Cardiology. Guidelines on the prevention, diagnosis and treatment of infective endocarditis. *Eur Heart J*. 2009; **30**(19): 2369–413.

95. Kulchycki LK, Edlow JA. Geriatric neurologic emergencies. *Emerg Med Clin North Am.* 2006; **24**(2): 273–98.

96. Weisfelt M, van de Beek D, Spanjaard L, *et al.* Community-acquired bacterial meningitis in older people. *J Am Geriatr Soc.* 2006; **54**(10): 1500–7.

97. Puxty JAH, Fox RA, Horan MA. The frequency of physical signs attributed to meningeal irritation in elderly patients. *J Am Geriatr Soc.* 1983; **31**(10): 590–2.

98. Mace SE. Central nervous system infections as a cause of an altered mental status? What is the pathogen growing in your central nervous system? *Emerg Med Clin North Am.* 2010; **28**(3): 535–70.

99. Thwaites G, Fisher M, Hemingway C, *et al.* British Infection Society Guidelines for the diagnosis and treatment of tuberculosis of the central nervous system in adults and children. *J Infect.* 2009; **59**(3): 167–87.

100. Brouwer MC, McIntyre P, de Gans J, *et al.* Corticosteroids for acute bacterial meningitis. Cochrane Database Syst Rev. 2010; 9: CD 004405.

101. Solomon T, Michael BD, Smith PE, *et al.* Management of suspected viral encephalitis in adults: Association of British Neurologists and British Infection Association National Guidelines. *J Infect.* 2012; **64**(4): 347–73.

102. Cunha BA. Distinguishing bacterial from viral meningitis: the critical importance of the CSF lactic acid levels. *Intensive Care Med.* 2006; **32**(8): 1272–3.

103. Townend BS, Hanson JA, Sturm JW, *et al.* Stroke or encephalitis? *Emerg Med Australas.* 2005; **17**(4): 401–4.

104. Riera-Mestre A, Requena A, Martinez-Yelamos S, *et al.* Herpes simplex encephalitis in older adults. *J Am Geriatr Soc.* 2010; **58**(1): 201–2.

105. Bell DJ, Suckling R, Rothburn MM, *et al.* Management of suspected herpes simplex encephalitis in adults in a UK teaching hospital. *Clin Med.* 2009; **9**(3): 231–5.

106. Phoenix G, Das S, Joshi M. Diagnosis and management of cellulitis. *BMJ.* 2012; **345**: e4955.

107. Kish TD, Chang MH, Fung HB. Treatment of skin and soft tissue infections in the elderly: a review. *Am J Geriatr Pharmacother.* 2010; **8**(6): 485–513.

108. Wong CH, Khin LW, Heng KS, *et al.* The LRINEC (Laboratory Risk Indicator for Necrotising Fasciitis) score: a tool for distinguishing necrotising fasciitis from other soft tissue infections. *Crit Care Med.* 2004; **32**(7): 1535–41.

109. Sultan HY, Boyle AA, Sheppard N. Necrotising fasciitis. *BMJ.* 2012; **345**: e4274.

110. Perl B, Gottehrer NP, Raveh D, *et al.* Cost effectiveness of blood cultures for adult patients with cellulitis. *Clin Infect Dis.* 1999; **29**(6): 1483–8.

111. Kilburn SA, Featherstone P, Higgins B, *et al.* Interventions for cellulitis and erysipelas. Cochrane Database Syst Rev. 2010; 6: CD004299.

112. Cavanagh PR, Lipsky BA, Bradbury AW, *et al.* Treatment for diabetic foot ulcers. *Lancet.* 2005; **366**(9498): 1725–35.

CHAPTER 8

Cerebrovascular disease

Strokes and transient ischaemic attacks (TIAs) cause a *sudden onset* of *focal neurological symptoms* (or signs). This fact is of key importance when diagnosing cerebrovascular events. The two conditions are arbitrarily distinguished by the duration of symptoms, being more than 24 hours with stroke but less than 24 hours with TIA. However, they have the same underlying causes and both carry a similarly elevated risk of future stroke. The diagnosis of stroke is not always straightforward. A collateral history is very important, especially for those with reduced consciousness or cognitive impairment. Around 20% of patients initially classified as having had a stroke by emergency physicians are subsequently found to have an alternative diagnosis (e.g. post-ictal states, cerebral tumours, and toxic/metabolic disorders).[1] Subarachnoid haemorrhage, which is usually classified as a type of stroke, is discussed on page 272.

STROKE

Stroke, like many other conditions, can present atypically in the frail elderly (i.e. non-specific functional or cognitive decline). However, on careful evaluation a persisting focal neurological deficit will be detectable. Brain imaging can show an acute lesion to support the diagnosis, but this is not always the case and depends on the timing and modality (CT vs MRI) of the scan.

The deficit caused by a stroke is usually maximal at the time of onset and gradually improves thereafter. But this recovery can take days to weeks and many will be left with some degree of residual impairment. The symptoms caused by mimic conditions, such as brain tumours, tend to get worse over time. Occasionally the deficit caused by a stroke can appear to worsen over the first few days after onset. This can be due to the development of cerebral oedema, haemorrhage or an intercurrent illness. The symptoms of stroke are typically 'negative' – that is, loss of function such as reduced vision, weakness or impaired sensation. 'Positive' symptoms, such as jerking movements, tingling sensations or seeing flashing lights, suggest an alternative pathology such as focal seizures or migraine. However, these general rules are not absolute.[2]

Strokes are divided into those caused by a blocked blood vessel (termed 'ischaemic') and those caused by a bleed into the brain tissue (termed 'haemorrhagic'). Ischaemic and haemorrhagic strokes can only reliably be distinguished by brain imaging. Headache can occur in both conditions but vomiting at symptom onset is more suggestive of haemorrhagic aetiology.

TRANSIENT ISCHAEMIC ATTACK

TIAs do not cause non-focal symptoms such as confusion or unconsciousness.

TIA can sometimes be confused with either focal seizures or migraine aura. Symptoms of TIA are typically maximal at onset but may spread or worsen over a few seconds. Symptoms of seizures or migraine are typically of a more gradual onset and may spread or worsen over several minutes. These latter conditions are more likely to produce 'positive' symptoms. Focal weakness (termed 'Todd's paresis') may be present after a seizure. A history of multiple recurrent stereotypical events is less suggestive of TIA. Very brief symptoms lasting just seconds are very unlikely to be caused by TIA.

TIAs are traditionally thought to differ from stroke by not causing an area of irreversible brain damage. Although defined as lasting less than 24 hours, in reality detailed brain imaging (e.g. diffusion-weighted MRI) will often show areas of brain infarction when symptoms have lasted more than 3 hours. TIAs are exclusively caused by ischaemic not haemorrhagic events, because symptoms with this latter pathology do not resolve within 24 hours.

Clots within the retinal arteries can cause episodes of transient painless monocular blindness (termed 'amaurosis fugax'). Patients usually experience complete blackness in one eye that lasts from seconds to minutes. As this condition has similar underlying mechanisms and elevated risk of future stroke, it is typically considered much like a TIA.

Assessment

Any reported neurological symptoms should be clarified. Vague terms such as 'my arm was dead' can sometimes be used to describe either motor or sensory loss. A witness history should be obtained if possible, especially if unconsciousness is reported or seizures are suspected. Dysphasia can be mistaken for confusion.

Patients with significant neglect may lack insight into the extent of their neurological deficit. Patients should be systematically asked about any weakness or sensory disturbance in the face, arm and leg on each side, changes in their speech or vision, and any headache. Activities at the time of onset of the symptoms may suggest alternative pathologies (e.g. postural change causing presyncope). The history should identify vascular risk factors – that is, smoking, hypertension, diabetes, other vascular disorders (including previous stroke) and atrial fibrillation (AF). Residual neurological deficits from a prior stroke may become more prominent during times of acute illness. This should be suspected when a very similar deficit to a previous stroke recurs.

Examination

A detailed neurological examination is crucial to assessment in those who have had a suspected cerebrovascular event. However, in the case of TIA the neurological signs will usually have resolved prior to assessment. The key components of examination are shown in Table 8.1.

TABLE 8.1 Important elements of examination for patients with suspected stroke

Examination	Comment
Motor system	Pronator drift (the downward movement of an outstretched arm or elevated leg while the eyes are closed) can uncover subtle motor impairments. In the frail elderly it is important to appreciate a difference between the patient's left and right sides rather than compare their strength to yours. Despite usually causing an upper motor neuron deficit, strokes typically cause early limb flaccidity and only develop spasticity later.
Sensory system	Sensory inattention suggests a parietal lobe lesion. It is tested for by asking the patient to close their eyes with their hands placed in front of them. The patient is told to inform the examiner where they feel being touched. The hands are then touched individually in turn, followed by both together. A patient with intact sensation but sensory inattention will correctly report the individual hands being touched but will only report the hand of the unaffected side when both are touched together.
Visual fields	Formal confrontation technique to assess visual fields is not always possible (e.g. in the presence of reduced consciousness, dysphasia or dementia). In such a situation the absence of a blink response to a threatening stimulus from the side (e.g. the examiner's hand brought rapidly towards the patient's face) suggests homonymous hemianopia. Visual inattention is assessed by standing in front of the patient with your arms outstretched, then asking the patient to look directly at your nose and point at any hand that moves. The fingers of each outstretched hand are then wiggled in turn, followed by both hands together. The patient with visual inattention will correctly identify the individual movements but when both are moved together they will only report movement in the unaffected field.

(continued)

Examination	Comment
Neglect	Neglect can be caused by lesions in the parietal lobe on either side of the brain, but tend to be more severe when affecting the non-dominant hemisphere. The patient's functional impairment may be out of proportion with the degree of motor or sensory loss. Simple techniques for detecting neglect include the Clock Drawing Test (*see* p. 55).
Speech	Asking the patient to obey commands tests comprehension of speech (i.e. identify receptive dysphasia). These should initially be one-stage commands (e.g. 'close your eyes') and then more complex sequences (e.g. 'point to the door then touch the bed'). Expressive dysphasia can be detected by asking the patient to name objects (e.g. pen and watch, then the smaller components of each, such as the nib, hands, etc.). Subtle dysarthria may be detected by asking the patient to repeat difficult phrases, such as 'West Register Street', 'baby hippopotamus' and 'biblical criticism'.
Swallow	The assessment of swallowing is important in all patients who have sustained a stroke. Formal assessment is best performed by speech and language therapists; however, a rapid bedside guide can be initiated by asking the patient to swallow a teaspoon of water and observing for any coughing or choking. If tolerated, then the next step is to observe the patient taking a sip of water from a cup, and so on.
Gait	Gait should be examined in patients able to safely stand. This can reveal subtle deficits in coordination or motor function that were not obvious when the patient was lying down.
Consciousness	The Glasgow Coma Scale score should be recorded in patients with reduced consciousness.
Vascular system	The examination of the vascular system should look for evidence of atrial fibrillation and hypertension. Auscultation over the carotid arteries for the detection of carotid bruits is an unreliable way to detect carotid stenosis and of little value.

Investigations

Basic blood tests include glucose (to identify underlying diabetes and exclude hypoglycaemia as a cause of symptoms), cholesterol, erythrocyte sedimentation rate (to exclude vasculitis) and an international normalised ratio if the patient is on warfarin. An ECG should be performed, particularly looking for AF.

Brain imaging is vital for distinguishing between haemorrhagic and ischaemic strokes. Occasionally it will identify an alternative cause for the patient's symptoms (e.g. a brain tumour). Current guidelines recommend that imaging should occur within 1 hour if thrombolysis is being considered, and always within 12 hours.[3] Some clinical situations necessitate more rapid brain imaging, for example:

➤ current anticoagulant use
➤ reduced level of consciousness
➤ progressive or fluctuating symptoms

➤ severe headache, neck stiffness, papilloedema or fever
➤ head trauma.

CT scanning is widely available, quick to perform and well tolerated, but it may not show abnormalities when performed immediately after the onset of an ischaemic stroke.[4] Early changes can be subtle – such as loss of grey–white matter differentiation, loss of definition of the lentiform nucleus, sulcal effacement and loss of the insular ribbon (*see* Figure 8.1).[5] Sometimes a blood clot can be visualised within the middle cerebral artery – called the 'dense middle cerebral artery sign' (*see* Figure 8.2). After hours to days, hypodense (dark grey or black) areas develop due to oedema followed by cell death and breakdown (*see* Figure 8.3). Bleeding is readily identified on CT straight after an event, as blood appears hyperdense (white) and remains so for approximately 10 days (*see* Figure 8.4). After this time the blood is gradually broken down to intermediary products, which become isodense (grey-like brain tissue) and finally hypodense. So CTs are unable to reliably distinguish haemorrhages and infarcts if delayed beyond 1 week from symptom onset.

MRI scans give better definition than CT scans and are more likely to detect acute infarcts. This is particularly true when 'diffusion-weighted' images are

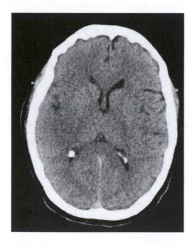

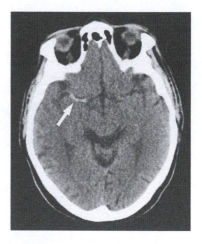

FIGURE 8.1 Subtle changes are seen in the patient's right hemisphere on a CT scan done soon after the onset of symptoms (there is reduced definition between the areas of grey and white matter, and the sulci are less clear)

FIGURE 8.2 The dense middle cerebral artery sign – a blood clot (light grey) can be seen in the patient's right middle cerebral artery (arrow)

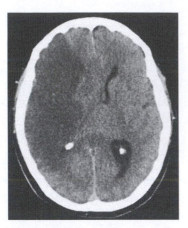 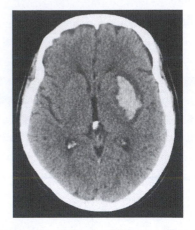

FIGURE 8.3 A brain CT scan showing an extensive right middle cerebral artery infarct (dark grey) with oedema causing compression of the lateral ventricles

FIGURE 8.4 A brain CT scan showing an acute haemorrhage (white) in the left basal ganglia with a small amount of surrounding oedema (dark grey)

obtained. On these scans acute infarcts appear hyperdense (*see* Figure 8.5). Acute haemorrhage is typically less distinct on MRI scans than on CT scans, but it can be made more apparent with the 'gradient-echo' technique. MRI is also capable of detecting the breakdown products of blood (haemosiderin), which allows the distinction of haemorrhagic and ischaemic strokes well beyond 1 week after the event. A proportion of patients are unable to undergo MRI either because they are unable to tolerate the noisy and claustrophobic procedure or because of metallic implants (e.g. a cardiac pacemaker).

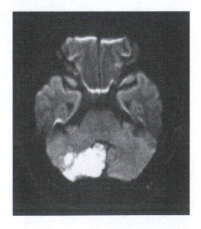

FIGURE 8.5 A diffusion-weighted MRI showing an acute infarct (white) in the right cerebellar hemisphere

Classification

The vascular territory involved can classify stroke and TIA. This is usually as affecting the left or right internal carotid artery (anterior circulation) or affecting the vertebrobasilar system (posterior circulation). This distinction helps when selecting appropriate patients for carotid surgery (*see* p. 217).

As well as being defined as ischaemic or haemorrhagic, stroke can also be classified according to the constellation of clinical features, which provides some prognostic information. The most-commonly used classification in the UK is as set out in Table 8.2; each type occurs in roughly equal numbers.[6] It can be seen that the prognosis for total anterior circulation infarcts is much worse than the other subtypes.

TABLE 8.2 The classification of stroke subtypes and associated prognosis

Stroke type	30-day mortality (%)	Independent at 1 year (%)
Lacunar stroke	2	60
The stroke affects subcortical fibres in the internal capsule or thalamus to give a unilateral pure motor or sensory deficit. As the fibres are closely packed together in these brain regions, the stroke affects a large bodily area (at least two of the face, arm and leg).		
Total anterior circulation stroke	39	4
This type of stroke affects a large area of the middle cerebral artery distribution leading to hemiplegia, sensory loss, hemianopia and other cortical signs such as inattention. When affecting the dominant hemisphere (the left for over 95% of people) there will also be dysphasia. The large area affected and subsequent brain oedema often results in reduced conscious level.		
Partial anterior circulation stroke	4	55
This stroke type also affects the brain cortex but it involves a smaller area than that of a total anterior circulation stroke. Typically there will be some degree of unilateral weakness plus either hemianopia, inattention (visual and/or sensory) or dysphasia (if affecting the dominant hemisphere). Partial anterior circulation stroke can also cause isolated dysphasia or a motor and/or sensory deficit affecting a smaller bodily area than seen with lacunar stroke (because of a small lesion within the motor/sensory cortex).		
Posterior circulation stroke	7	62
Stroke in this region can cause a range of clinical presentations. These include isolated hemianopia (lesion in occipital lobe), cerebellar signs and cranial nerve disorders (brainstem lesions). Given the close relationship of structures in the brainstem and cerebellum it is likely that a lesion here will cause a spectrum of signs rather than any one in isolation.		

ISCHAEMIC STROKE AND TRANSIENT ISCHAEMIC ATTACK

Cerebral blood vessels can become blocked because of clots formed locally or embolised from elsewhere. The commonest cause is thought to be emboli from atheroma on the walls of large blood vessels (i.e. the aorta and carotid arteries). Around a third of events in patients aged over 80 years are associated with AF due to clot formation within the left atrium.[7] Occasionally cardiac emboli can result from other structures (e.g. artificial heart valves or a hypokinetic left ventricular wall). Next most common in the frail elderly is intracranial thrombus formation. Other causes are rare in the elderly. This is represented in Figure 8.6.

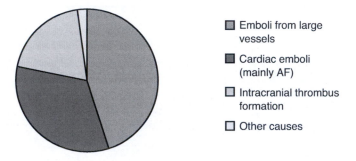

■ Emboli from large vessels

■ Cardiac emboli (mainly AF)

□ Intracranial thrombus formation

□ Other causes

FIGURE 8.6 The approximate breakdown of causes of ischaemic cerebrovascular events in the frail elderly

The key risk factors are:
➤ hypertension
➤ atrial fibrillation
➤ smoking
➤ diabetes
➤ history of previous vascular disease (including stroke).

Thrombolysis for acute ischaemic stroke

Recombinant tissue plasminogen activator acts by converting plasminogen to plasmin, which breaks down the fibrin polymers that form clots. It has been found to reduce the risk of the combined end point of death or dependency following ischaemic stroke when compared with placebo (odds ratio, 0.80; 95% confidence interval (CI), 0.69–0.93).[8] Its benefit seems to extend to 4.5 hours from onset of symptoms.[9] There is an associated risk of symptomatic intracranial haemorrhage that can be fatal. Given this risk, it is important to select the patients most likely to benefit.

Appropriate patients have a persisting neurological deficit (i.e. not rapidly improving) that is not so severe that they are unresponsive. They have not had recent surgery or a bleeding disorder (within 3 weeks) and they have not had a prior stroke (within 3 months). They did have a reasonable level of function prior to the event (e.g. not a nursing home resident). Blood pressure >180/105 mmHg, blood sugar >22 mmol/L and any seizures since onset are contraindications. A large area of hypodensity on the pretreatment brain CT scan suggests that the patient will not do well with thrombolysis. Initial criteria suggested a cut-off age limit of 80 years. However, data are emerging that suggest thrombolysis may still be beneficial in some older patients.[10–12] Many stroke physicians would consider patients aged over 80 who previously functioned well and who meet other criteria as suitable for thrombolysis.

Stroke units

Stroke patients should be transferred to a specialist stroke unit as soon as possible. The basic concept of a stroke unit is that care is based around multidisciplinary rehabilitation delivered by specialist staff in a ward that is geographically discrete from the rest of the hospital. When compared with non-specialised care, stroke units have been found to be associated with a reduction in 1-year mortality and the combined outcome of death and institutionalisation with no net increase in length of stay.[13]

Secondary prevention of ischaemic stroke and transient ischaemic attack
Antiplatelet drugs
Aspirin at a dose of 300 mg per day for the first 2 weeks following stroke is associated with improved outcomes.[14] It can be given rectally in those who cannot swallow. The most significant side effect is an increased risk of gastrointestinal bleeding. Dipyridamole (modified release 200 mg twice daily) when added to aspirin has been shown to have an additional benefit in reducing longer-term adverse vascular outcomes following stroke or TIA.[15] However, it does have some additional side effects, including headache, which leads to discontinuation in around 10% of patients. Clopidogrel has been compared with the combination of aspirin and dipyridamole following stroke and was associated with a similar risk of recurrent stroke (8.8% vs 9.0%; 95% CI, 0.92–1.11) but a lower risk of major haemorrhagic events (3.6% vs 4.1%; 95% CI, 1.00–1.32) over a mean period of 2.5 years.[16]

Based on this evidence, the National Institute for Health and Clinical Excellence recommends aspirin 300 mg daily for the first 2 weeks following stroke (or up to the point of hospital discharge).[17] After that time, clopidogrel is recommended first line for the prevention of stroke.[18] The combination of aspirin and dipyridamole is currently recommended first line for the prevention of TIA.

Anticoagulation

Warfarin is mainly used to prevent stroke in patients who have AF. The prevalence of AF is discussed on page 231. It is associated with an elevated risk of stroke because of embolus formation with the left atrium. The actual size of the risk of stroke varies from patient to patient depending on other clinical features. Several rating scales have been developed to help stratify patients; one example is the CHADS2.[19] Here one point is given for each of a history of **C**ongestive cardiac failure, **H**ypertension, **A**ge over 75 years and **D**iabetes, and a history of **S**troke scores **2** points, leading to a total score between 0 and 6. The estimated annual risk of stroke without blood-thinning treatment ranges from 1.9% for a score of 0 to 18.2% for a score of 6.

Warfarin reduces the relative risk of stroke by around 65%.[20,21] This benefit seems to be preserved in patients aged over 75 years.[22] The main adverse effect is an increased risk of bleeding. Intracranial bleeds occur at a rate of around 0.3%–1% per year, depending on patient characteristics.[23] An increased risk of bleeding is seen in those with excessive alcohol intake, renal impairment, liver disease, non-steroidal anti-inflammatory drug use or an underlying diagnosis of cancer.[24] Risks are also higher in patients who fail to obtain stable blood level readings (international normalised ratio values) or those with cognitive impairment who lack assistance to take the medication as prescribed. Evidence suggests that the patient's risk of falling should not have a major influence on the decision to warfarinise.[25]

As there is an increased risk of bleeding into an area of infarcted brain tissue immediately following an ischaemic stroke, guidelines currently recommend that warfarin is not given in the initial 2 weeks (although shorter time intervals may be appropriate in some patients following non-disabling stroke and a period of one week is recommended for those with prosthetic heart valves). An antiplatelet agent should be used in the interim (e.g. aspirin 300 mg daily).[3]

Dabigatran, a direct thrombin inhibitor, is a newer alternative to warfarin. It seems to be as effective as warfarin in preventing stroke but may have a lower risk of major bleeding.[26] It has the advantage of being a standardised dose that does not need titrating or monitoring. The two potential limitations are the higher cost and the inability to rapidly reverse the anticoagulation effect. Similarly, apixaban, a direct factor Xa inhibitor, has recently been found to be associated with lower rates of stroke or major bleeding in patients with AF than in those receiving warfarin.[27] The use of such drugs is likely to increase in the future.

Cholesterol reduction

Studies of people with a history of vascular disease (including stroke) suggest a relative risk reduction of around 20%–25% for statins over a 5-year period.[28-30] The typical recommended drug in the UK at present is simvastatin 40 mg daily.[3]

Blood pressure control

The Joint British Societies' Guidelines recommend a blood pressure target of better than 130/80 mmHg for all patients following stroke.[31] Currently it is recommended that treatment for high blood pressure should be delayed until 2 weeks after the stroke onset or until the time of hospital discharge (whichever occurs sooner) unless there are other clinical reasons why tighter control would be worthwhile (e.g. hypertensive encephalopathy).[3]

Control of blood sugar

Diabetic patients who have had a stroke should have their future blood sugar control optimised. The acute management of diabetes in the frail elderly is discussed on page 265. Guidelines recommend maintaining a blood glucose concentration between 4 and 11 mmol/L in the immediate phase following acute stroke.[3]

Smoking cessation

Smokers should be educated on the benefits of quitting. While in hospital, nicotine patches may be required to reduce the incidence of withdrawal symptoms. After discharge, information should be provided regarding local services to help support cessation.

Carotid endarterectomy

It is believed that emboli originating from atheromatous plaques on the carotid arteries cause 15%–20% of ischaemic strokes.[32] Carotid endarterectomy is a surgical technique that removes atheroma from the blood vessel surface. It is relevant for patients who have sustained an ischaemic stroke or TIA within the last 2 weeks affecting the associated carotid territory (i.e. anterior circulation).[33] Atheroma on the blood vessel walls causes vessel narrowing, which can be detected by carotid ultrasound or angiography studies (including CT or MRI modalities). The benefits of this procedure are most noted in those with a vessel narrowing of 70%–99%.[34-36] It may also be of value in selected patients with stenoses of 50%–70%. Those with completely occluded vessels are not thought to benefit from surgery. The benefits of carotid endarterectomy are most marked in older patients. The absolute risk reduction over 2 years has been calculated as 29% in those aged 75 and over, compared with 15% for those aged 65–74 and 10% for those aged below 65.[37] The finding of significant stenosis is more common in the elderly. Despite these observations, patients aged over 80 years are less likely to be referred for carotid imaging.[38]

Prognosis

The prognosis varies depending on the subtype of stroke sustained (*see* Table 8.2). The overall figure is that 10% will die within the first month and 23% will be dead by 1 year.[39] The risk of recurrent stroke following either a minor stroke or TIA is similar and is highest immediately following an acute event, being 8%–12% in the first week, 12%–15% in the first month and 17%–19% within 1 year.[40] However, this risk can be dramatically reduced by rapid assessment and commencement of appropriate treatment following an event.[41]

The 'ABCD2' is a scoring tool that aims to stratify patients following a suspected TIA into groups according to risk of stroke (*see* Table 8.3). The total score ranges from 0 to 7. Those with a score less than 4 have a 1.2% risk of stroke within the next 7 days, but this rises to 5.9% with a score of 4 or 5, and 11.7% with a score over 5.[42] This can allow selection of the highest-risk patients for more rapid assessment where resources are limited.

TABLE 8.3 Calculating the ABCD2 score

Criteria	Points scored
Age 60 or over	1
Blood pressure	
• systolic >140 mmHg or diastolic >90 mmHg	1
Clinical features – one of	
• unilateral weakness	2
• speech disturbance	1
Duration	
• 60 minutes or more	2
• 10–59 minutes	1
• less than 10 minutes	0
Diabetes	1

INTRACEREBRAL HAEMORRHAGE

Intracranial bleeding causes around 15% of strokes. This is mainly due to intracerebral haemorrhage (ICH), but subarachnoid haemorrhage is also possible. Around 80% of ICH is related to either hypertension or cerebral amyloid angiopathy.[43,44] Alternative pathologies include arteriovenous malformations, aneurysms, tumours and coagulopathy (including warfarin use).

➤ *Hypertension*: bleeding is usually located 'deep' in the brain – i.e. the basal ganglia, brainstem or cerebellum. High blood pressure can damage the walls of the small perforating blood vessels in these regions.

➤ *Cerebral amyloid angiopathy*: bleeding is usually 'lobar' – that is, located in or adjacent to the cerebral cortex. It is due to beta-amyloid deposition in the blood vessel walls. It is more likely to lead to recurrent events and there may be a history of previous bleeds or multiple lesions on brain scanning (these are best visualised by gradient-echo MRI). It occurs to some extent in many older patients, but it is more common in those with neurodegenerative conditions such as Alzheimer's disease.

The presentation of ICH is usually very similar to ischaemic stroke – that is, a sudden onset of a focal neurological deficit. It is distinguished from ischaemic stroke by brain imaging. Patients should be transferred to an acute stroke unit. Guidance for the treatment for blood pressure is the same as that for ischaemic strokes. Patients on warfarin should have their anticoagulation reversed. This is most effectively achieved by giving a combination of prothrombin complex concentrate and vitamin K intravenously.[45] Antiplatelet drugs should be withheld. Cases of ICH are occasionally suitable for neurosurgical intervention. It is usually appropriate to obtain a specialist surgical opinion but the overall evidence for benefit of surgery is unclear.[46] Guidelines recommend early blood pressure intervention for those with ICH plus a systolic value over 200 mmHg (e.g. with parenteral medication).[3]

The prognosis for ICH is less favourable than that of ischaemic stroke. The mortality rate is 30%–50% in the first 30 days and many of the survivors will be left with a neurological deficit.[47] The prognosis is even worse for older patients. When ICH is associated with warfarin use, the mortality rate is around 70%.[48] The risk of recurrent ICH is higher for lobar bleeds (15% per year) than for deep bleeds (2% per year).[49] This is mainly because of the association with cerebral amyloid angiopathy. Angiography, typically MRI modality, can be used to look for underlying structural abnormalities such as vascular malformations in selected patients. Identifying and then treating such lesions can reduce the risk of recurrent ICH.

> **KEY POINTS**
>
> - Stroke and TIA cause a sudden onset of focal neurological symptoms or signs.
> - Non-focal symptoms such as dizziness are unlikely to be due to a cerebrovascular event.
> - Stroke causes 'negative' symptoms (e.g. loss of power, loss of sensation, impaired vision and/or reduced speech).
> - Be careful not to mistake dysphasia for confusion.
> - Patients with unilateral neglect may have a functional limitation that is greater than would be predicted by their degree of motor impairment.
> - Stroke patients should have their swallow assessed early in their admission.
> - The benefit of thrombolysis for acute stroke probably extends to patients aged over 80 years and so very old patients who previously functioned well should be urgently assessed for suitability.
> - Patients who have had a stroke should be cared for on a specialised stroke unit.
> - Smokers may require nicotine patches to prevent withdrawal symptoms while in hospital.
> - Anticoagulation should be considered for patients who have had a cerebrovascular event and are in AF.
> - Following ischaemic stroke or TIA, elderly patients should be considered for carotid imaging, as they are more likely to have a vessel narrowing and are more likely to benefit from surgery.
> - The risk of a recurrent event is highest immediately following the index one; for this reason, patients should be assessed as soon as possible and have relevant secondary prevention commenced.
> - ICH: bleeding around the basal ganglia is most likely to be caused by hypertension, whereas bleeding in the cortex is most likely to be related to cerebral amyloid angiopathy.
> - ICH carries a worse prognosis than ischaemic stroke.

REFERENCES

1. Libman RB, Wirkowski E, Alvir J, *et al.* Conditions that mimic stroke in the emergency department: implications for acute stroke trials. *Arch Neurol.* 1995; **52**(11): 1119–22.
2. De Freitas GR. Borderlands of transient ischemic attacks, seizures and other transient neurological deficits. Commentary on de Reuck and van Maele: transient ischemic attacks and inhibitory seizures in elderly patients (*Eur Neurol.* 2009; **62**: 344–8). *Eur Neurol.* 2010; **63**(1): 60–1.
3. Intercollegiate Stroke Working Party. *National Clinical Guideline for Stroke.* 4th ed. London: Royal College of Physicians; 2012. Available at: www.rcplondon.ac.uk/sites/default/files/national-clinical-guidelines-for-stroke-fourth-edition.pdf (accessed 25 January 2013).

4. Wardlaw JM, Farrall AJ. Diagnosis of stroke on neuroimaging: 'scan all immediately' strategy improves outcomes and reduces cost. *BMJ*. 2004; **328**: 655–6.

5. Wardlaw JM, Mielke O. Early signs of brain infarction at CT: observer reliability and outcome after thrombolytic treatment – systematic review. *Radiology*. 2005; **235**(2): 444–53.

6. Bamford J, Sandercock P, Dennis M, *et al*. Classification and natural history of clinically identifiable subtypes of cerebral infarction. *Lancet*. 1991; **337**(8756): 1521–6.

7. Wolf PA, Abbott RD, Kannel WB. Atrial fibrillation: a major contributor to stroke in the elderly: the Framingham study. *Arch Intern Med*. 1987; **147**(9): 1561–4.

8. Wardlaw JM, del Zoppo G, Yamaguchi T, *et al*. Thrombolysis for acute ischaemic stroke. Cochrane Database Syst Rev. 2003; 3: CD000213.

9. Hacke W, Kaste M, Bluhmki E, *et al*. Thrombolysis with alteplase 3 to 4.5 hours after acute ischaemic stroke. *N Engl J Med*. 2008; **359**(13): 1317–29.

10. Engelter ST, Bonati LH, Lyrer PA. Intravenous thrombolysis in stroke patients of >80 versus <80 years of age: a systematic review across cohort studies. *Age Ageing*. 2006; **35**(6): 572–80.

11. Ford GA, Ahmed N, Azevedo E, *et al*. Intravenous alteplase for stroke in those older than 80 years old. *Stroke*. 2010; **41**(11): 2568–74.

12. Mishra N, Ahmed A, Anderson G, *et al*. Thrombolysis in very elderly people: controlled comparison of SITS International Stroke Thrombolysis Registry and Virtual International Stroke Trials Archive. *BMJ*. 2010; **341**: c6046.

13. Stroke Trialists' Collaboration. Collaborative systematic review of the randomised trials of organised inpatient (stroke unit) care after stroke. *BMJ*. 1997; **314**(7088): 1151–9.

14. International Stroke Trial Collaborative Group. The International Stroke Trial (IST): a randomised trial of aspirin, subcutaneous heparin, both, or neither among 19435 patients with acute ischaemic stroke. *Lancet*. 1997; **349**(9065): 1569–81.

15. ESPRIT Study Group. Aspirin plus dipyridamole versus aspirin alone after cerebral ischaemia of arterial origin (ESPRIT): randomised controlled trial. *Lancet*. 2006; **367**(9523): 1665–73.

16. Sacco RL, Diener H, Yusuf S, *et al*. Aspirin and extended-release dipyridamole versus clopidogrel for recurrent stroke. *N Engl J Med*. 2008; **359**(12): 1238–51.

17. National Institute for Health and Clinical Excellence. Stroke: diagnosis and initial management of acute stroke and transient ischaemic attack (TIA); Nice guideline 68. London: NIHCE; 2008. Available at: www.nice.org.uk/nicemedia/live/12018/41331/41331.pdf (accessed 25 January 2013).

18. National Institute for Health and Clinical Excellence. Clopidogrel and Modified-release Dipyridamole for the Prevention of Occlusive Vascular Events: NIHCE guideline 90. London: NICE; 2010. Available at: www.nice.org.uk/nicemedia/live/13285/52030/52030.pdf (accessed 25 January 2013).

19. Gage BF, Waterman AD, Shannon W, *et al*. Validation of clinical classification schemes for predicting stroke: results from the national registry of atrial fibrillation. *JAMA*. 2001; **285**(22): 2864–70.

20. Atrial Fibrillation Investigators. Risk factors for stroke and efficacy of antithrombotic therapy in atrial fibrillation: analysis of pooled data from five randomized controlled trials. *Arch Intern Med*. 1994; **154**(13): 1449–57.

21. Hart RG, Halperin JL, Pearce LA. Lessons from the Stroke, Prevention in Atrial Fibrillation trials. *Ann Intern Med*. 2003; **138**(10): 831–8.

22. Mant J, Hobbs FD, Fletcher K, *et al*. Warfarin versus aspirin for stroke prevention in an elderly community population with atrial fibrillation (the Birmingham Atrial Fibrillation

Treatment of the Aged Study, BAFTA): a randomised controlled trial. *Lancet*. 2007; **370**(9586): 493–503.

23. Hart RG, Boop BS, Anderson DC. Oral anticoagulants and intracranial haemorrhage: facts and hypotheses. *Stroke*. 1995; **26**(8): 1471–7.

24. Gage BF, Fihn SD, White RH. Warfarin therapy for an octogenarian who has atrial fibrillation. *Ann Intern Med*. 2001; **134**(6): 465–74.

25. Man-Son-Hing M, Nichol G, Lau A, *et al*. Choosing antithrombotic therapy for elderly patients with atrial fibrillation who are at risk for falls. *Arch Intern Med*. 1999; **159**(7): 677–85.

26. Connolly SJ, Ezekowitz MD, Yusuf S, *et al*. Dabigatran versus warfarin in patients with atrial fibrillation. *N Engl J Med*. 2009; **361**(12): 1139–51.

27. Lopes RD, Al-Khatib SM, Wallentin L, *et al*. Efficacy and safety of apixaban compared with warfarin according to patient risk of stroke and of bleeding in atrial fibrillation: a secondary analysis of a randomised controlled trial. *Lancet*. 2012; **380**(9855): 1749–58.

28. Collins R, Armitage J, Parish S, *et al*. Effects of cholesterol-lowering with simvastatin on stroke and other major vascular events in 20,536 people with cerebrovascular disease or other high-risk conditions. *Lancet*. 2004; **363**(9411): 757–67.

29. Baigent C, Keech A, Kearney PM, *et al*. Efficacy and safety of cholesterol-lowering treatment: prospective meta-analysis of data from 90,056 participants in 14 randomised trials of statins. *Lancet*. 2005; **366**(9493): 1267–78.

30. Amarenco P, Bogousslavsky J, Callahan A, *et al*. High-dose atorvastatin after stroke or transient ischemic attack. *N Engl J Med*. 2006; **355**(6): 549–59.

31. British Cardiac Society, British Hypertension Society, Diabetes UK, *et al*. JBS2: Joint British Societies' guidelines on prevention of cardiovascular disease in clinical practice. *Heart*. 2005; **91**(Suppl. 5): v1–52.

32. Chaturvedi S, Bruno A, Feasby T, *et al*. Carotid endarterectomy – an evidence-based review: report of the Therapeutics and Technology Assessment Subcommittee of the American Academy of Neurology. *Neurology*. 2005; **65**(6): 794–801.

33. Rothwell PM, Eliaszew M, Gutnikov SA, *et al*. Endarterectomy for symptomatic carotid stenosis in relation to clinical subgroups and timing of surgery. *Lancet*. 2004; **363**(9413): 915–24.

34. North American Symptomatic Carotid Endarterectomy Trial Collaborators. Beneficial effect of carotid endarterectomy in symptomatic patients with high-grade carotid stenosis. *N Engl J Med*. 1991; **325**(7): 445–53.

35. Barnett HJM, Taylor DW, Eliasziw M, *et al*. Benefit of carotid endarterectomy in patients with symptomatic moderate or severe stenosis. *N Engl J Med*. 1998; **339**(20): 1415–25.

36. European Carotid Surgery Trialists' Collaborative Group. Randomised trial of endarterectomy for recently symptomatic carotid stenosis: final results of the MRC European Carotid Surgery Trial (ECST). *Lancet*. 1998; **351**(9113): 1379–87.

37. Alamowitch S, Eliasziw M, Algra A, *et al*. Risk, causes, and prevention of ischaemic stroke in elderly patients with symptomatic internal-carotid-artery stenosis. *Lancet*. 2001; **357**(9263): 1154–60.

38. Fairhead JF, Rothwell PM. Underinvestigation and undertreatment of carotid disease in elderly patients with transient ischaemic attack and stroke: comparative population based study. *BMJ*. 2006; **333**(7567): 525–7.

39. Bamford J, Sandercock P, Dennis M, *et al*. Classification and natural history of clinically identifiable subtypes of cerebral infarction. *Lancet*. 1991; **337**(8756): 1521–6.

40. Coull AJ, Lovett JK, Rothwell PM. Population based study of early risk of stroke after

transient ischaemic attack or minor stroke: implications for public education and organisation of services. *BMJ*. 2004; **328**(7435): 326.

41. Rothwell PM, Giles MF, Chandratheva A, *et al*. Effect of urgent treatment of transient ischaemic attack and minor stroke on early recurrent stroke (EXPRESS study): a prospective population-based sequential comparison. *Lancet*. 2007; **370**(9596): 1432–42.

42. Johnston SC, Rothwell PM, Nguyen-Huynh MN, *et al*. Validation and refinement of scores to predict very early stroke risk after transient ischaemic attack. *Lancet*. 2007; **369**(9558): 283–92.

43. Qureshi AI, Tuhrim S, Broderick JP, *et al*. Spontaneous intracerebral hemorrhage. *N Engl J Med*. 2001; **344**(19): 1450–60.

44. Thanvi B, Robinson T. Sporadic cerebral amyloid angiopathy: an important cause of cerebral haemorrhage in older people. *Age Ageing*. 2006; **35**(6): 565–71.

45. Hankey JP. Warfarin reversal. *J Clin Pathol*. 2004; **57**(11): 1132–9.

46. Mendelow AD, Gregson BA, Fernandes HM, *et al*. Early surgery versus initial conservative treatment in patients with spontaneous supratentorial intracerebral haematomas in the International Surgical Trial in Intracerebral Haemorrhage (STICH): a randomised trial. *Lancet*. 2005; **365**(9457): 387–97.

47. Brott T, Broderick J, Kothari R, *et al*. Early hemorrhage growth in patients with intracerebral hemorrhage. *Stroke*. 1997; **28**(1): 1–5.

48. Steiner T, Rosand J, Diringer M. Intracerebral hemorrhage associated with oral anticoagulant therapy: current practices and unresolved questions. *Stroke*. 2006; **37**(1): 256–62.

49. Eckman MH, Rosand J, Knudsen KA, *et al*. Can patients be anticoagulated after intracerebral haemorrhage? A decision analysis. *Stroke*. 2003; **34**(7): 1710–16.

CHAPTER 9

Chest pain and shortness of breath

The two common presenting complaints of chest pain and shortness of breath have been covered together as a number of conditions can present with either or both of these symptoms. A wide range of disorders can precipitate chest pain or shortness of breath and so we have concentrated on the more common serious causes. Pneumonia is another possibility – this is discussed on page 179.

ACUTE CORONARY SYNDROMES

Acute coronary syndrome (ACS) is a term covering both acute myocardial infarction (MI) and unstable angina. Like many conditions it becomes more common in older age and outcomes are typically less favourable. Currently the mean age of onset of MI is approximately 70 years.[1] Around 33% of ACS events occur in people aged over 75, and 60% of deaths occur in this group.[2] Following an MI the mortality rate for patients aged 85 and over is around 26%–30%, compared with 3%–4% for those aged <65.[1,3]

Presentation

As discussed in previous chapters, almost any medical illness in the frail elderly can present as 'off legs', falls or confusion. It has long been recognised that older people with ACS are more likely to present in an atypical fashion than younger people. A study of patients with an acute MI found that presenting with any-thing other than chest pain, discomfort, heaviness or pressure occurred in 33% of those aged 75 or over, compared with 27% of those aged 65–74, and 12% of those aged 35–64 years.[4] Another study found that chest pain was present in 90% of ST segment elevation MI patients and 77% of ACS patients aged <65 years, but only 57% and 40% of those aged 85 and over, respectively.[3,5] In a different population, chest pain was the chief complaint in 68% of patients aged 75 and over with ACS, compared to 79% of those aged below 75.[6] Elderly patients who complained of pain in the left arm were more likely to have ACS. Another group found that MI presented with typical chest pain in 62% of those aged over 85, 72% aged 75–84, 78% aged 65–74 and 85% of those below the age of 65.[1] Eleven per cent of those aged over 85 presented with cardiogenic shock, compared with less than 2% of those aged below 65 years. An additional cohort of ACS patients found that 86% of those aged below 65 years, 79% of those aged 65–74 and 68% of those aged 75 or over presented with typical anginal chest pain.[7] These data are summarised in Table 9.1.

TABLE 9.1 Percentage of patients of different ages presenting without classical cardiac chest pain

	Age (years)			
	<65	**65–74**	**75–84**	**85+**
ACS	14–23	21	32	60
MI	10–15	22–27	28–33	38–43

Abbreviations: ACS = acute coronary syndrome, MI = myocardial infarction

Heart failure is a more common initial presentation of MI in the frail elderly (45% of those aged 85 and over vs 12% aged <65).[3] Dyspnoea (49%), diaphoresis (26%), nausea and vomiting (24%), and syncope (19%) are more common presentations of ACS in the elderly.[5] A smaller proportion of elderly patients have the classical ECG changes of ST segment elevation in acute MI (31% of those aged over 85 vs 51% of those below 65 years).[1] This is partly due to the higher rate of left bundle branch block in older people (8%–34% of those aged 85 and over vs 2%–5% of those under 65 years).[1,3] Left ventricular hypertrophy is also common. ECG changes can occur in response to medications (e.g. digoxin). It is important to obtain an old ECG whenever possible to determine the presence of new changes. A normal ECG does not exclude ACS. Many ACS events will be detected only by elevated cardiac troponins after hours or even days from the onset of symptoms. Of course, troponins can also be elevated in several other conditions and therefore should be used in the appropriate clinical context to ensure correct interpretation and diagnosis.

Treatment

The higher incidence of atypical presentations in the old promotes delays in treatment and higher mortality rates.[8,9] It is necessary to have a high index of suspicion, especially in those with new or worsened heart failure or ECG changes. Other factors influencing treatment decisions include contraindications (e.g.

warfarin use – unless anticoagulant effects are reversed) and co-morbidities (e.g. dementia). Elderly patients are less likely than younger patients to receive aspirin, beta-blockers, percutaneous coronary intervention or thrombolysis following an ACS.[1,10–13]

The higher risk of recurrent events in the elderly leads to a higher absolute chance of benefit from many treatments. The available evidence seems to suggest that treatments used in younger people are still effective in the old. Beta-blockers, angiotensin-converting enzyme (ACE) inhibitors and statins are associated with improved outcomes following MI.[3] The use of percutaneous coronary intervention and beta-blockers in patients aged over 80 years with MI are associated with reduced mortality rates.[14] Mortality rates after 30 days for primary angioplasty following MI are higher in those aged over 75 than in those aged 65–75 or <65 (13% vs 5% and 3%, respectively).[15] However, this is still an effective treatment compared with thrombolysis in older patients who are more likely to benefit.[2] In addition, it reduces the risk of haemorrhagic stroke, which occurs in 1%–2% of patients aged over 65 receiving thrombolytic drugs. In general the same treatment protocols used in younger adults are still appropriate for the elderly.

Cardiac surgery

Even in non-elective (urgent or emergency) cardiac surgery in patients aged over 80 years, early mortality rates of 6%–11% have been observed, and 5-year survival rates around 50%.[16,17] Similar to non-cardiac surgery, functional ability can be used to predict likely outcomes from surgery. Those with slower gait speeds (taking 6 or more seconds to walk 5 metres) have a threefold higher risk of mortality and morbidity.[18] Transcatheter aortic valve implantation is a new, less invasive technique for the treatment of aortic valve disease in those unable to undergo open procedures on cardiopulmonary bypass.

KEY POINTS

- 33%–60% of frail elderly patients with ACS do not have classical chest pain.
- ACS may present as heart failure/shortness of breath, sweating, nausea and vomiting.
- The mortality rate after MI is much higher in the elderly.
- Older patients usually benefit from the same treatment protocols as used in younger adults.

HEART FAILURE

Heart failure is defined as the heart being no longer able to pump sufficient blood to meet the body's metabolic requirements. Its prevalence rises from around 1% in adults in their 50s, to around 10% in those aged in their 80s.[19] This is due to age-related changes of the cardiovascular system (*see* p. 4) and higher prevalence of cardiovascular disease, such as hypertension, which can precipitate heart failure. The prognosis is poor, with survival rates around 60%–80% at 1 year and just 30% at 5 years, with the oldest patients having the worst prospects.[20,21]

'Diastolic heart failure' is a term for patients with the clinical features of heart failure but with a normal ejection fraction on echocardiography. This is caused by increased stiffness of the myocardium due to increased collagen deposition and reduced amounts of elastin, which are associated with ageing. Diastolic heart failure may account for half of cases of heart failure in the frail elderly.[22,23] The relevance of this condition is that standard echocardiographic assessment of left ventricular systolic function is an unreliable way to diagnose cardiac impairment. Available evidence suggests that the treatment of diastolic heart failure should be the same as that for systolic heart failure.

Assessment

Left ventricular impairment causes pulmonary oedema, which presents as breathlessness. Right ventricular impairment causes peripheral oedema, which is usually noted as swelling of the ankles. Congestive cardiac failure is the combination of left and right ventricular impairment.

It is important to assess the whole patient rather than individual clinical signs. Bibasal chest crackles may be caused by other pathologies (e.g. pulmonary fibrosis). Pulmonary oedema may cause wheezing to be heard in the chest ('cardiac asthma'). Leg oedema may also be caused by low albumin, venous insufficiency, reduced mobility and drugs (e.g. calcium channel blockers, alpha-blockers, dopamine agonists or pioglitazone). Non-steroidal anti-inflammatory drugs promote fluid retention and may precipitate heart failure. There is evidence that such unhelpful drugs are commonly given to the frail elderly with heart failure.[24] Clearly, a review of current medications is a part of the assessment process. A raised jugular venous pressure and, when present, a third heart sound ('gallop rhythm') also suggest heart failure.

At the time of an acute presentation with heart failure, consideration should be given to the underlying precipitant (*see* Table 9.2). This could be an acute MI, atrial fibrillation (AF), a change in medication or poor adherence to prescribed drugs. The patient may also have deteriorated because of a superimposed illness such as a chest infection or pulmonary embolism.

An ECG may show signs of cardiac enlargement, such as left ventricular hypertrophy, and possibly previous ischaemia or AF. A chest X-ray is likely to show cardiac enlargement, upper lobe venous congestion, and possibly pulmonary oedema and effusions. Blood tests should look for hypoalbuminaemia, electrolyte disturbances (especially sodium, potassium and magnesium) and exclude anaemia and hyperthyroidism (causes of 'high output' cardiac failure). Brain natriuretic peptide has been proposed as a marker of cardiac failure that can be measured from blood samples.[25] However, it is a non-specific test, as levels may rise with other cardiac and non-cardiac conditions (e.g. pulmonary emboli and even normal ageing). A negative test result makes heart failure less likely, but its clinical value in the frail elderly is unclear. Cardiac troponins can be used to detect a recent MI as the precipitant. Echocardiography is able to identify valvular lesions and distinguish between diastolic and systolic dysfunction.

TABLE 9.2 Common reasons for patients to present with exacerbations of heart failure

Reason	Comment
Worsening of underlying condition	Cardiac failure is a progressive incurable condition
New cardiac problem	For example, myocardial infarction or atrial fibrillation
Non-adherence to medications	*See* p. 307
Prescription of unhelpful drug	For example, NSAIDs, calcium channel blockers or pioglitazone
Superimposed illness	For example, chest infection or pulmonary embolism

Abbreviation: NSAID = non-steroidal anti-inflammatory drug

Treatment

As with all chronic diseases, patient education is important and helps improve medication concordance. If adherence to a treatment regime is suboptimal, then other measures may also be appropriate (*see* p. 307). Other precipitating factors should be addressed. Unhelpful medications should be reduced or stopped whenever possible.

In the acute setting hypoxia should be corrected with oxygen therapy. Non-invasive ventilatory support with continuous positive airway pressure may be useful in severe cases.[26] Nitrates can be given intravenously to reduce cardiac load, but hypotension may limit their use.

Loop diuretics (e.g. furosemide or bumetanide) provide symptomatic relief from fluid overload. Initial intravenous administration may be more effective in those with bowel oedema because of right heart failure. Patients with renal impairment may need large doses for a therapeutic effect. Thiazide diuretics (e.g.

bendroflumethiazide) can have a potent additional effect in resistant cases, but caution is needed, as there is a high risk of hyponatraemia and hypokalaemia. Spironolactone is a potassium-sparing diuretic that inhibits the action of aldosterone. At low doses (25 mg per day) it is associated with a reduction in mortality rates in patients with heart failure on standard treatment.[27] This effect may be mediated by avoiding cardiac arrhythmias induced by hypokalaemia, but serious hyperkalaemia develops in 2% of patients.

Beta-blockers are of proven benefit in reducing mortality in younger adults with heart failure. Evidence suggests that this benefit is also seen in the elderly.[28–30] Low doses should be used initially and slowly titrated up with monitoring for adverse effects. Similarly, ACE inhibitors and angiotensin receptor blockers have been shown to reduce mortality in younger age groups and seem to be as effective in older populations.[31] ACE inhibitors are usually considered first line and angiotensin receptor blockers used only if the patient is intolerant (e.g. because of dry cough that occurs in 5%–10% of those on ACE inhibitors). Doses should be started low and gradually increased. Careful monitoring is required, particularly looking for hypotension, renal impairment and hyperkalaemia.

Digoxin is sometimes used in the treatment of heart failure on the basis it may provide positive inotropic benefits to cardiac contraction. At doses of 250 mcg per day it has been associated with lower rates of hospitalisation, but no reduction in mortality.[32] The risk of toxicity from digoxin is elevated in the frail elderly (*see* p. 305). It is unlikely that these patients could tolerate such a high dose. It should not be considered usual therapy, but might be appropriate if ACE inhibitors or beta-blockers are not tolerated. Cardiac resynchronisation might be suitable for those with sinus rhythm plus bundle branch block on their ECG.[33] Implantable cardioverter-defibrillators can reduce the risk of sudden death in patients with heart failure plus cardiac arrhythmias.[34]

Secondary prevention strategies typically include antiplatelets, statins and blood pressure control. Those in AF should be considered for anticoagulation and rhythm/rate control (*see* p. 231). Smokers should be advised to stop. Given the poor prognosis it is necessary to consider appropriate palliative care strategies for those with advanced heart failure.

KEY POINTS

- Heart failure affects around 10% of people in their 80s.
- In the elderly it is often due to diastolic failure, which can make echocardiography results misleading.

- A number of commonly used drugs can precipitate heart failure – especially calcium channel blockers and non-steroidal anti-inflammatory drugs.
- Beta-blockers and ACE inhibitors can improve survival in the frail elderly.

CARDIAC ARRHYTHMIAS

Cardiac arrhythmias in the elderly are usually associated with structural abnormalities of the heart, but they can also be provoked by imbalances of electrolytes, especially hypokalaemia and hypomagnesaemia. These disturbances are discussed on page 79. In addition, many drugs can be implicated, including those that prolong the QT interval (*see* Table 5.2) and cholinesterase inhibitors (donepezil, rivastigmine and galantamine). The common clinically significant problems of AF and ventricular tachycardia (VT) are discussed shortly. Cardiac arrhythmias can sometimes present as syncope (*see* p. 133).

Traditionally anti-arrhythmic drugs have been used for tachyarrhythmias and pacemaker insertion recommended for those with bradyarrhythmias. The newer technique of radiofrequency catheter ablation is an alternative approach. It is associated with good outcomes in the treatment of a number of arrhythmias in selected elderly patients.[35]

Atrial fibrillation

AF is more common in older than younger people, affecting less than 2% of those below and 6% of those over the age of 65.[36] Over 80 years of age the prevalence rises to between 7% and 14% of the population. These figures may underestimate the actual prevalence of AF, as non-sustained (paroxysmal) episodes are likely to be missed. Patients with any cardiac abnormality (e.g. previous MI, left ventricular impairment or atrial enlargement) are more likely to develop it. Only 15% of AF occurs in people with structurally normal hearts.[37] AF may be asymptomatic if the heart rate is within the normal range but it may induce shortness of breath and chest pain when tachycardia is present.

Anticoagulation

A major problem with AF is the associated increased risk of stroke due to the formation of emboli with the left atrium. This risk can be reduced significantly with anticoagulant drugs such as warfarin (*see* p. 216).

Rhythm control

Trying to convert the patient back to sinus rhythm is usually not attempted in elderly people who have reasonable rate control and are asymptomatic.

Anti-arrhythmic medications are often ineffective and many have a risk of significant side effects, especially in this patient group. Cardioversion can be used but the risk of AF recurrence is high. Catheter ablation for AF is being more frequently used although appropriate patient selection is important and this may not be appropriate for the frail elderly. A longer duration of AF and the presence of left atrial enlargement make the chances of restoring sinus rhythm less likely. Studies that have compared patients randomly assigned to either attempted sinus rhythm restoration or rate control alone did not find any long-term benefit from the former approach.[38,39] A different approach may be adopted for atrial flutter. This rhythm also confers an increased stroke risk but rate control is often more difficult to achieve than in patients with AF. This rhythm can be cured in the majority of cases with catheter ablation and this option should be explored if the patient is suitable. However, it should be noted that many of these patients develop AF in the future, although this may be easier to manage conservatively.

Rate control

Targeting a pulse rate below 110 beats per minute seems to be at least as effective as tighter rate control.[40] Beta-blockers are the drug of choice as they are effective at controlling heart rate both in those with persistent and paroxysmal AF. They may also be beneficial to those with heart failure that often co-exists in the frail elderly. Sotalol has a wider range of actions on the heart (beta-blocker and class III type) and is associated with a greater pro-arrhythmogenic tendency and so should be avoided in older patients. Amiodarone (class III) is an effective anti-arrhythmic drug but has many potential side effects with long-term use, including thyroid disorders, pulmonary fibrosis, hepatic impairment, polyneuropathy and photosensitivity. It also has many potential drug interactions. Digoxin has many limitations in the frail elderly and is only indicated in a few clinical situations (*see* p. 305). Some calcium channel blockers (e.g. diltiazem) can be used to control heart rate. However, they may impair cardiac function and so are typically less suitable for older patients.

Ventricular tachycardia

VT can be described as sustained (lasting 30 seconds or more) or non-sustained (lasting less than 30 seconds). Sustained VT is likely to present as acute chest pain, breathlessness, syncope or cardiac arrest. Non-sustained VT is common and usually asymptomatic in the elderly, being found on around 4% of 24-hour ECG recordings of those without a history of cardiac disease.[41] Such patients and those with multiple ventricular ectopic beats also without a history of heart disease do not appear to have an increased risk of cardiac events. Starting anti-arrhythmic medication in this situation is not advised. However, patients with episodes of sustained VT or those with underlying heart disease plus non-sustained VT have a better prognosis if treated with anti-arrhythmic drugs.

Beta-blockers are effective in reducing the risk of VT, sudden death (including ventricular fibrillation) and recurrent MI.[41] They are the usual recommended therapy. Sotalol seems no more effective yet has higher risks of adverse effects, including arrhythmias, and is seldom suitable. Amiodarone is effective at reducing VT but is associated with many side effects, as mentioned earlier. It is less suitable for the frail elderly. Class I drugs (e.g. quinidine, lidocaine and flecanide) and calcium channel blockers are neither safe nor effective and should not be used for this purpose.[41] Calcium channel blockers are also less likely to be appropriate in the frail elderly due to a high incidence of left ventricular impairment.

Implantable cardio-defibrillators are effective for terminating life-threatening VT or ventricular fibrillation. They do not reduce the incidence of these rhythms and so are typically used in combination with anti-arrhythmic drugs. Suitable patients include those with episodes of sustained VT or those with non-sustained VT who also have ischaemic heart disease plus left ventricular impairment. However, patient selection is important, as some older individuals have a greater risk of non-arrhythmic death.[42] Other treatment options include coronary revascularisation procedures for those with ischaemia-induced VT and radiofrequency ablation.

AORTIC DISSECTION

Aortic dissection is caused by a tear in the aortic intimal layer, which leads to passage of blood into a false luminal channel between the intima and inner media. The Stanford classification system refers to all dissections affecting the ascending aorta as type A, and those that only affect the descending aorta as type B.

Aortic dissection is a less common cause of chest pain (0.3% of admissions with chest pain), but is frequently misdiagnosed leading to avoidable adverse outcomes.[43] It becomes commoner in older age, particularly in those with a history of hypertension. It also occurs more frequently in people who have had an aortic valve replacement or recent cardiac catheterisation.

The classical presentation is with pain. This is typically localised in the chest or back, of sudden onset, severe and described as 'sharp' or 'tearing' in character. There may be variability in palpated pulse pressures (radial, carotid and femoral) or recorded blood pressures in differing limbs (>20 mmHg). Patients may present with hypotension or shock. The murmur of aortic incompetence (early diastolic) is found in less than a third of patients. It can cause distal organ malperfusion or ischaemia that can lead to other clinical features – for example, focal neurological deficits, renal/hepatic dysfunction or limb ischaemia. Cardiac malperfusion can lead to ECG changes and rises in troponin blood levels. These may all hamper the diagnosis.

A chest X-ray may show evidence of mediastinal widening, but can be normal. A posterior–anterior projection is most useful, but these are often not performed in emergency situations. In addition, other changes in X-rays in older patients (e.g. unfolding of the aorta) may make them harder to interpret. D-dimer levels are usually elevated but this is a non-specific finding. The diagnostic test of choice is CT angiography, but MRI or transoesophageal echocardiography are also useful.

Detected cases should be discussed with a cardiothoracic surgeon. Type A lesions are typically repaired surgically, which changes the prognosis from a 10% survival rate untreated to a 75%–90% survival rate with surgery.[43] A review of surgery for type A dissections in patients aged over 75 years found an in-hospital mortality rate of 13%, compared with 10% for younger cases.[44] This suggests that surgery is still the best management option in selected older patients. Type B lesions are usually managed non-operatively. The in-hospital mortality rate for patients aged over 70 years with a type B dissection has been found to be 16% (compared with 10% for younger cases).[45] Pain should be controlled with analgesia, and hypertension, when present, can be reduced by intravenous beta-blockers.[43]

KEY POINTS

- Cardiac arrhythmias can be provoked by electrolyte disturbances and some medications.
- AF affects around 10% of people aged over 80 years and is associated with an increased risk of stroke.
- Rate control (preferably with beta-blockers) is typically a more effective strategy than trying to restore sinus rhythm in the frail elderly.
- Sustained VT is a serious condition that requires control with drugs (preferably beta-blockers) and possibly an implantable defibrillator, coronary revascularisation or radiofrequency ablation.
- Non-sustained VT is common, typically asymptomatic and requires no treatment in patients without underlying heart disease.
- Aortic dissection is a less common cause of chest pain but is frequently misdiagnosed.
- Type A dissections are usually managed surgically, whereas type B lesions are usually managed non-operatively.

PULMONARY EMBOLISM

Pulmonary embolism (PE) is typically caused by thrombus formation within the leg veins that embolises to the pulmonary vasculature. The elderly have multiple reasons for being at increased risk (*see* Figure 9.1). PE is more common following a period of reduced mobility, including hospitalisation. This emphasises the point that early mobilisation of elderly patients is beneficial. Patients with reduced leg movement following a stroke or lower limb fracture are at particular risk. Hypercoagulability may be more common with advanced age and also some disease states including dehydration and having an underlying cancer. Some medications can also increase the risk. These include strontium ranelate and raloxifene that are sometimes used in the treatment of osteoporosis. The classic symptoms of PE are shortness of breath, pleuritic chest pain and haemoptysis. There may also be signs of deep vein thrombosis in a limb. But a range of clinical manifestations can occur from being asymptomatic to presenting as sudden death.

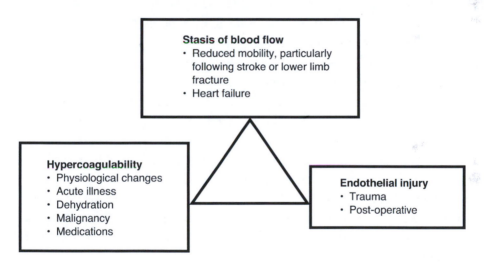

FIGURE 9.1 Typical risk factors for pulmonary embolus seen in elderly patients (based on Virchow's triad)

Comparing older patients (age 65 or over) and younger ones (age <65) with confirmed PE, dyspnoea occurred at a similar frequency (85% vs 76%), but pleuritic chest pain was less common in the older patients (48% vs 79%).[46] There were fewer with haemoptysis (7% vs 21%), but more presenting as syncope (28% vs 10%). Such differences may be more pronounced in the frail elderly. Another study also found similar rates of dyspnoea in those aged 70 and over compared with those aged under 40 (78% vs 82%), but less pleuritic pain (51% vs 70%) and haemoptysis (8% vs 32%).[47] Twenty-eight per cent presented as isolated shortness of breath and 10% presented as either shock or syncope. Tachypnoea (20 breaths per minute or more) was present in 74% and tachycardia (>100 bpm) was present in 29% of the older group. Ninety-four per cent of the old had at least one of dyspnoea, tachypnoea or pleuritic chest pain at presentation.

Findings on ECG recordings are most often non-specific, such as changes in the ST segments or T waves. Around 21% have a normal ECG.[47] The reported 'classic' ECG changes of PE occur infrequently: right axis deviation (7%), right bundle branch block (5%) and '$S_1Q_3T_3$' (5%).[46] Chest X-rays occasionally show an effusion or wedge infarction but typically look unremarkable. D-dimer levels are usually raised, but this is a non-specific finding. A negative d-dimer makes PE less likely. When this is coupled with a low clinical probability, then PE is effectively excluded.[48] Hypoxia is likely to be present on oxygen saturation monitors and arterial blood gas sampling. CT pulmonary angiography (CTPA) has become the diagnostic investigation of choice. Ventilation–perfusion scans may be used in some cases (e.g. severe renal impairment due to the risk of contrast-induced kidney injury with CTPA), but the high prevalence of co-morbidities (e.g. chronic obstructive pulmonary disease (COPD) or heart failure) in the elderly make them harder to interpret reliably.

There should be a high index of suspicion of PE if hypoxia and/or an elevated respiratory rate are present that are not explained by chest X-ray findings. Patients with massive PE (i.e. in shock) aged 75 and over seem to have similar benefits to younger patients when given thrombolysis (approximately a 10% improvement in perfusion lung scanning after 2 days, rising to around 30% at 1–3 weeks).[49] The standard treatment of non-massive PE is subcutaneous low-molecular-weight heparin followed by a period of oral anticoagulation with warfarin. The duration of warfarin therapy may be influenced by the presence of any ongoing risk factors or previous thromboembolic events, but a typical time scale would be 3 months.

KEY POINTS

- Elderly patients who are less mobile during periods of acute illness are at an elevated risk of developing a PE.
- Compared with younger patients, the old are equally likely to report shortness of breath but less likely to complain of pleuritic chest pain or haemoptysis.
- ECG and chest X-ray findings are unreliable. The diagnostic test of choice is CTPA.

CHRONIC OBSTRUCTIVE PULMONARY DISEASE

COPD is a progressive disease of airflow obstruction. It is often accompanied by chronic bronchitis, a disorder of excess mucus production, and emphysema (dilated airways). It is also characterised by acute exacerbations. It is estimated that elderly patients with COPD experience two to three of these per year, each lasting around 12 days.[50] It usually develops secondary to cigarette smoke exposure, but some industrial dusts and alpha 1 antitrypsin deficiency underlie a few cases. Some of the clinical features overlap with those of asthma and these conditions can co-exist.

The prevalence of COPD increases with advancing age. It rises from about 4%–5% of the population aged 60 to a peak around 16% of men and 8% of women in their late 70s.[51] The spirometry definition of COPD is to have a forced expiratory volume in 1 second to forced vital capacity ratio (FEV_1/FVC) of less than 70%. However, changes in the lungs of older people (*see* p. 5) may make this less reliable. Among those who have never smoked, 35% of healthy people aged over 70 years, and 50% of those over 80 have an FEV_1/FVC ratio less than 70%.[52] In those with limited physical capacity an FEV_1/FEV_6 (forced expiratory capacity in 6 seconds) ratio can be used as an alternative reasonable estimate.[50]

Long-term treatment

Patients with COPD usually take treatments to control symptoms outside acute exacerbations. Unfortunately there is little evidence that these have any role in reducing long-term lung function decline.[53] The first line of therapy is inhaled bronchodilators, which act by relaxing smooth muscle in the airway walls.[54] The most commonly used agents are beta-agonists and anticholinergics, often in combination.

Inhaled beta-agonists come in short-acting (e.g. salbutamol) and long-acting forms (e.g. salmeterol). There is some evidence that this latter class can reduce the frequency of acute exacerbations and overall mortality.[54] Potential side effects include tachycardia, the precipitation of cardiac arrhythmias, tremor and hypokalaemia.

Inhaled anticholinergic drugs have few systemic side effects due to poor absorption. They can cause dry mouth and occasionally precipitate urinary retention in men with prostatic enlargement.[54] Tiotropium, which is taken once a day, is the usual preferred agent. A meta-analysis of studies comparing inhaled anticholinergics to placebos or other active drugs associated them with an increased rate of cardiovascular death, MI or stroke (1.8% vs 1.2%; relative risk, 1.58; 95% confidence interval, 1.21–2.06).[55] Therefore these drugs should only be continued in those who have significant symptomatic benefits.

Inhaled steroids have fewer side effects than oral preparations, but oropharyngeal deposition can result in local irritation, candidiasis, and some systemic absorption. A review of trials of inhaled steroids in stable COPD failed to show a survival benefit, and there was an associated increased risk of pneumonia (relative risk, 1.34; 95% confidence interval, 1.03–1.75).[56] But a trial comparing inhaled fluticasone and salmeterol, alone or in combination, with placebo in patients (mean age, 65 years) over a 3-year period did find a reduced number of exacerbations and improved health status and spirometry values in those on the combined treatment.[57] They are usually considered suitable for those with severe disease or recurrent exacerbations.[50]

Inhaled medications may be less effective in the frail elderly because of poor inhaler technique. This can be due to poor timing of actuation and inhalation, impaired cognition or weakness of the hands (e.g. arthritis). The use of dry powder devices is not dependent on timing or muscle strength, but some elderly patients do not generate sufficient inspiratory flow for the medication to reach the lower respiratory tract. In a study of older adults (mean age, 74 years) with COPD, 46% reported finding a metered-dose inhaler difficult to use, but only 17% found a dry powder device difficult to use.[58] Spacer devices can increase intrapulmonary drug delivery, with reduced oropharyngeal deposition, leading to increased efficacy. However, some older adults provided with spacer devices do not use them. A randomised trial of the elderly found a greater frequency of correct use of either breath-actuated aerosol devices or dry powder inhalers than of metered dose inhalers with spacers.[59] Despite this knowledge, older people infrequently have their inhaler technique checked.

Oral theophylline has also been used as a bronchodilator in COPD. Possible side effects include precipitating seizures and cardiac arrhythmias. Toxicity is increased in older adults, even at similar blood levels to younger individuals. It has several important drug interactions (see p. 300). This class of drug is rarely a good option in the frail elderly.[54]

Smoking results in accelerated decline in lung function and increases mucous viscosity, which increases the risk of acute exacerbations. Those who stop smoking have a rate of lung function decline that is half that of continued smokers.[60] Discontinuing smoking is very important, even in older patients, but smoking cessation advice is rarely given to the elderly.[61,62] It is important to consider prescribing nicotine patches to patients while in hospital, to prevent withdrawal symptoms.

Long-term oxygen improves survival and quality of life in advanced COPD plus hypoxia (probably by reducing pulmonary artery pressure and increasing cardiac output). The typical indication is a value for partial pressure of oxygen in arterial blood that is below 8.0 kPa when well. This may be required at the time of hospital discharge. Pulmonary rehabilitation can benefit those with moderate to advanced disease. This is particularly true if there is evidence of de-conditioning, weight loss, depression and social isolation. It can increase muscle mass and exercise tolerance, with reduced breathlessness. The effects in older people seem to be similar to those seen in younger age groups.[63] So referral to such a service should be considered.

Acute exacerbations

Acute exacerbations are associated with worsening of shortness of breath, more sputum production, sputum purulence, increased cough and signs of infection (fever, tachycardia and delirium). They can be due to environmental factors or poor medication concordance, but around 80% are caused by infections with either bacteria (e.g. *Haemophilus influenzae*, *Pseudomonas aeruginosa*, *Streptococcus pneumoniae*, *Moraxella catarrhalis*, *Mycoplasma* species, or *Chlamydia pneumoniae*) or viruses (e.g. rhinoviruses, influenza, or parainfluenza).[64] They may lead to further declines in lung function, loss of independence or death. Expiratory wheeze typically accompanies acute exacerbations, but this can be caused by other conditions, such as heart failure (termed 'cardiac asthma').

A combination of nebulised salbutamol and ipratropium is the standard treatment for acute exacerbations. Oxygen should be administered at a specific concentration via a Venturi mask, typically starting at 28% unless there is severe hypoxia. The concentration given should be judged by measurement of oxygen saturations (aiming for >90%) and blood gas sampling (to detect rising carbon dioxide levels). Antibiotics improve outcomes in patients with at least two of the following: increased shortness of breath, increased sputum production or purulent sputum.[53] The choice of agent will be guided by illness severity and local prescribing guidelines. The use of systemic steroids in acute exacerbations is associated with a reduction in length of hospital stay. Recurrent courses increase the risk of osteoporosis and these patients should be considered for appropriate treatment (*see* p. 165). In those who produce large amounts of viscous sputum, mucolytic agents (e.g. carbocisteine) may be of benefit, but there is no randomised controlled trial evidence of efficacy in acute exacerbations.

During severe exacerbations the use of non-invasive ventilation can help selected patients. Those suitable typically have a rising partial pressure of carbon dioxide and acidosis despite usual initial therapy. It reduces the need for intubation and can cut both mortality and length of stay. It appears to be similarly tolerated and effective in both the elderly and younger adults.[65]

KEY POINTS

- Spirometry has reduced diagnostic ability in the elderly.
- Check the inhaler technique of the frail elderly with COPD, and consider alternative devices or formulations if it is poor.
- Even elderly smokers should be advised to stop.
- Nicotine replacement therapy can prevent withdrawal symptoms while in hospital.
- Non-invasive ventilation can be an effective component of the treatment of severe exacerbations in the old.
- Consider the need for long-term oxygen and pulmonary rehabilitation prior to discharge from hospital.

REFERENCES

1. Boucher J, Racine N, Thanh TH, *et al*. Age-related differences in in-hospital mortality and the use of thrombolytic therapy for acute myocardial infarction. *CMAJ*. 2001; **164**(9): 1285–90.
2. Jokhadar M, Wenger NK. Review of the treatment of acute coronary syndrome in elderly patients. *Clin Interv Aging*. 2009; **4**: 435–44.
3. Alexander KP, Newby LK, Armstrong PW, *et al*. Acute coronary care in the elderly, part II: ST-segment–elevation myocardial infarction. *Circulation*. 2007; **115**(19): 2570–89.
4. Then KL, Rankin JA, Fofonoff DA. Atypical presentation of acute myocardial infarction in 3 age groups. *Heart Lung*. 2001; **30**(4): 285–93.
5. Alexander KP, Newby LK, Cannon CP, *et al*. Acute coronary care in the elderly, part I: non-ST-segment–elevation acute coronary syndromes. *Circulation*. 2007; **115**(19): 2549–69.
6. Han JH, Lindsell CJ, Hornung RW, *et al*. The elder patient with suspected acute coronary syndromes in the emergency department. *Acad Emerg Med*. 2007; **14**(8): 732–9.
7. Stern S, Behar S, Leor J, *et al*. Presenting symptoms, admission electrocardiogram, management, and prognosis in acute coronary syndromes: differences by age. *Am J Geriatr Cardiol*. 2004; **13**(4): 188–96.
8. Grossman SA, Brown DFM, Chang Y, *et al*. Predictors of delay in presentation to the ED in patients with suspected acute coronary syndromes. *Am J Emerg Med*. 2003; **21**(5): 425–8.
9. Coronado BE, Pope JH, Griffith JL, *et al*. Clinical features, triage, and outcome of patients presenting to the ED with suspected acute coronary syndromes but without pain: a multicenter study. *Am J Emerg Med*. 2004; **22**(7): 568–74.
10. Giugliano RP, Camargo CA, Lloyd-Jones DM, *et al*. Elderly patients receive less aggressive medical and invasive management of unstable angina. *Arch Intern Med*. 1998; **158**(10): 1113–20.
11. Rathore SS, Mehta RH, Wang Y, *et al*. Effects of age on the quality of care provided to older patients with acute myocardial infarction. *Am J Med*. 2003; **114**(4): 307–15.
12. Magid DJ, Masoudi FA, Vinson DR, *et al*. Older emergency department patients with acute myocardial infarction receive lower quality of care than younger patients. *Ann Emerg Med*. 2005; **46**(1): 14–21.
13. Schoenenberger AW, Radovanovic D, Stauffer J, *et al*. Age-related differences in the use

of guideline-recommended medical and interventional therapies for acute coronary syndromes: a cohort study. *J Am Geriatr Soc.* 2008; **56**(3): 510–6.

14. Kashima K, Ikeda D, Tanaka H, *et al*. Mid-term mortality of very elderly patients with acute myocardial infarction with or without coronary intervention. *J Cardiol.* 2010; **55**(3): 397–403.

15. De Boer M, Ottervanger JP, Suryapranata H, *et al*. Old age and outcome after primary angioplasty for acute myocardial infarction. *J Am Geriatr Soc.* 2010; **58**(5): 867–72.

16. Ghanta RK, Shekar PS, McGurk S, *et al*. Nonelective cardiac surgery in the elderly: is it justified? *J Thorac Cardiovasc Surg.* 2010; **140**(1): 103–9.

17. Speziale G, Nasso G, Barattoni MC, *et al*. Short-term and long-term results of cardiac surgery in elderly and very elderly patients. *J Thorac Cardiovasc Surg.* 2011; **141**(3): 725–31.

18. Afilalo J, Eisenberg MJ, Morin J, *et al*. Gait speed as an incremental predictor of mortality and major morbidity in elderly patients undergoing cardiac surgery. *J Am Coll Cardiol.* 2010; **56**(20): 1668–76.

19. Kannel WB, Belanger AJ. Epidemiology of heart failure. *Am Heart J.* 1991; **121**(3 Pt. 1): 951–7.

20. Nieminen MS, Harjola V. Definition and epidemiology of acute heart failure syndromes. *Am J Cardiol.* 2005; **96**(6A): 5–10G.

21. Bhatia RS, Tu JV, Lee DS, *et al*. Outcome of heart failure with preserved ejection fraction in a population-based study. *N Engl J Med.* 2006; **355**(3): 260–9.

22. Aurigemma GP, Gaasch WH. Clinical practice: diastolic heart failure. *N Engl J Med.* 2004; **351**(11): 1097–105.

23. Hogg K, Swedberg K, McMurray J. Heart failure with preserved left ventricular systolic function. *J Am Coll Cardiol.* 2004; **43**(3): 317–27.

24. Klarin I, Fastbom J, Wimo A. The use of angiotensin-converting enzyme inhibitors and other drugs with cardiovascular effects by non-demented and demented elderly with a clinical diagnosis of heart failure: a population-based study of the very old. *Eur J Clin Pharmacol.* 2006; **62**(7): 555–62.

25. De Denus S, Pharand C, Williamson DR. Brain natriuretic peptide in the management of heart failure the versatile neurohormone. *Chest.* 2004; **125**(2): 652–68.

26. Gupta R, Kaufman S. Cardiovascular emergencies in the elderly. *Emerg Med Clin North Am.* 2006; **24**(2): 339–70.

27. Pitt B, Zannad F, Remme WJ, *et al*. The effect of spironolactone on morbidity and mortality in patients with severe heart failure. *N Engl J Med.* 1999; **341**(10): 709–17.

28. Dulin BR, Haas SJ, Abraham WT, *et al*. Do elderly systolic heart failure patients benefit from beta blockers to the same extent as the non-elderly? Meta-analysis of >12,000 patients in large-scale clinical trials. *Am J Cardiol.* 2005; **95**(7): 896–8.

29. Flather MD, Shibata MC, Coats AJS, *et al*. Randomized trial to determine the effect of nebivolol on mortality and cardiovascular hospital admission in elderly patients with heart failure (SENIORS). *Eur Heart J.* 2005; **26**(3): 215–25.

30. Kramer JM, Curtis LH, Dupree CS, *et al*. Comparative effectiveness of beta-blockers in elderly patients with heart failure. *Arch Intern Med.* 2008; **168**(22): 2422–8.

31. Mangoni AA, Jackson SHD. The implications of a growing evidence base for drug use in elderly patients. Part 2. ACE inhibitors and angiotensin receptor blockers in heart failure and high cardiovascular risk patients. *Br J Pharmacol.* 2006; **61**(5): 502–12.

32. Digitalis Investigation Group. The effect of digoxin on mortality and morbidity in patients with heart failure. *N Engl J Med.* 1997; **336**(8): 525–33.

33. Cleland JGF, Daubert J, Erdmann E, *et al*. The effect of cardiac resynchronization on morbidity and mortality in heart failure. *N Engl J Med*. 2005; **352**(15): 1539–49.

34. Bardy GH, Lee KL, Mark DB, *et al*. Amiodarone or an implantable cardioverter-defibrillator for congestive heart failure. *N Engl J Med*. 2005; **352**(3): 225–37.

35. Dagres N, Piorkowski C, Kottkamp H, *et al*. Contemporary catheter ablation of arrhythmias in geriatric patients: patient characteristics, distribution of arrhythmias, and outcome. *Europace*. 2007; **9**(7): 477–80.

36. Feinberg WM, Blackshear JL, Laupacis A, *et al*. Prevalence, age distribution, and gender of patients with atrial fibrillation: analysis and implications. *Arch Intern Med*. 1995; **155**(5): 469–73.

37. Peters NS, Schilling RJ, Kanagaratnam P, *et al*. Atrial fibrillation: strategies to control, combat, and cure. *Lancet*. 2002; **359**(9306): 593–603.

38. Page RL. Clinical practice: newly diagnosed atrial fibrillation. *N Engl J Med*. 2004; **351**(23): 2408–16.

39. Roy R, Talajic M, Nattel S, *et al*. Rhythm control versus rate control for atrial fibrillation and heart failure. *N Engl J Med*. 2008; **358**(25): 2667–77.

40. Van Gelder IC, Groenveld HF, Crijns HJ, *et al*. Lenient versus strict rate control in patients with atrial fibrillation. *N Engl J Med*. 2010; **362**(15): 1363–73.

41. Aronow WS. Treatment of ventricular arrhythmias in the elderly. *Cardiol Rev*. 2009; **17**(3): 136–46.

42. Healey JS, Hallstrom AP, Kuck K, *et al*. Role of the implantable defibrillator among elderly patients with a history of life-threatening ventricular arrhythmias. *Eur Heart J*. 2007; **28**(14): 1746–9.

43. Ranasinghe AM, Strong D, Boland B, *et al*. Acute aortic dissection. *BMJ*. 2011; **343**: 317–19.

44. Kawahito K, Adachi H, Yamaguchi A, *et al*. Early and late surgical outcomes of acute type A aortic dissection in patients aged 75 years and older. *Ann Thorac Surg*. 2000; **70**(5): 1455–9.

45. Mehta RH, Bossone E, Evangelista A, *et al*. Acute type B aortic dissection in elderly patients: clinical features, outcomes, and simple risk stratification rule. *Ann Thorac Surg*. 2004; **77**(5): 1622–9.

46. Kokturk N, Oguzulgen IK, Demir N, *et al*. Differences in clinical presentation of pulmonary embolism in older vs younger patients. *Circ J*. 2005; **69**(8): 981–6.

47. Stein PD, Gottschalk A, Saltzman HA, *et al*. Diagnosis of acute pulmonary embolism in the elderly. *J Am Coll Cardiol*. 1991; **18**(6): 1452–7.

48. Lucassen W, Geersing G, Erkens PMG, *et al*. Clinical decision rules for excluding pulmonary embolism: a meta-analysis. *Ann Intern Med*. 2011; **155**(7): 448–60.

49. Gisselbrecht M, Diehl J, Meyer G, *et al*. Clinical presentation and results of thrombolytic therapy in older patients with massive pulmonary embolism: a comparison with nonelderly patients. *J Am Geriatr Soc*. 1996; **44**(2): 189–93.

50. Hanania NA, Sharma G, Sharafkhaneh A. COPD in the elderly patient. *Semin Respir Crit Care Med*. 2010; **31**(5): 596–606.

51. Van Durme YMTA, Verhamme KMC, Stijnen T, *et al*. Prevalence, incidence, and lifetime risk for the development of COPD in the elderly: the Rotterdam Study. *Chest*. 2009; **135**(2): 368–77.

52. Hardie JA, Buist AS, Vollmer WM, *et al*. Risk of over-diagnosis of COPD in asymptomatic elderly never-smokers. *Eur Respir J*. 2002; **20**(5): 1117–22.

53. Hayes D, Meyer KC. Acute exacerbations of chronic bronchitis in elderly patients. *Drugs Aging*. 2007; **24**(7): 555–72.

54. Dzierbia AL, Jelic S. Chronic obstructive pulmonary disease in the elderly: an update on pharmacological management. *Drugs Aging.* 2009; **26**(6): 447–56.
55. Singh S, Loke YK, Furberg CD. Inhaled anticholinergics and risk of major adverse cardio-vascular events in patients with chronic obstructive pulmonary disease: a systematic review and meta-analysis. *JAMA.* 2008; **300**(12): 1439–50.
56. Drummond MB, Dasenbrook EC, Pitz MW, *et al.* Inhaled corticosteroids in patients with stable chronic obstructive pulmonary disease: a systematic review and meta-analysis. *JAMA.* 2008; **300**(20): 2407–16.
57. Calverley PMA, Anderson JA, Celli B, *et al.* Salmeterol and fluticasone propionate and survival in chronic obstructive pulmonary disease. *N Engl J Med.* 2007; **356**(8): 775–89.
58. Jarvis S, Ind PW, Shiner RJ. Inhaled therapy in elderly COPD patients: time for re-evaluation? *Age Ageing.* 2007; **36**(2): 213–18.
59. Jones V, Fernandez C, Diggory P. A comparison of large volume spacer, breath-activated and dry powder inhalers in older people. *Age Ageing.* 1999; **28**(5): 481–4.
60. Scanlon PD, Waller LA, Altose MD, *et al.* Smoking cessation and lung function in mild-to-moderate chronic obstructive pulmonary disease. The Lung Health Study. *Am J Respir Crit Care Med.* 2000; **161**(2 Pt. 1): 381–90.
61. Ruse CE, Molyneux AWP. A study of the management of COPD according to established guidelines and the implications for older patients. *Age Ageing.* 2006; **34**(3): 299–301.
62. Gellert C, Schottker B, Brenner H. Smoking and all-cause mortality in older people: systematic review and meta-analysis. *Arch Intern Med.* 2012; **172**(11): 837–44.
63. Katsura H, Kanemaru A, Yamada K, *et al.* Long-term effectiveness of an inpatient pulmonary rehabilitation program for elderly COPD patients: comparison between young-elderly and old-elderly groups. *Respirology.* 2004; **9**(2): 230–6.
64. Sethi S. Infectious etiology of acute exacerbations of chronic bronchitis. *Chest.* 2000; **117**(5 Suppl. 2): 380–5S.
65. Balami JS, Packham SM, Gosney MA. Non-invasive ventilation for respiratory failure due to acute exacerbations of chronic obstructive pulmonary disease in older patients. *Age Ageing.* 2006; **35**(1): 75–9.

CHAPTER 10

Other presentations

This section contains a range of conditions and syndromes that commonly present acutely to medical services in the elderly. Each has its own spectrum of traditional clinical features but, of course, a non-specific or covert presentation is also possible in the frail. The topics covered are:

➤ dizziness
➤ acute gastrointestinal (GI) haemorrhage
➤ Parkinson's disease (PD)
➤ depression
➤ diabetes
➤ headache
➤ acute back pain
➤ acute joint inflammation
➤ elder abuse
➤ palliative care.

DIZZINESS

Dizziness is a vague term that can cover a number of clinical presentations and diagnoses. It is important to distinguish between vertiginous (a sensation of movement of the patient or their surroundings) and non-vertiginous varieties. Non-vertigo symptoms include light-headedness (presyncope or wooziness) and disequilibrium (imbalance or unsteadiness) sensations. But some patients will describe a combination of these symptoms and some will describe symptoms that are hard to classify.

In a community-based population of older adults, the complaint of any form of dizziness was reported by 33% of patients aged 70, rising to 51% of patients aged 90 years.[1] Symptoms occurring on a daily frequency were reported by 5% of those aged 70, rising to 25% of those aged 90 years. In a study of elderly patients in primary care who reported dizziness for at least 2 weeks, presyncope was judged to be the commonest type of dizziness affecting 69% of patients, but 44% had more than one subtype.[2] Vertigo was present in 41%, dysequilibrium in 40% and a small number of cases were deemed unclassifiable. Another study recruiting unselected dizzy older patients found light-headedness or unsteadiness to be reported by around two-thirds with only one-third describing vertigo.[3] When dizzy patients were subjected to both specialist ear, nose and throat and neurocardiovascular assessments, 28% were diagnosed with a cardiovascular condition compared to 18% diagnosed with a peripheral vestibular disorder.[4]

The maintenance of balance is dependent on a complex array of sensory and motor systems (*see* Figure 10.1). In the elderly there may be an impairment of multiple systems all contributing to the complaint of dizziness (e.g. age-related macular degeneration, degenerative changes in the inner ear and peripheral neuropathy).

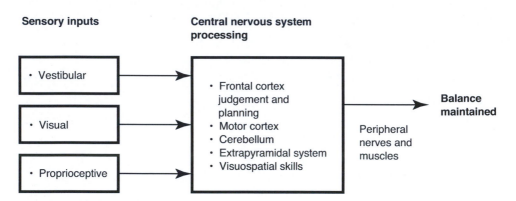

FIGURE 10.1 The interplay between different sensory and motor systems in the maintenance of balance

Vertigo

With vertigo, patients typically complain of a sensation of rotation of their surroundings. It is caused by problems that affect the inner ear, eighth cranial nerve, vestibular nuclei or the cerebellum. Lesions of the inner ear or eighth cranial nerve are termed peripheral causes, whereas lesions of the vestibular nuclei or cerebellum are termed central causes. Table 10.1 shows clinical features that can help distinguish between these groups of causes.

TABLE 10.1 Typical clinical features that can distinguish between peripheral and central causes of vertigo

	Peripheral cause	Central cause
Nystagmus	Horizontal – fast phase away from affected side	Horizontal – fast phase towards affected side
	Unidirectional	May be multidirectional or have vertical and rotatory components
	Reduced by optic fixation	
Nausea or vomiting	More severe	Less severe
Effect of head movement	Symptoms increased	No change
Imbalance	Less severe	More severe
Auditory symptoms	Common	Uncommon
Other neurological signs	No	Likely
Head thrust test	Positive	Negative

Peripheral vertigo

With a peripheral cause of vertigo patients are more likely to have marked nausea and vomiting, symptoms may be worse in certain head positions, and auditory symptoms (deafness, tinnitus and a feeling of fullness in the ear) are more likely. A positive 'head thrust test' (also called the 'head impulse test') result suggests a peripheral cause. In this test the patient's head is moved quickly to one side while the patient tries to maintain their gaze on a fixed object. In a positive test the patient's eyes have to make a corrective saccade (sensitivity around 63%, specificity 93%).[5] The value and safety of this test in the frail elderly is unknown and so we do not recommend its routine use. Occasionally, ototoxic drugs such as gentamicin can precipitate vertigo.

Benign paroxysmal position vertigo (BPPV) is caused by debris within the semicircular canals of the labyrinthine structures, which inappropriately activate the sensory cells. Typically, this causes brief episodes of vertigo (seconds) provoked by positional change such as rolling over in bed. It can be diagnosed by the Hallpike test.

Ménière's disease is a poorly understood degenerative disorder of the inner ear. The vertigo lasts minutes to days. It is associated with hearing loss, tinnitus and a sensation of aural fullness. There is likely to be a history of recurrent attacks over several years.

Vestibular neuritis is thought to be caused by a viral infection of the vestibular pathway. It results in continual vertigo lasting hours to days, with spontaneous gradual resolution. There may be preceding symptoms consistent with a viral illness. Sometimes it is associated with reduced hearing.

Central vertigo

Vertigo of a central cause is typically associated with other neurological signs (e.g. ataxia, ipsilateral Horner's syndrome, facial weakness, unilateral deafness, diplopia, dysphagia or dysarthria). Nystagmus that is vertical or in all directions of gaze and not resolving on optical fixation suggests a central cause. When related to cerebellar pathology there are likely to be other signs of cerebellar dysfunction (e.g. dysarthria, nystagmus, incoordination and ataxic gait).

The most important central cause of vertigo is cerebrovascular disease. A study found that 10% of cerebellar strokes confirmed by MRI findings presented as isolated vertigo.[6] On examination all cases were found to have nystagmus (spontaneous or gaze-evoked) and most had an unsteady gait. Of patients aged over 44 years (mean age, 69 years) presenting to an emergency department (ED) with dizziness (including vertigo and imbalance), 3.2% were diagnosed as having had a stroke, over 80% of these patients had other symptoms (e.g. weakness, sensory loss, speech or visual symptoms).[7] Just 0.5% of patients presenting with dizziness in isolation were diagnosed as having had a stroke. Symptoms typically last for several hours to days. Stroke in the elderly is usually associated with vascular risk factors.

Vertigo can also be associated with a form of migraine (termed 'migrainous vertigo' or 'vestibular migraine'). Typically, it gradually worsens over a 5-minute period and then resolves within an hour. There is usually the characteristic severe throbbing headache of migraine following the vertigo. There may be predictable trigger factors such as fatigue, stress or certain foods.

Management

The management of vertigo depends on the underlying cause. BPPV can be treated by the Epley manoeuvre, which is a specific series of movements aimed at getting the causative debris out of the inner ear. Relevant patients should be referred to an ear, nose and throat service for consideration for this procedure. Histamine receptor antagonists that cross the blood–brain barrier (e.g. cyclizine (acting at H_1 receptors) and betahistine (H_3)) have a role in the short-term management of some cases of peripheral vertigo but prolonged use should be avoided.[8] Some of these drugs can have anticholinergic side effects including sedation, confusion and dizziness. Patients with central vertigo should be managed according to the underlying cause.

Light-headedness

Light-headedness can also be described as wooziness or presyncope. It is usually caused by a transient global reduction in cerebral blood flow. This is due to neurocardiovascular (e.g. orthostatic hypotension (OH)) or cardiac (e.g. arrhythmia) conditions. When episodes are more severe or prolonged this can lead to syncope. The causes and management of these conditions are discussed on page 132.

Atherosclerotic disease affecting the vertebrobasilar arteries can make this more likely to occur. This can provoke multiple similar transient ischaemic attack-like episodes.[9] These events can be triggered by anything that further reduces cerebral blood flow, such as orthostatic hypotension on standing. They may also be provoked at rest by posterior circulation emboli or by cardiac dysrhythmias. The most common complaints caused are light-headedness, blurred vision, and ataxia which is usually short-lived.[10] Patients presenting with these symptoms who have risk factors for vascular disease should be considered for secondary prevention measures such as antiplatelet and statin therapy (*see* p. 215).

Dysequilibrium

Dysequilibrium is a sensation of reduced balance and unsteadiness on walking. It has multiple potential causes – examples are outlined here.

➤ Gait and balance disorders:
  − brain pathology – ischaemia, degeneration (e.g. PD)
  − musculoskeletal (e.g. osteoarthritis)
➤ Sensory loss:
  − hearing, vision, peripheral neuropathy
➤ Medications:
  − for example, opiates, psychotropics and anti-epileptics.

Just as light-headedness can be viewed as the precursor to syncope, disequilibrium can be viewed as the precursor to non-syncopal falls. The underlying causes are similar and so the patient evaluation should also be much the same (*see* p. 125).

Non-specific dizziness

Non-specific dizziness (or 'chronic subjective dizziness') is a term for the group of symptoms for which a diagnosis is difficult to achieve. The described symptoms may be vague, such as 'muzziness', and hard to classify. Hypoglycaemia, following head trauma, and psychiatric disorders (including anxiety and depression) may present with this symptom. Typically, patients do not have vertigo but are hypersensitive to movement and feel off-balance when walking. In the frail elderly it may be associated with widespread small vessel cerebrovascular changes seen on brain imaging.

- Dizziness is a vague term – try to classify as vertigo, light-headedness or disequilibrium sensations.
- Peripheral and central causes of vertigo can usually be distinguished by clinical features.
- Common peripheral causes of vertigo are BPPV, Ménière's disease and vestibular neuritis.
- The most important central cause is cerebrovascular disease.
- Light-headedness should be considered a milder form of syncope and investigated and treated in a similar way.
- Disequilibrium should be viewed as the precursor to non-syncopal falls and investigated and treated in a similar way.
- Some patients will describe combinations of symptoms and some will describe symptoms that are hard to classify.

ACUTE GASTROINTESTINAL HAEMORRHAGE

Upper gastrointestinal tract bleeding

Upper GI bleeding typically presents as melaena, vomiting bright red blood (haematemesis) or partially digested blood (termed 'coffee grounds'), or a mixture of these. Occasionally it can present as orthostatic hypotension or syncope in the absence of overt blood loss. There may be associated symptoms such as dyspepsia, but older patients are more likely to be asymptomatic prior to an upper GI bleed. In a series of patients with peptic ulcers found on endoscopy, pain was not reported by 29% of those aged over 60, compared with 7% of those aged <50 years.[11]

It is more common in elders because of higher rates of non-steroidal anti-inflammatory drug (NSAID) use (including aspirin), *Helicobacter pylori* infections and a higher prevalence of gastro-oesophageal reflux disease, which can lead to erosive oesophagitis. Selective serotonin reuptake inhibitors (SSRIs), bisphosphonates and corticosteroids can also all increase the risk of upper GI bleeding. The severity of bleeding is likely to be worse if on anticoagulant or antiplatelet medications.

History should include enquiring about alcohol intake and prior hepatic disease. Examination should include assessment for signs of chronic liver disease. These factors may give clues to underlying hepatic cirrhosis and raise the suspicion of a bleed from oesophageal or gastric varices. The pulse and blood pressure should be checked. A postural drop in blood pressure can be caused by significant blood loss. Blood tests should include looking for anaemia and an elevated urea (a sign of dehydration or digestion of blood in the gut).

Management begins with appropriate fluid resuscitation. Once stabilised, an upper GI endoscopy should be performed in the majority of patients as soon as possible.

Occasionally very frail or cognitively impaired patients may be unable to safely undergo endoscopy. In other situations the urgency of endoscopy can be guided by the risk of re-bleeding, which can in turn be estimated by the Glasgow–Blatchford bleeding score or pre-endoscopy Rockall score (*see* Table 10.2). The Glasgow–Blatchford bleeding score is calculated by adding the scores for blood parameters (urea and haemoglobin levels), clinical features (blood pressure, pulse, presentation with malaena or syncope) and additional marks if hepatic disease or cardiac failure co-exist.[12] A pre-endoscopy Rockall score of zero suggests a low risk of re-bleeding. As our patients will at least score points for old age, an urgent endoscopy is typically appropriate. Patients with suspected variceal bleeding require urgent endoscopy.

TABLE 10.2 The Rockall score pre-endoscopy (calculated by adding the numbers for age, vital signs and co-morbidity together – total score 0–7)

Clinical feature	Rockall score			
	0	1	2	3
Age (years)	<60	60–79	80+	
Vital signs	Normal	Pulse >100	Systolic BP <100	
Co-morbidity	Nil major		Major co-morbidity (e.g. heart failure or ischaemic heart disease)	Renal or liver failure, metastatic cancer

Abbreviation: BP = blood pressure

Studies have found the commonest causes of upper GI bleeding in the elderly to be peptic ulcers (42%–73%), gastritis (7%–28%), oesophagitis or oesophageal ulcers (7%–18%), oesophageal or gastric varices (2%–11%), Mallory–Weiss tears (2%–4%) and upper GI malignancies (1%–4%).[13] However, there may be some difference between the 'young' old and the oldest old. Compared with people aged 65–74, people aged 75 and over have been found to be more likely to present with mental status change but less likely to report dizziness, and NSAID use was less commonly associated (16% vs 35%).[14] The younger group were more likely to have a duodenal (28% vs 9%) or gastric (49% vs 25%) ulcer on endoscopy, with gastritis (21%), oesophagitis (30%) and normal endoscopy (27%) found more commonly in the older group.

Peptic ulceration may be amenable to endoscopic intervention (e.g. epine-phrine injection or vessel clipping). Following the procedure patients should be prescribed a proton pump inhibitor (PPI) drug. The patient should be tested for the presence of *H. pylori* infection – this is usually done by using a rapid urease test on a biopsy sample taken during endoscopy. Those with a positive result should have *H. pylori* eradication – typically, a combination of a PPI plus clarithromycin and amoxicillin (or metronidazole if penicillin allergic) for 1 week. Patients with re-bleeding may require surgical intervention. Bleeding peptic ulcers carry a worse mortality risk in the elderly. A study found a 30-day mortality rate around 10% for patients aged 65–79, which rose to 17% for people aged over 80, compared with just 4% for those 64 and below.[15] Gastritis and oesophagitis is managed with PPI drugs plus avoidance of potential precipitants (e.g. NSAIDs). Stress-related gastric mucosal injury can occur during the time of any severe illness.

A variceal bleed should be suspected in cases where there are signs of chronic liver disease, known hepatic cirrhosis or a history of previous variceal bleeding. These patients should be given an intravenous (iv) antidiuretic hormone (e.g. terlipressin) or somatostatin analogue (e.g. octreotide) to reduce splanchnic blood flow. An upper GI endoscopy should be urgently arranged. Endoscopic treatment typically involves banding of the varices. Long-term beta-blocker medication can reduce the risk of future bleeding.

Lower gastrointestinal tract bleeding

Lower GI bleeding is more common in older people. In Western countries it is most commonly due to diverticular disease (*see* p. 157).[16] Other frequent causes include colonic angiodysplasia, tumours, haemorrhoids, inflammatory bowel disease and ischaemic colitis (*see* p. 158). The typical presenting symptom is the reporting of passing bright red blood per rectum (termed 'haematochezia'), but bleeding into the right colon can occasionally present as melaena.[16]

Bleeding from diverticular disease is usually painless and settles spontane-ously.[17] Colonic angiodysplasia is caused by degeneration of blood vessels. The bleeding is often occult, presenting as iron deficient anaemia, but can cause hae-matochezia in some individuals. Although inflammatory bowel disease usually presents in younger people, around 15% of cases develop their first symptoms after the age of 65.[18] Massive bleeding can be caused by bowel neoplasia if there is invasion into a blood vessel. There may be an associated history of change in bowel habit and weight loss. Haemorrhoids typically cause recurrent small volume bleeds associated with passing stools. Lower GI bleeding can follow polypectomy or post-irradiation colitis (typically after treatment for prostate, genitourinary or gynaecological malignancies). It can also be associated with infectious diarrhoea caused by campylobacter, salmonella, shigella or *Escherichia coli* food poisoning. Nicorandil can cause intestinal ulceration and rectal bleeding.

The usual investigation of choice is colonoscopy, which also offers an opportunity to control the bleeding by methods such as thermal coagulation, clipping or the injection of sclerosing agents. If the bleeding cannot be controlled, then surgical intervention may be required.

KEY POINTS

- Upper GI bleeding is more common in elders due to higher rates of NSAID use, *H. pylori* infections and a higher prevalence of gastro-oesophageal reflux disease.
- SSRIs, bisphosphonates and corticosteroids can also all increase the risk of upper GI bleeding.
- Patients with a history of excess alcohol intake, prior hepatic disease or signs of chronic liver disease on examination should be suspected of having a variceal bleed – they should be commenced on a drug to reduce splanchnic blood flow (e.g. terlipressin).
- Assessment tools such as the Rockall score can help judge the urgency of endoscopy in non-variceal bleeding.
- The commonest causes of upper GI bleeding in the elderly are peptic ulcers, gastritis, oesophagitis and oesophageal ulcers.
- Lower GI bleeding in Western countries is most commonly due to diverticular disease. The investigation of choice is colonoscopy.

PARKINSON'S DISEASE

PD is a progressive neurodegenerative condition resulting from the death of dopamine-producing cells mainly in the substantia nigra (within the basal ganglia). It is increasingly common with advancing age with a prevalence of around 2%–3% in those aged 75 years and over.[19] It can cause both motor (including falls and immobility) and non-motor symptoms (e.g. confusion, depression and pain). It is also associated with other co-morbidities, which can all result in hospital admission. Idiopathic PD is distinct from other conditions that can cause a Parkinsonian syndrome or Parkinsonism (*see* Table 10.3). Unfortunately, there is no completely reliable test to diagnose PD.[20] The following clinical criteria are used in making a diagnosis:

➤ bradykinesia (slow movements) is essential, plus a least one of . . .
  – rigidity – increased tone, typically 'lead pipe' plus 'cog-wheeling'

— tremor – at rest, characteristically 'pill-rolling'
— postural instability – reduced ability to maintain balance following a
  backwards jerk of the shoulders.

TABLE 10.3 Conditions other than idiopathic Parkinson's disease that can cause
Parkinsonism in the elderly

Condition	Comments
Vascular Parkinsonism	Due to accumulated damage from multiple subcortical infarcts
	Patients tend not to have tremor but do have increased leg tone and a Parkinsonian gait ('lower body Parkinsonism')
	Often associated with cognitive impairment and vascular risk factors
	Vascular lesions are seen on brain imaging
Drug-induced Parkinsonism	Due to use of antidopamine medications (e.g. antipsychotics, prochlorperazine or metoclopramide)
	May not improve on drug withdrawal if use has been over a long time period
Dementia with Lewy bodies	Parkinsonism plus fluctuating cognitive impairment and visual hallucinations
	Patients tend to be very sensitive to antidopamine medication (*see* also p. 116)
Progressive supranuclear palsy	Parkinsonism plus cognitive impairment, early falls, and impaired up and down gaze
	Patients may develop dysarthria and dysphagia
Multiple system atrophy	Parkinsonism plus any of autonomic neuropathy, cerebellar signs or pyramidal tract signs
	Autonomic neuropathy can present with orthostatic hypotension, urinary incontinence or impotence
	Patients often develop dysarthria, dysphagia or stridor

The assessment of bradykinesia is outlined on page 47. PD typically affects gait, initially causing reduced arm swing but progressing to small steps and shuffling. In more advanced disease a 'festinating' pattern may be seen – starting slowly but gradually increasing speed. Patients with idiopathic PD usually have a slowly progressive condition that starts unilaterally. Occasionally, essential tremor can be mistaken for PD (*see* Table 2.1). Getting an accurate diagnosis aids management. PD patients are more likely to respond well to dopaminergic medication and suffer problems if it is discontinued abruptly. Falls and cognitive impairment in the first year after diagnosis make other causes of Parkinsonism more likely. The multiple pathologies and polypharmacy of old age magnify the disability and handicap of PD and make old people more prone to complications. The key treatments used in PD are shown in Table 10.4. Levodopa has only a short duration of action and needs to be given at specific times through the day. Check with the patient when they take their medication and prescribe it accurately. Advanced PD is associated with complex motor symptoms (i.e. dyskinesias, gait freezing and 'on-off' phenomena).

TABLE 10.4 Commonly used medications for the management of Parkinson's disease (PD)

Drug	Mechanism of action	Comments
Levodopa	Converted to dopamine within the brain (dopamine does not cross the blood–brain barrier) Given with a peripheral decarboxylase inhibitor (as co-beneldopa or co-careldopa) to limit side effects	Best available medication but can induce dyskinesias after prolonged use Available in standard-release (given three to five times a day), dispersible and slow-release formulations This latter version is typically used to combat symptoms overnight Dispersible forms have a rapid onset of action and can help get PD patients going in the morning They may also be helpful for those with a poor swallow
Entacapone	A peripherally acting COMT inhibitor that blocks the breakdown of levodopa	Needs to be used in conjunction with levodopa Can cause an orange discolouration of urine and occasionally diarrhoea Preparations combining levodopa, a decarboxylase inhibitor and entacapone are available
Dopamine agonists	Direct action at post-synaptic dopamine receptors	Key potential side effects are somnolence, hallucinations and leg oedema Non-ergot drugs (e.g. ropinirole and pramipexole) are preferred Rotigotine can be given as a transdermal patch Apomorphine is usually given by sub-cutaneous injection
MAOIs	MAOIs (type B) block the breakdown of dopamine within the brain	Could provoke the serotonin syndrome (especially if used with antidepressants) Selegiline is also available in a form that dissolves on the tongue, which may be suitable for those with an impaired swallow
Amantadine	NMDA receptor blocking action within the brain	Typically used to treat dyskinesias in advanced PD Side effects include confusion, hallucinations and leg oedema
Anticholinergics	Reduce anticholinergic activity within the brain	Associated with many side effects (*see* p. 302) and very rarely appropriate for use in the frail elderly

Abbreviations: COMT = catechol-O-methyltransferase, MAOIs = monoamine oxidase inhibitors, NMDA = N-methyl-D-aspartate

Acute presentations

Patients with PD are very likely to be admitted to acute hospitals, either because of the disease itself or due to its many complications.[21] They often do badly in hospital where they may be looked after by non-specialists. This is particularly true if their condition is not recognised, they do not receive their usual medication on time, and any complications are not anticipated and treated correctly. Patients with PD are prone to infections (especially pneumonia and urinary tract infections (UTIs)), falls, swallowing problems, delirium and dementia.[21,22] Rarely, they may also develop life-threatening complications such as neuroleptic malignant-like syndrome (NMLS).

Motor symptoms

Older patients with PD are more troubled with gait and balance problems leading to falls and immobility. Dyskinesias and severe motor fluctuations, apart from 'end of dose' deterioration are less commonly seen in older patients. Occasionally, however, dyskinesias may precipitate hospital admission and take the form of chorea (jerking), athetosis (writhing) or myoclonus (twitching). This may be precipitated by medication changes and intercurrent illness. Dyskinesias may even sometimes be misdiagnosed as severe tremors, or even seizures. Management is to treat the intercurrent illness and careful adjustment (reduction) of the levodopa medication, preferably under the guidance of a specialised doctor or nurse. End-of-dose deterioration may respond to the fractionation of levodopa into smaller, more frequent doses or the addition of another agent (such as entacapone), or a dopamine agonist (such as ropinirole or pramipexole). Unfortunately, none of the many medications for PD seem to help with balance problems and for this a multidisciplinary approach with the help of a physiotherapist and occupational therapist is most useful. The provision of walking aids may also be beneficial. Wheeled frames tend to help patients with PD maintain gait rhythm more than those without wheels. Sticks can be unhelpful, as PD patients tend to have reduced arm swing.

Autonomic symptoms

Autonomic function, involving both the sympathetic and parasympathetic systems, is often impaired in PD. Disabling symptoms that can result in admission to hospital include light-headedness and syncope due to OH or arrhythmias, bladder problems and constipation. Ageing, with its decline in autonomic function and multiple pathology and polypharmacy, is an additional factor leading to symptoms.[23] Although autonomic dysfunction is common in PD, severe symptoms within 2 years of diagnosis (e.g. severe postural hypotension) should raise the suspicion of multiple system atrophy.

OH is defined as a fall in blood pressure of 20 mmHg or more systolic, or 10 mmHg or more diastolic, from lying to standing. In PD patients it is often secondary to autonomic failure and side effects of drugs. It is found in around 50% of PD patients who are ill.[24] The management of OH in PD is similar to that in other patients (*see* p. 135). In addition it should be considered whether possible to reduce incriminating anti-Parkinsonian drugs such as levodopa. Domperidone may help with drug-induced OH.

Bladder problems occur in up to 75% of people with PD.[20] Nocturia, daytime urgency and frequency are common. The mechanism is usually detrusor over-activity, but an atonic bladder with urinary retention and overflow should also be considered. A UTI should be excluded (unlikely if symptoms for more than a week). Management can include bladder retraining (*see* p. 88). Anticholinergic drugs may help, but they should be used with caution in patients with PD because of the risk of adverse effects such as delirium.

Constipation is common in PD. Faecal incontinence may occur due to faecal impaction. Patients should be encouraged to keep their fluid intake up (e.g. eight glasses of water per day) and regular laxatives may be required. Abdominal pain and subacute bowel pseudo-obstruction due to colonic dysmotility are a frequent reason for patients with PD to be admitted to surgical wards (*see* p. 156).

Falls in Parkinson's disease

Falls are common in PD, with two-thirds of patients falling per year.[25] Causes include poor PD control with medication, postural instability and OH. Falls in PD can result in significant morbidity and mortality or in loss of confidence, a loss of mobility and increased dependence. They require a multidisciplinary assessment and rehabilitation plan similar to that for falls in other older people (*see* Chapter 5). Early onset of falls in patients with PD may indicate an alternative diagnosis, such as progressive supranuclear palsy.[26]

Swallowing problems

Swallowing dysfunction occurs from the earliest stages of PD.[27] All phases of swallowing can be affected (oral, pharyngeal and oesophageal).[22] Dysphagia in PD results from catecholamine degeneration and Lewy body formation within the brain stem and within pharyngeal muscles, and unfortunately does not always respond to levodopa.[27] It can also be precipitated by acute illness, which can lead to aspiration pneumonia.[28] Dysphagia can lead to a reduced ability to take PD medications, which may further worsen swallowing. This acute withdrawal of dopaminergic drugs could trigger NMLS (*see* p. 259).[29]

A reduced oral intake can also cause problems around the time of surgical operations.[30] For elective procedures the advice of a specialist PD team should be sought in advance. When delayed gastric emptying or an ileus is likely to occur post-operatively it is more appropriate to temporarily switch to transdermal or subcutaneous medication formulations.

Swallowing assessment is very important as silent aspiration can result in recurrent chest infections and multiple hospital admissions. When a problem is detected, early referral to a speech and language therapist is appropriate. They may do additional assessments and advise the patient on techniques to improve swallowing.[28] It is very important that patients with PD continue their usual medication regimen when they are admitted to hospital to optimise function (including swallowing). If they are not able to reliably take their usual medication for any reason (e.g. dysphagia or impaired consciousness) then they can be switched to an equivalent dose of levodopa, which can be given as a dispersible preparation, or via a nasogastric tube. Equivalent doses are given in Table 10.5. If a nasogastric tube is not possible then an alternative is a dopamine agonist transdermal patch (rotigotine) or a subcutaneous apomorphine infusion. Advice from a specialist should be obtained as soon as possible.

TABLE 10.5 Approximate equivalent levodopa daily doses[30]

Drug	Adjustment
Levodopa	None
Levodopa controlled release	Dose in milligrams × 0.7
Levodopa + COMT inhibitor	Dose in milligrams × 1.3
Pergolide	Dose in milligrams × 100
Lisuride	
Pramipexole (base)	
Carbergoline	
Ropinirole	Dose in milligrams × 20
Rotigotine	
Bromocriptine	Dose in milligrams × 10
Apomorphine	

Abbreviation: COMT = catechol-O-methyltransferase

Psychotic symptoms

Psychotic symptoms affect up to 40% of patients with PD, often leading to hospital admission.[31] Visual hallucinations are the most common, but auditory hallucinations and paranoid delusions may also occur.[32] Hallucinations and dementia are two major risk factors for patients with PD ending up in a nursing home.[33] The aetiology of psychotic symptoms is complex and requires careful evaluation. They may arise as part of the neurotransmitter disturbance of PD, but can also be caused by any of the drugs used to treat motor symptoms, or they may arise as part of delirium, which is common in PD. The management is the same as that for other delirium – search for and treat any underlying infective or metabolic causes while maintaining a supportive rehabilitative environment (*see* p. 112).[34] Delirium in PD differs from the usual delirium in older people in that medication is much more likely to be a contributory cause.

If PD medication is thought to be the cause then the usual practice is to stop the last medication prescribed before the symptoms arose ('last in, first out' approach). Otherwise, the recommended order for stopping medications is anticholinergic, monoamine oxidase inhibitor, amantadine, dopamine agonist, entacapone and then levodopa.[35] However, this may be at the cost of worsening motor symptoms. Antipsychotics, especially haloperidol, should be avoided because of the extra-pyramidal side effects and the prognosis is considerably worse in terms of mortality and progressing to dementia.[36] A safer option may be to use benzodiazepines, such as lorazepam. As a last resort, quetiapine (which is an antipsychotic with less extra-pyramidal side effects) may be used, but starting at very low doses and being alert for any adverse reaction.[37] Finally, cholinesterase inhibitors, such as rivastigmine, may be of benefit in patients with co-existent dementia,[38] but should only be prescribed under specialist supervision, can worsen motor symptoms and may take several weeks to be effective.

Neuroleptic malignant-like syndrome

NMLS is fortunately a rare complication of PD, but it can be life-threatening, especially if not recognised promptly. It is usually due to withdrawal of dopaminergic drugs, but it has also been reported upon sudden withdrawal of non-dopaminergic drugs, including amantadine and anticholinergics.[39,40] Because of possible deterioration of motor function and the risk of NMLS, it is essential that patients with PD do not have their medication inadvertently delayed, or even discontinued, on admission to hospital. This can happen all too easily in a busy admission unit and can be prevented by writing up the initial doses as a stat prescription and also making sure PD drugs are easily available on admission wards at short notice. NMLS is clinically indistinguishable from neuroleptic malignant syndrome (*see* p. 303), which is due to an idiosyncratic reaction to antipsychotic medication and which may also occur in PD.[41] Patients with NMLS present with fever, rigidity and decreased level of consciousness.

This may lead to rhabdomyolysis (*see* p. 73), aspiration pneumonia and thromboembolism. The mortality is high (around 20%). The main differential diagnosis is neuroleptic malignant syndrome, heat stroke, severe infection, serotonin syndrome (*see* next section) and toxicity due to other drugs.[39] The key to management is early recognition, dopaminergic replacement (either by levodopa orally or via nasogastric tube, or by a subcutaneous apomorphine infusion) and supportive treatment with iv fluids and fever reduction.

Serotonin syndrome

The serotonin syndrome is a toxic reaction to pro-serotinergic agents. Clinical features range from mild cases of tremor, tachycardia and diarrhoea to severe cases of potentially fatal neuromuscular rigidity, clonus, hyperthermia, hyper- or hypotension and delirium.[42] It can lead to rhabdomyolysis, acidosis and disseminated intravascular coagulation. Causative agents include all antidepressants, but especially SSRIs and monoamine oxidase inhibitors (which can also be used in the treatment of PD). Some other drugs, such as tramadol, have pro-serotinergic activity. It is more likely to occur with combinations of these serotinergic drugs possibly in the presence of agents that block their hepatic degradation, such as erythromycin or sodium valproate. Appropriate management is to discontinue the causative agent(s), and give iv fluids and benzodiazepines. Severe cases may need ventilation, and iv beta-blockers can be used to control hypertension and tachycardia.

KEY POINTS

- Ascertain the exact diagnosis – for example, idiopathic PD with a good response to levodopa or a form of Parkinsonism.
- PD does not only cause motor symptoms – common non-motor problems include confusion, depression and pain.
- Look for intercurrent infection (e.g. chest, urinary) as a cause of functional decline.
- Ensure essential medication is administered at correct times – for example, write up stat doses and consider nasogastric tube insertion. Acute withdrawal of medication can have disastrous consequences. Symptom control can be tricky in the perioperative period.
- Check cognition and consider delirium.
- Check the safety of swallowing.
- Avoid antipsychotics, especially haloperidol and other drugs that have extrapyramidal side effects (e.g. metoclopramide and prochlorperazine).

- Encourage mobility and independence of patients with PD – refer to physiotherapy and occupational therapy.
- Discuss progress with family and carers – they may be able to supply information about previous mobility and medication regimen.
- Plan discharge well in advance in conjunction with multidisciplinary team members.
- Ask for specialist advice early (e.g. specialist nurse or consultant).

DEPRESSION

The term depression encompasses a range of clinical syndromes from minor mood disorders to major depression. The prevalence of major depression among people aged over 75 in the community is estimated to be around 5%–9%, and is higher in those with chronic co-morbid disease.[43] Its detection at the time of acute hospital admission can be more difficult, as symptoms of physical disease (e.g. loss of energy) can be mistaken as evidence of depression. One study found the prevalence of depression in ED patients aged 70 and over (mean age, 78 years) to be 17%.[44] In another study of patients aged over 65 (mean age, 75 years) without dementia presenting to an ED, 27% had evidence of depression (24% of those who lived in the community and 47% of those who lived in nursing homes).[45] Depression was not detected in any of the patients by the attending emergency physician. When ED physicians were asked if the patient they had just assessed had depression, detection rates were poor (sensitivity 27%, specificity 75%).[46] Estimates of prevalence rates for major depression among the hospitalised elderly vary widely. One study found a rate of 14% in one hospital and 45% in another.[47] A systematic review of studies found a mean prevalence of 20%.[48] A more recent study of patients aged 70 and over on hospital wards found a prevalence of possible major depression of 24% and definite major depression of 8%.[49]

Depression negatively impacts on older people in hospital (*see* Table 10.6) and is the commonest cause of suicide and self-harm. It is particularly common in older patients with a chronic physical health problem, especially cancer, heart disease, diabetes, PD and stroke.[50] Unfortunately, depression accompanying physical illness is often poorly recognised and poorly managed.[51,52] Key clinical features include low mood, loss of interest (anhedonia) and worthlessness. There may be a coexistent anxiety disorder. Clues to the diagnosis include being more functionally restricted or not progressing as expected. Somatic complaints in the depressed commonly include reduced energy, reduced appetite, weight loss and insomnia. This can lead to wasting time and resources searching for an underlying physical illness.

TABLE 10.6 The potential consequences of depression in older people in hospital

Potential consequence
Longer inpatient stays
Higher readmission rates
Increased use of outpatient services
Poor mental health of carers
Increased functional impairment and disability
Reduced quality of life
Increased risk of nursing home placement
Increased morbidity and mortality

Diagnosis

Depression is really a clinical syndrome rather than a specific diagnosis. There is no gold standard test available and the diagnosis is usually made on the basis of operational criteria, such as International Classification of Diseases (10th Edition).[53] Simple screening tests are discussed on page 57. To diagnose depression, two of the core symptoms must be present, plus at least two of the remaining symptoms, for at least 2 weeks (Table 10.7). In moderate depression, five to six symptoms are present, and in severe depression, seven or more symptoms.

TABLE 10.7 International Classification of Diseases (10th Edition) (ICD-10) criteria for the diagnosis of depression

ICD-10 criteria
Depressed mood*
Loss of interest*
Reduction in energy*
Loss of confidence or self-esteem
Unreasonable feelings of self-reproach or inappropriate guilt
Recurrent thoughts of death or suicide
Diminished ability to think/concentrate or indecisiveness
Change in psychomotor activity with agitation or retardation
Sleep disturbance
Change in appetite with weight change

Note: *Core symptoms

The diagnosis of depression in older people with physical illnesses may be difficult, especially as older people with depression tend to present with more somatic symptoms.[54] Many drugs such as steroids, benzodiazepines, beta-blockers and alcohol can cause depression.[50] It is important to have a low index of suspicion and take a collateral history from relatives and carers. Nursing staff are often more alert than medical staff to symptoms of depression, because they see patients for longer periods between ward rounds.

Patients with hypoactive delirium (*see* p. 107) may clinically resemble depression, and this latter diagnosis cannot be made reliably during a delirious episode. In a study evaluating older hospital in-patients (mean age, 71 years) referred to a psychiatry service with suspected depression, 42% were subsequently diagnosed with delirium.[55] Classical depression symptoms, both psychiatric and physical, were common in those with delirium (approximately two-thirds of cases). Those with delirium were more likely to have a history of acute cognitive decline and perform poorly on mental test scores. The patients with delirium had worse outcomes than the non-delirious. Some patients will have both depression and delirium, and this group tend to do the least well.[56]

Suicide

The elderly have the highest risk of completed suicide.[43,57] The majority have an underlying psychiatric disorder, most commonly major depression (affecting around 80%).[57] Identified risk factors in older people include male sex, depression, living alone or social isolation, bereavement, chronic disability, drug or alcohol problems, low educational level and a history of previous psychiatric treatment or suicide attempt.[43,57,58] Such patients should be screened for suicidal ideation. In addition, ask patients directly about hallucinations and delusions and also look for bipolar disorder by questioning whether mania or hypomania has occurred earlier in life.

Treatment

Antidepressant medications are not routinely recommended for those with only mild depression, where other interventions such as cognitive behavioural therapy may be more appropriate.[59] These patients should be referred on to their general practitioner on discharge for reassessment and treatment in primary care, including possible psychological interventions. It is important to follow up mild depression, as it is a risk factor for severe depression.

Patients with moderate or severe depression should be considered for treatment with antidepressants. There is little to choose between the second-generation antidepressants, and it makes sense to prescribe a generic SSRI, such as sertraline or citalopram, in the first instance.[60] It may take at least 2 weeks to see a response. These drugs increase the risk of upper GI bleeding. Of the SSRIs, citalopram and sertraline tend to have fewer drug interactions. It had become accepted knowledge that tricyclic antidepressants had more anticholinergic effects and should be avoided in the elderly. However, a recent observational study has suggested that SSRIs are associated with a higher risk of falls and hyponatraemia than other antidepressants, and non-SSRI, non-tricyclic antidepressants (trazadone, mirtazepine and venlafaxine) with a higher risk of cerebrovascular disease, fractures and seizures.[61] However, these differences may simply be due to prescribing bias. Patients should be followed up to monitor response to treatment. Most depression can be managed in primary care, but referral to a psychiatrist should be considered in some situations (*see* Table 10.8).

TABLE 10.8 Criteria for referral of depressed elderly patients to a psychiatrist

Criteria
Severe depression
Psychotic depression
Bipolar disorder
Significant suicide risk
Diagnosis in doubt
Inadequate response to initial therapy
Cognitive impairment
Complex requirements
Condition deteriorating

Depression, cerebrovascular disease and dementia

Depression is a risk factor for dementia, and depression is present in 20% of patients with Alzheimer's dementia.[60] Treatment of depressive symptoms in dementia can be rewarding as they may contribute to behavioural symptoms. However, antidepressant medication may not be effective.[62] All patients with depression should have a cognitive assessment. Similarly, there is an overlap with cerebrovascular disease. The prevalence of post-stroke major depression in hospital is around 20%.[63] The concept of vascular depression arises from the observation that white matter hyperintensities on MRI of the brain are often present in older people with depressive symptoms.[64,65] Vascular depression is associated with vascular risk factors and patients tend to have greater disability, cognitive impairment, apathy and psychomotor retardation. Management is by the control of vascular risk factors as well as anti-depressants, but these patients tend to respond less well and have a poorer prognosis.

KEY POINTS

- Around 10% of elderly patients on hospital wards have major depression.
- Depression often goes unrecognised and can lead to longer lengths of stay, worse functional outcomes and increased mortality rates.
- Somatic complaints of depression can be wrongly interpreted as evidence of a physical illness.
- Simple screening tests should be used to detect depression.
- In moderate to severe depression the use of SSRI drugs (usually citalopram or sertraline) is recommended.
- Complex cases should be referred to specialist psychiatry services.

DIABETES

The goals of treatment in diabetes for the frail elderly who are likely to have multiple co-morbidities (e.g. heart failure and dementia) will be different from those of an otherwise fit older person. The aim of strict plasma glucose control is to reduce vascular complications such as retinopathy and stroke. The evidence is that approximately 8 years of tight glycaemic control is necessary before decreases in vascular outcomes occur.[66] In the frail elderly tight glycaemic control can lead to a substantial burden with dietary restriction, frequent finger stick testing, frequent insulin injections, polypharmacy and an increased risk of hypoglycaemia. Moreover, many of these patients have a life expectancy less than 8 years. There is evidence that admissions to hospital with hypoglycaemia increase the risk of developing dementia.[67] On the other hand, moderate glycaemic control may have other benefits in the frail elderly, such as decreased symptomatic hyperglycaemia, improved cognition, improved continence and possibly less predisposition to falls.[68] The level of glycaemic control to achieve these benefits is less than that to obtain long-term vascular benefits. For this reason, guidelines for the management of diabetes in the frail elderly recommend moderate rather than tight control of plasma glucose, for example aiming for glycosylated haemoglobin levels between 60 and 69 mmol/mol (7.6%–8.5%).[69]

Diabetes in older people is usually type 2. Non-obese elderly persons with type 2 diabetes differ from younger patients with type 2 diabetes in that they show a marked impairment in insulin release with only mild insulin resistance, as opposed to marked insulin resistance in the presence of adequate levels of insulin.[70] Frailty and sarcopenia are both linked to diabetes and are common in older diabetics.[71] Older people with diabetes therefore commonly present as geriatric emergencies, especially with delirium, falls, immobility and adverse consequences of drugs described elsewhere in this book, as well as presenting with the typical diabetic emergencies of diabetic ketoacidosis (DKA), hyperosmolar hyperglycaemic state (HHS) and hypoglycaemia. In frail older patients the aim is to minimise geriatric syndromes (falls, delirium, immobility and side effects of medication) and their complications, as well as prevent and treat diabetic complications, and comprehensive geriatric assessment is an essential part of management.[71]

Diabetic emergencies

Diabetes and its complications are common causes for admission to acute hospital. People in hospital with diabetes are, on average, older than other patients (in England, median age of 75 years, compared with 65 years for all other patients).[72] Patients with diabetes are also more likely to be admitted as an emergency compared to the general population and have longer lengths of stay. Over 90% of diabetic patients are admitted for problems other than the management of their diabetes. Of the patients with type 2 diabetes that do come to hospital specifically for the management of their diabetes, around half are admitted with active foot disease, 18% with hypoglycaemia, 16% with hyperglycaemia (not DKA or HHS), 10% with HHS and 3% with DKA.[72]

Although diabetic emergencies are generally common, junior doctors are not always confident in their management. For example, a survey of 2149 trainee doctors showed that only 27% were fully confident in diagnosing and managing DKA compared with 66% and 65% for managing angina and asthma, respectively.[73] There are excellent guidelines available and most hospitals have specialist diabetic teams to provide advice. Managing diabetic emergencies correctly can be life saving as well as very satisfying.

Diabetic ketoacidosis

DKA is a common life-threatening complication of type 1 diabetes but can also affect those with type 2 diabetes. It is defined as the existence of the biochemical triad of ketonaemia, hyperglycaemia and acidaemia. The mortality has dropped in the last 20 years to less than 5% in experienced centres.[74] Age, however, remains the most significant risk factor for a poor outcome.[75] Complications include hypokalaemia and hyperkalaemia, hypoglycaemia, cerebral oedema and pulmonary oedema. The diagnosis of DKA and assessment of severity is based on the biochemical parameters listed in Table 10.9.[76] The commonest cause in patients of all ages is infection followed by inadequate insulin.[74]

The main aims of management of DKA are rehydration (often a fluid deficit of over 6 L), potassium replacement, resolution of ketoacidosis, prevention of complications and the treatment of any underlying cause. There are well-established

UK modern management guidelines, but despite this, many hospitals use out of date protocols and errors in patient care are common.[77] The new key recommendations in management based on the Joint British Diabetes Society 2010 guidelines are listed in Table 10.10.[78] Patients with severe DKA should be managed on an intensive therapy unit.

TABLE 10.9 Diagnostic criteria for diabetic ketoacidosis (DKA) and hyperglycaemic hyperosmolar state (HHS)

	Mild DKA	Moderate DKA	Severe DKA	HHS
Blood glucose (mmol/L)	≥14	≥14	≥14	>33
Blood pH	7.25–7.35	7.0–7.24	<7.0	>7.3
Blood bicarbonate (mmol/L)	15–18	10–14	<10	>15
Urine ketones	>++	>++	>++	≤+
Blood ketones[a] (mmol/L)	>1.0	>3.0	>5.0	<1.0
Serum osmolarity[b] (osmol/L)	Variable	Variable	Variable	>320
Anion gap[c] (mmol/L)	>10	>12	>14	Variable
Mental state	Alert	Alert or drowsy	Coma	Delirium or coma

Notes: [a]Measured as beta-hydroxyl butyrate; [b]estimated by the following equation: 2 × [sodium + potassium] + urea + glucose (units all as millimoles per litre); [c]estimated by the following equation: sodium − [chloride + bicarbonate] (units all as millimoles per litre)

TABLE 10.10 Modern recommendations for management of diabetic ketoacidosis

1	The best method for monitoring the response to treatment is to measure bedside capillary blood ketones using a ketone meter (e.g. hourly measurements)
2	If it is not possible to measure blood ketones, then venous pH and bicarbonate should be used alongside bedside glucose monitoring to assess the response to treatment
3	Venous blood should be used in blood gas analysers rather than arterial blood (unless co-existent respiratory problems would make this more useful)
	This can be used to assess pH and electrolytes (e.g. every 2 hours)
4	It is only necessary to intermittently perform laboratory confirmation of pH, bicarbonate and electrolytes (e.g. every 4 hours)
5	Insulin should be given intravenously at a weight-based fixed rate until resolution of the ketosis has been achieved
6	Ten per cent dextrose should be given in addition once the blood glucose falls below 14 mmol/L, which allows the fixed-rate insulin to be continued
7	Patients already taking long-acting insulin analogues, such as insulin glargine, should continue these in the usual doses alongside other treatment
8	The diabetes specialist team should be involved as soon as possible

Insulin is given intravenously at a fixed rate 0.1 units/kg/hour. When the plasma glucose drops below 14 mmol/L, then 10% dextrose is given at a rate of 125 mL/hour alongside normal saline fluid resuscitation with potassium replacement. Fixed-rate insulin, along with iv 10% dextrose, is given until the ketosis resolves. Resolution is defined as a venous pH >7.3 or ketones <0.3 mmol/L. As soon as the patient's ketosis has resolved and the patient is ready and able to eat, then he or she should be converted to subcutaneous insulin in consultation with the local specialist diabetes liaison team. Frail older people often require more judicious fluid replacement than younger patients – for example, 2 L over 4 hours; 1 L over 4 hours; then 3 L over the next 24 hours.

Hyperosmolar hyperglycaemic state

HHS (also known as 'hyperosmolar non-ketotic hyperglycaemia') is one of the most serious acute complications of diabetes, with significant morbidity and a mortality of around 15%.[74] It is defined as blood glucose >33 mmol/L, pH >7.3, bicarbonate >15 mmol/L and serum osmolarity >320 (osmol/L) but a small amount of ketones may also be present (*see* Table 10.9).

TABLE 10.11 Symptoms of hypoglycaemia – but note these may be absent or diminished in frail older people

Autonomic	Sweating, palpitations, shaking, hunger
Neuroglycopenia	Confusion, drowsiness, odd behaviour, speech difficulty, incoordination, seizures
General	Headache, nausea

HHS is a complication of type 2 diabetes and may be the first presentation. It is commoner in older people.[75] Unlike DKA, which presents usually within 24 hours, in HHS the history may be several days, or even weeks. There is often underlying sepsis. Subacute deterioration occurs with severe dehydration, hypernatraemia and uraemia. Delirium is common and is more related to the hyperosmolarity than the high plasma glucose. The fluid deficit is high, often around 10 L. Treatment is similar to DKA except patients with HHS are more sensitive to insulin, and infusion rates of 1–3 units per hour are sufficient. Higher rates of insulin infusion can result in rapid osmotic changes and can be dangerous. Maintain serum potassium in the range of 4–5 mmol/L. Fluid replacement should be cautious – 3 L in the first 12 hours. Thromboembolic complications are common and prophylaxis with low-molecular-weight heparin is essential.

Hypoglycaemia

The risk of severe hypoglycaemia rises with age because the physiological and autonomic response to hypoglycaemia diminishes. Older patients also have less time between the development of sympathetic symptoms and neuroglycopenia than younger patients.[79] Risk factors include frailty, renal impairment, co-morbidity, social isolation and living in a care home. Admission to hospital with a hypoglycaemic attack considerably increases the risk of future dementia.[67]

Hypoglycaemia is a lower than normal level of blood glucose – any reading below 4.0 mmol/L should be treated.[80] The symptoms of hypoglycaemia are listed in Table 10.11. Focal neurological symptoms or signs may be misdiagnosed as stroke. Hypoglycaemia may go unrecognised and it is essential to check blood glucose in any unwell known diabetic. Hypoglycaemia is most common in type 1 diabetes as a result of mismatch of insulin, carbohydrate intake and carbohydrate utilisation. Prolonged hypoglycaemia can also occur in type 2 diabetics if they are taking hypoglycaemic agents, particularly sulphonylureas. In patients who are conscious and able to swallow then treatment is 15–20 g quick acting carbohydrate, such as 200 mls of fruit juice.[80] This can be repeated until blood glucose is above 4 mmol/L and then followed up by a long-acting carbohydrate, such as a glass of milk. In an unconscious patient, iv 20% or 10% glucose is preferred because of the risk of extravasation injury with 50% glucose. Glucagon 1 mg intramuscularly is an alternative if venous access is difficult.

Hypoglycaemia may be more prolonged in older people and is more likely to recur. There should be a low threshold for hospital admission. Older patients admitted with hypoglycaemia should be referred to the local specialist diabetes team and followed up as recurrent episodes of hypoglycaemia are particularly damaging to the vulnerable older brain.

KEY POINTS

- HSS can be recognised by a blood glucose of greater than 33, a raised plasma osmolarity >320 and a pH >7.30.
- HSS can present with delirium, stupor or coma and mortality is high (15%).
- HSS should be treated with low-dose insulin infusion (one to three units per hour) to prevent rapid shifts in osmolarity and sodium concentrations.
- Hypoglycaemia may be more prolonged in older people and is more likely to recur – have a low threshold for hospital admission.
- Recurrent hypoglycaemia can lead to dementia.
- Always check blood glucose in any unwell patient who is diabetic.

HEADACHE

Although headache is a less common presenting complaint in older adults, it is much more likely to be due to a serious underlying disorder.[81] Around half of patients aged over 65 report having at least one headache per year, with the majority being either tension-type or migraine.[82] Table 10.12 shows the commonest causes of headache detected in patients over age 65 presenting to a hospital neurology service.[81] Most headaches in the elderly are caused by conditions that are not life-threatening, but around 15%–30% that present to emergency services do have a serious underlying disorder.[83,84] Headaches are also more likely to be associated with serious underlying pathology if they are described as acute onset, occipitonuchal (posterior) in location or associated with any positive findings on neurological examination.[85]

TABLE 10.12 The commonest causes of headache in patients over age 65 presenting to a hospital neurology service

Cause	Rate (%)
Tension type	43
Idiopathic trigeminal neuralgia	19
Subarachnoid haemorrhage	8
Temporal arteritis	6
Brain tumour	4
Cervical spine disorder	3
Post-herpetic trigeminal neuralgia	3
Cluster headache	2

Note: Data obtained from Pascual and Berciano[81]

Headache can be divided into primary and secondary forms depending on whether or not they are caused by a primary neurological disorder or an alternative underlying pathology. Examples of primary headaches are migraine, tension-type headache (TTH) and cluster headache. These are not life-threatening conditions. Examples of secondary headaches are those caused by intracranial bleeding, meningitis, brain tumours or temporal arteritis. These conditions are potentially very serious, making accurate diagnosis imperative.

Primary causes of headache

Tension-type headache

TTH is the commonest form of headache, but its prevalence is lower in older age, affecting around 25% of people.[84] It is described as a continual band of tightening or pressing pain across the forehead. It may be provoked by emotional stress or lack of sleep. It does not usually affect ability to perform daily activities and is not usually associated with other symptoms (e.g. no nausea, vomiting or photophobia).

Migraine

The prevalence of migraine is lower in old age, affecting around 5% of people aged over 80 years (women more than men).[84] Only a small proportion of people (1%–2%) have a first attack of migraine in old age.[81] The characteristics of migraine attacks tend to change with advancing age. Headaches without aura become more similar to the pain of TTH, and some migraines with aura may lose the headache component.[84] This latter phenomenon can cause confusion with transient ischaemic attack (*see* p. 208). Patients typically have a history of prior attacks, but occasionally classic migraine can present for the first time in late life. Migraine headache is characterised as unilateral, pulsing or throbbing in nature and often associated with nausea, vomiting and photophobia. The headache is of gradual onset and lasts from hours to days. Aura precedes the headache by around 30 minutes and lasts for several minutes. Most commonly they are visual in nature (e.g. flashing lights) but can occasionally cause other neurological symptoms such as hemiparesis or vertigo (*see* p. 248). Typically patients want to lie down in a quiet room during periods of headache.

Other primary headaches

➤ Cervicogenic headache is a term for a headache secondary to a cervical spine disorder causing compression of the C2 or C3 nerve roots. The pain is located on the back of the head and may be made worse by movement.
➤ Trigeminal neuralgia is a cause of severe facial pain. This is typically described as unilateral shock-like pains in the distribution of the trigeminal nerve.
➤ Cluster headache is less common in the elderly.[84] Patients usually report a severe unilateral periorbital pain that lasts between 15 minutes and 3 hours.[86] It is likely that there will be associated ipsilateral autonomic symptoms – lacrimation, redness of eye, rhinorrhoea, ptosis or miosis. Classically attacks are described as occurring in 'clusters' with periods of remission in between.
➤ Hypnic headaches are more common in later life. They cause a moderate bilateral pain of variable frequency, lasting around 15 minutes, which wakes the patient from sleeping.[84] The cause is unknown but they are thought to be benign and they often disappear after several years.

Secondary causes of headache

Secondary headaches can be caused by life-threatening underlying conditions. However, they can also be caused by less serious problems, including medication-induced headaches – for example, nifedipine and isosorbide preparations or following the chronic use of analgesic drugs ('medication overuse headache'). Other possible serious causes of headache discussed elsewhere in this book include subdural haematoma (*see* p. 168) and meningitis/encephalitis (*see* p. 194).

Subarachnoid haemorrhage

Subarachnoid haemorrhage (SAH) has been found to be present in 1%–4% of patients presenting to ED with headache.[83] It is more common in women than men, has a mean age of onset of 55 years and is associated with hypertension, smoking, excessive alcohol intake and cocaine use.[87] However, around 10% of SAH occurs in people over the age of 75 years.[88] In 85% of cases the underlying cause is a ruptured intracranial aneurysm.[89]

Typically, patients complain of a sudden onset (over seconds) of the worst headache they have ever experienced, but only around 25% of such patients will have SAH.[90] There may or may not be associated neck pain, photophobia, nausea/vomiting, confusion or reduced consciousness. Neck stiffness is not universally present and may not develop until 3 or more hours after the onset of headache.[89] Fundoscopy may reveal intraocular haemorrhages due to increased cerebrospinal fluid pressure. Focal neurological deficits can be present because of expansion of the aneurysm, intracerebral blood or localised vasospasm triggered by blood in the subarachnoid space.

Urgent CT scanning performed within 12 hours of onset will detect around 95% of SAH. If the CT is negative, a lumbar puncture is indicated. This should be performed after a period of at least 6, but preferably 12, hours has passed since symptom onset.[89] This will allow the direct measurement of bilirubin concentration (which cannot be caused by a traumatic tap). A study found a misdiagnosis rate for SAH of 12% and this was associated with worse outcomes.[91] Patients more likely to be missed were those with normal mental status and smaller areas of bleeding on the CT scan. Hypertension, hypoxia and ECG changes can be associated with SAH and lead to diagnostic difficulty.[89]

Following diagnosis a neurosurgical opinion should be sought, and most patients will be transferred to a neurosurgical unit. Treatment usually involves endovascular embolisation with coiling of the aneurysm in order to lower the risk of re-bleeding. A worse outcome is associated with vasospasm, which reduces cerebral blood flow. Nimodipine, a calcium channel blocker, is typically given to reduce the risk of vasospasm.[92] Aneurysmal SAH has a poor prognosis, with a 50% fatality rate, and around one-third of survivors require long-term care.[87] In a series of patients aged 75 and over, just 15% were independent at the time of hospital discharge.[88]

Temporal arteritis

Temporal arteritis is an inflammatory process of medium to large sized cranial vessels. It typically presents with headache, fever, malaise and weight loss. Patients may also complain of jaw claudication (50% of cases), scalp tenderness (50%) and visual loss (20%).[93] Clinical examination may reveal tenderness, enlargement or reduced pulsation within the affected temporal artery. It is an emergency as any resultant visual loss is typically irreversible. Blood tests show an erythrocyte sedimentation rate (ESR) >50 mm/hour. A temporal artery biopsy (ideally before steroids, but may be positive up to 2 weeks after their commencement) may reveal a characteristic pattern of vasculitis (e.g. monocyte infiltration and granuloma formation). The artery may only show segmental involvement, so a 2 cm length sample is required. Treatment is with steroids, typically prednisolone initially at a dose of 40–60 mg per day, which is gradually reduced over several months.[93] Patients with visual symptoms should be referred urgently to an ophthalmologist. Symptoms typically improve quickly (within 48 hours) once treatment is commenced.

Brain tumours

Brain tumours can present as headache, slowly progressive neurological deficits, seizures, signs of raised intracranial pressure, or cognitive impairment. Patients may describe a generalised headache, gradually worsening over time and exacerbated by bending or coughing. It might be described as worse in the morning and it may waken them from sleep, but none of these features are universally present. In the later stages there can be associated vomiting, transient visual loss on postural change, reduced consciousness and papilloedema.

The majority of brain tumours detected in the elderly are secondary metastatic deposits of extra-cranial tumours. The commonest primary sites are lung (50%–60%), breast (15%–20%), melanoma (5%–10%), and GI tract (4%–6%).[94] Around half of primary brain tumours are of glial cell origin. In the elderly, low-grade gliomas (e.g. astrocytomas and oligodendrogliomas) are uncommon. Unfortunately, high-grade 'glioblastoma multiforme', which has signs of necrosis, haemorrhage and oedema on imaging, is common. This type of tumour has around a 30% 1-year survival when untreated. Other possibilities include meningiomas (around 25%), pituitary adenomas (20%), vascular lesions (e.g.

angiomas) and, rarely, lymphomas. Diagnosis is based on brain imaging – usually plain CT scans, but contrast-enhanced images or MRI may provide additional information. When there is significant surrounding oedema the patient should be commenced on dexamethasone. A neurosurgical or oncological opinion should be urgently sought.[95]

Acute glaucoma

Acute glaucoma usually causes a sudden onset of a severe unilateral headache. There is likely to be associated blurred vision and conjunctival erythema, possibly with nausea and vomiting. The cornea may appear cloudy. However, atypical presentations can occur in the old and a delay in diagnosis, which can lead to lasting visual loss, is common.[96] Suspected patients should be referred to an ophthalmologist for measurement of intraocular pressures.

KEY POINTS

- The majority of headaches are due to non-serious pathologies such as TTH and migraine, but older patients are more likely to have a serious underlying disorder (15%–30% of headaches presenting to emergency services).
- SAH is often missed in older people and this adversely affects the outcome – it should be suspected in all patients who complain of a sudden onset of a severe headache.
- Always consider temporal arteritis as a cause for any headache in an older person, particularly if there are systemic symptoms. Blood tests should include an ESR.
- Brain tumours (primary or secondary) can sometimes present as headache.
- Acute glaucoma can cause a sudden onset of a severe unilateral headache. There might be associated blurred vision and conjunctival erythema.

ACUTE BACK PAIN

Back pain is a common symptom in adults. It is estimated that over 90% of cases are due to a non-serious underlying condition.[97] There is some evidence that severe or disabling back pain is more prevalent in the elderly.[98,99] A number of 'red flag' criteria have been identified to help detect patients most likely to have a serious underlying diagnosis (*see* Table 10.13) and these include onset in patients over the age of 50 years.[97] Therefore, all back pain should be assessed for the possibility of a serious underlying diagnosis in the frail elderly. The first step is to take a detailed history and perform an examination, including the neurological system. Blood tests should include a full blood count, alkaline phosphatase, C-reactive protein (CRP), ESR and serum calcium level. X-rays in the frail elderly are likely to show degenerative changes, caution is required to ensure these changes are not wrongly assumed to be the cause of the patient's symptoms. Serious causes of back pain seen more commonly in the frail elderly are discussed here.

TABLE 10.13 Red flag symptoms to look out for when assessing frail older patients with back pain

Patient characteristics	Age >50 years
	History of malignancy or immunosuppression
	Recent procedure that may cause bacteraemia
Nature of the pain	Gradual onset
	Thoracic location
	Duration >6 weeks
	Recent trauma
	Worse at rest or overnight
	Poor relief from analgesia
	Associated fever, rigors, sweating or weight loss
Physical findings	Systemically unwell
	Fever
	Hypotension or hypertension
	Pulsatile abdominal mass
	Differential blood pressure/pulse between limbs
	Spinal tenderness
	Focal neurological signs
	Urinary retention

Aortic emergencies

Abdominal aortic aneurysms (AAAs) classically present with abdominal pain (*see* p. 158), but they can also present as acute back pain. In the event of aneurysm rupture, physical signs of shock may be absent at first presentation. Abdominal examination may not reveal an abnormality. The sensitivity to detect a pulsatile mass is just 80% in patients with aneurysms up to 5 cm in diameter.[100] Back pain has been found to be the primary complaint in 4% of patients with AAA rupture. Aortic dissection, especially when affecting the descending aorta, can also present as acute back pain (*see* p. 233).

Spinal cord compression

Spinal cord compression is most commonly caused by epidural metastases, but epidural abscesses (*see* 'Spinal infections') or haematomas (especially if anticoagulated) are also possible.[100] Back pain characteristically precedes the onset of neurological deficits. Cord compression should be considered in all cancer patients presenting with new back pain. In women, breast cancer is the most likely underlying cause. Weakness, sensory loss and bladder dysfunction may only develop later. The prognosis after the onset of neurological deficits is limited. With appropriate treatment, only 15%–22% of patients who have become immobile will regain the ability to walk.[100] X-rays are usually unhelpful in making a diagnosis. MRI scanning is the test of choice. Treatment is with immediate steroids and urgent consultation with oncology or neurosurgery for consideration of radiotherapy and/or surgical intervention.

Cauda equina syndrome

Cauda equina syndrome is due to compression of the spinal nerves below the level of the termination of the spinal cord. It typically presents with perineal sensory loss plus urinary and faecal incontinence or retention.[100] There may also be sciatica and bilateral foot or quadriceps weakness. Symptoms are usually of rapid onset. The most common cause is lumbar spinal disc herniation, but infections or malignant aetiologies are possible. MRI is the test of choice. Patients should be urgently referred to a neurosurgeon.

Spinal infections

Epidural abscesses are most commonly caused by *Staphylococcus aureus*, but other organisms, including tuberculosis, are also possible. Risk factors include immunocompromise (e.g. the human immunodeficiency virus, diabetes, alcohol abuse and steroid use), degenerative spinal disease or a source of infection elsewhere in the body.[100] Blood tests may show an elevated white cell count (WCC) and inflammatory markers, but these are unreliable. Blood cultures should be obtained. MRI is the investigation of choice. Alternative options include CT or nuclear medicine bone scans. Percutaneous CT-guided or surgical drainage of the abscess should be considered. Broad-spectrum antibiotics offering good coverage of *S. aureus* and Gram-negative organisms should be continued for 4–6 weeks.

Vertebral osteomyelitis is the infection of a vertebral body but can also spread into the adjacent disc space. The organisms typically enter the body elsewhere and are distributed to the spine via the blood circulation. It is most commonly caused by *S. aureus*, but other organisms, including Gram-negative bacteria and tuberculosis, are also possible. Back pain may develop over weeks to months. The prognosis is less favourable if neurological deficits are present. Blood inflammatory markers are usually elevated. Blood cultures should be obtained. Plain X-rays show abnormalities in around 50% of cases, but MRI and CT scans are more sensitive.[100] A CT-guided biopsy (ideally performed before commencing treatment) aids choice of antibiotic, which will need to be given for 6–12 weeks.[100] Surgical intervention may be appropriate for those who fail to improve on medical therapy or who develop neurological signs.

Osteoporotic vertebral fractures

Osteoporotic vertebral fractures most commonly occur in the low thoracic to upper lumbar region. They can be asymptomatic or present as progressive spinal curvature with height loss (kyphosis), chronic back pain, or acute back pain following minor trauma. They are diagnosed by plain X-ray images (*see* Figure 10.2). The investigation and treatment of osteoporosis is discussed on page 165. Patients are also likely to require analgesia.

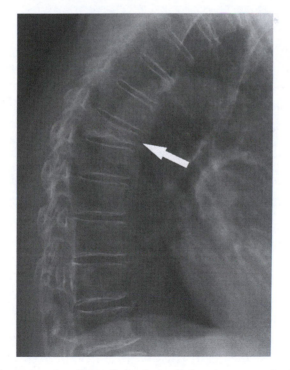

FIGURE 10.2 A thoracic spine X-ray (lateral view) showing a vertebral wedge fracture (white arrow)

Multiple myeloma

Multiple myeloma is an uncommon condition, but its incidence increases with advancing age. It is said to present with bone pain secondary to lytic bone lesions in around 70% of cases and this is most commonly in the back or lower ribs. The pain usually develops gradually and is made worse by movement. There may be features of bone marrow suppression (anaemia, bruising and increased infections), renal failure, hypercalcaemia (*see* p. 81) or hyperviscosity. Lytic bone lesions can lead to pathological fractures. Initial investigations should include a full blood count, ESR, renal function, calcium level and protein electrophoresis of serum and urine. Plain X-rays may show lytic bone lesions. Patients should be referred to a haematologist for further assessment.

KEY POINTS

- Back pain is less common in old age, but more likely to have a serious underlying cause.
- AAA rupture and aortic dissection can present as back pain.
- Always examine for signs of cord compression in any patient with cancer who presents with back pain.
- Cauda equina syndrome typically presents with perineal sensory loss plus urinary and faecal incontinence or retention.
- Raised serum WCC or inflammatory markers can suggest an underlying epidural abscess or osteomyelitis.
- Osteoporotic vertebral fractures can occur after only minor trauma in the frail elderly.
- Multiple myeloma is more common in older age and can present as back pain.

ACUTE JOINT INFLAMMATION

Acute joint inflammation may occur in a single or multiple joints. It typically presents with pain, swelling and reduced mobility. Here we consider only acutely inflamed joints of a non-traumatic aetiology. Studies of adult patients have suggested that the commonest causes of non-traumatic acutely inflamed joints are gout (15%–27%), septic arthritis (8%–27%), rheumatoid arthritis (11%–16%) and osteoarthritis (5%–17%), with no cause found in 16%–36% despite investigations.[101]

Assessment

As with other presentations the assessment should begin with taking a history and performing an examination. History should include any prior joint disease and risk factors for specific causes. Examination should include evaluation of other joints and looking for systemic signs (e.g. gouty tophi on the hands, elbows and ears). X-rays should be performed of the affected joint(s). The next step is aspiration of synovial fluid to look for crystals and organisms, and to send the fluid for culture. Blood tests often show elevated serum CRP, ESR and WCC, but these are of only minor help in distinguishing the possible underlying causes.[101] In selected cases further investigation with ultrasound, MRI or bone scanning may be warranted.

Septic arthritis

Risk factors for septic arthritis include age over 80 years, diabetes, rheumatoid arthritis, recent joint surgery, prosthetic joints and the presence of cellulitis.[101] Organisms can enter the joint space directly (e.g. in response to surgery or joint injections) or migrate from a different septic source (e.g. UTI or cellulitis). In patients aged over 80 years the commonest sites are the knee (40%), shoulder (18%) and hip (8%), and the commonest organisms are staphylococci (57%), streptococci (24%) and Gram-negative bacilli (14%).[102] Most patients have joint pain (85%) and swelling (78%), but the presence of fever is an unreliable clinical sign.[101]

In almost all cases, the CRP and ESR will be elevated, but around half of patients have a normal serum WCC.[102] The aspirated synovial fluid is likely to contain $>50 \times 10^9$/L white blood cells, with at least 90% neutrophils.[101] Ideally this joint aspiration should occur soon after presentation and prior to the commencement of antibiotics. Following this, the patient should be commenced on an iv antibiotic, in accordance with local guidance and likely causative organism, while awaiting laboratory results. A delay in diagnosis may lead to septicaemia and joint destruction, which increase the probability of disability, joint replacement surgery and death. Outcomes are less favourable in older patients. The mortality rate for those aged 60 or below is 0.7%, rising to 4.8% of those aged 60–79, and 9.5% of those aged 80 and above.[102]

Acute gout

Elderly-onset gout (first presenting in people aged over 65 years) is the most common inflammatory arthropathy in old age, with a prevalence of around 3%.[103] In this population it is at least as common in women as in men. Risk factors for gout include obesity, diabetes, hypertension, cardiac disease, renal disease, diuretic use and high alcohol intake. The clinical features suggesting acute gout include a rapid onset (maximal inflammation within 1 day of symptoms), redness over the joint and the presence of any tophi. Tophi are more commonly noted at presentation in the elderly and they may overly Heberden's or Bouchard's nodes of co-existent osteoarthritis.[103] There may be a history of previous similar episodes. It is also more likely if the affected joint is the first metatarsophalangeal, but it can affect any. The finding of elevated serum urate levels suggests that the patient is at higher risk of gout. However, not all people with an elevated serum urate will develop gout and those with an acute attack may have a serum level within the normal range. Therefore, serum urate is not a reliable test for the diagnosis of acute gout. Monosodium urate crystals are found within synovial fluid of patients with acute gout, but it may co-exist with septic arthritis and so fluid should also be sent for culture.

NSAIDs have traditionally been used to treat acute gout. However, they are associated with many potential adverse effects in the elderly (*see* p. 304). They may be cautiously used in selected patients for short periods of time. Consideration should be given to the concomitant use of a PPI to limit gastric toxicity. Another option, once septic arthritis has been excluded, is to use corticosteroids. These can be given by the oral, iv or intra-articular routes. A third choice is colchicine. This may cause diarrhoea and vomiting, which can lead to dehydration. Colchicine should only be given in low doses (e.g. 500 mcg twice daily) and be withdrawn once symptoms settle.[104] It is not suitable for patients with significant renal or hepatic impairment and can cause myopathy.

Urate-lowering medications (e.g. allopurinol) can prevent further acute episodes. These drugs should not be started during an acute attack, but patients already taking them can continue to do so. Allopurinol should be started at low doses (e.g. 100 mg daily) several weeks after symptom remission and can be gradually increased according to serum urate levels providing renal function is not severely impaired. The target is to lower serum urate to below 0.36 mmol/L.[104] It can cause side effects including rashes. In the management of gout it is also appropriate to look for and, where possible, address underlying risk factors such as obesity, medications and alcohol intake.

Pseudogout

Pseudogout presents similarly to acute gout but is more likely to affect the larger, more proximal joints of the shoulder, wrist or knee. The onset of inflammation may also be more gradual than that of gout. It can be associated with hypothyroidism, hyperparathyroidism, haemochromatosis or hypomagnesaemia. Calcium pyrophosphate crystals are found within the aspirated synovial fluid. Treatment is with analgesia only. It may take 2–4 weeks for the inflammation to settle.

Osteoarthritis

In people aged over 60 years osteoarthritis has a prevalence of around 12% at the knee and around 7% at the hip.[105] It is typically a chronic condition but it can occasionally present as acute joint swelling. In this situation there is likely to be crepitus on movement of the joint but palpable warmth is unlikey.[101] X-rays usually show characteristic changes (loss of cartilage, osteophyte formation plus bone sclerosis and cyst formation around the joint margins). Blood inflammatory markers are usually normal and synovial fluid will not show high levels of white blood cells.

Rheumatoid arthritis

Rheumatoid arthritis is a common inflammatory arthropathy in elderly people, affecting around 2% of this population.[106] Typically, the onset is in earlier age, but around 10%–20% presents in those aged over 60. When presenting in older age it is more likely to affect the proximal large joints – typically the shoulder and knee. There is usually a history of morning stiffness lasting more than 1 hour. The sicca syndrome (dry mouth and eyes) may be associated. X-rays may show juxta-articular erosive changes and joint space narrowing. Blood tests are likely to show raised inflammatory markers. Autoantibodies should also be tested. Rheumatoid factor and anti-cyclic citrullinated peptide (anti-CCP) are positive in around two-thirds of those with late onset rheumatoid arthritis.[107] Anti-CCP is less likely to give a false-positive result than rheumatoid factor. Patients should be referred to a rheumatologist for specialist management.

KEY POINTS

- The commonest causes of non-traumatic acutely inflamed joints in the elderly are gout, septic arthritis, rheumatoid arthritis and osteoarthritis.
- A key component of assessing an acutely inflamed joint is aspiration of synovial fluid to look for crystals and organisms, and to send the fluid for culture.
- A delay in diagnosis of septic arthritis may lead to septicaemia and joint destruction, which increase the probability of disability, joint replacement surgery and death.
- Elderly-onset gout is the most common inflammatory arthropathy in old age, with a prevalence of around 3%.

- A swollen joint due to osteoarthritis is not usually warm to touch, and it is associated with normal blood tests and characteristic X-ray appearances.
- Around 10%–20% of rheumatoid arthritis first presents in those aged over 60.

ELDER ABUSE

Older people are sometimes subjected to abuse. It can take the form of neglect or be physical, financial, psychological or sexual in its nature. It may be unintentional because of a lack of knowledge by the carer, or may be deliberate.[108] This may be a sign of carer stress. Abuse may occur in predictable patterns where abused partners or children become the abusers.[109] Risk factors for abuse include patient cognitive impairment and social isolation, carer alcohol consumption or depression, and poor pre-morbid relationships.[110–112] It can be difficult to detect because of lack of a precise definition or pathognomonic physical signs. Evidence may be subtle and many cases (perhaps 84%) go undetected.[113] Victims may feel embarrassed or guilty, or fear retaliation if they expose the culprit.

➤ Physical – injury with the intention of causing harm. It may range from hitting to inappropriate physical restraint.

➤ Sexual – any non-consensual sexual interaction. This may range from verbal innuendo to rape.

➤ Emotional/psychological – may be through verbal or physical acts. It may involve humiliation or threats to withdraw care or nutrition.

➤ Financial – theft or improper use of property or money. It may involve coercion to change a will.

➤ Neglect – for example inadequate nutrition, hydration or living environment. It may be unintentional.

Estimates of the proportion of community-dwelling elderly who have experienced some form of abuse are typically in the range 2%–10%, depending on the population studied and the definition used.[112,114] In a study of community-dwelling elders who were receiving respite care, 45% of their carers admitted to committing some form of abuse at home.[111] A Spanish study detected probable abuse in 29% of people over the age of 75 (mean age, 82 years) who lived in their own home.[115] An Israeli study of older adults (mean age, 79 years) admitted to hospital found that 6% of people disclosed experiencing abuse, 21% had signs of abuse, and 33% were judged to be at high risk of abuse.[116]

A UK report found psychological abuse to be the commonest (34%), followed by financial (20%), physical (19%), neglect (12%), and sexual (3%) forms, and some suffered more than one type.[117] Abusers were most often family members

(46%) but could be paid carers (34%). Male family members were more likely to be the perpetrators and women more likely to be the victims. Most abuse occurred within the person's own home (64%), with care homes (23%) and hospitals (5%) being the next most frequent settings. When it does occur in the victim's home they usually co-habit with the abuser (the exception being financial abuse where victims typically live alone).[112]

Most emergency physicians rarely ask patients direct questions about abuse and only half of detected cases are reported to authorities.[118] Common reasons for not reporting abuse include subtle signs, denial by the victim and physician uncertainty about procedures, definitions and legislation. It is difficult to comprehend the misery that older people trapped in such situations must endure. In addition, it is associated with reduced survival rates compared with the non-abused, even when corrections are made for co-morbidities.[119]

Assessment

It is necessary to have a high index of suspicion to detect the often subtle signs of abuse. The nature of assessment may be determined by the patient's cognition and so this also needs to be tested. Any intervention may also be influenced by the victim's mental capacity. A non-confrontational approach with good communication skills should be adopted. The patient should be assessed in the absence of their carer or other suspected abuser. Start with general questions such as, 'Do you feel safe where you live?'[108] If evidence of abuse is uncovered then its nature, frequency and any precipitating factors should be sought.[112] Confrontation with an alleged abuser should be avoided. An empathetic and non-judgemental approach is best.

Clues to diagnosis include delays in seeking medical help, multiple admissions, inconsistent stories, and evidence of emotional withdrawal. Commonly detected clinical findings that could indicate neglect include falls, malnutrition/dehydration, medication errors, pressure ulcers, poor personal hygiene and oversedation.[108] There may be signs of physical injury. Injuries that raise concerns are those in locations not commonly affected by accidental trauma – for example, inner thighs and arms, palms and soles, ear, posterior neck and axilla.[109] Large bruises (>5 cm diameter) and bruises on the head, neck, lateral right arm and back have been found to be more commonly associated with elder abuse.[120] The bruises are likely to be of varying ages. There could be unexplained fractures or untreated injuries. Such patients and their carers should be asked about the origin of the injury and any inconsistencies noted.

Intervention

The first steps are accurate documentation of injuries (ideally with photographs), appropriate medical attention, and the gathering of collateral information. Awareness of local vulnerable adult protection policies is required. The best course of action may be determined by a combination of patient acceptance of help and/or their mental capacity. Admission to hospital or alternative accommodation should be considered in order to remove the patient from an at-risk situation. In less serious cases a referral to social services may be more appropriate. A vulnerable adult meeting coordinated by social services is likely to be required. The police may need to be involved if a crime has been committed.

KEY POINTS

- Elder abuse can take the form of neglect or be physical, financial, psychological or sexual in its nature. It may be unintentional because of a lack of knowledge by the carer, or it may be deliberate.
- It is necessary to have a high index of suspicion to detect the often subtle signs of abuse.
- Clues to diagnosis include delays in seeking medical help, multiple admissions, inconsistent stories, and evidence of emotional withdrawal.
- When looking for evidence of abuse a non-confrontational approach should be adopted. The patient should be assessed in the absence of their carer or other suspected abuser. Start with general questions such as, 'Do you feel safe where you live?'
- The first steps in managing suspected abuse are accurate documentation of injuries, giving the patient the appropriate medical attention, and gathering collateral information.

PALLIATIVE CARE

Palliative care is an approach that improves the quality of life of patients and their families facing the problems associated with life-threatening illness, through the prevention and relief of suffering by means of early identification and impeccable assessment and treatment of pain and other problems, physical, psychological and spiritual.[121] Traditionally used in cases of incurable cancer, the approach is valuable in many other situations in the elderly – for example, in end-stage heart failure, PD, stroke and dementia. Although the majority of people in the UK are thought to want to die at home, over half die in hospital.[122] A book about emergency medicine in older people would be incomplete without a section on palliative care, as often older patients with terminal illness are admitted to hospital in their last few days as emergencies.

Triggers for emergency admissions of patients already known to community palliative care teams are new symptoms (e.g. infection, bleeding and dyspnoea) and poor control of existing symptoms (e.g. pain, constipation and nausea), rather than unavailability of care.[122] A common complaint by carers, relatives and older patients is that acute hospitals concentrate too much on curative treatment when no longer appropriate, instead of providing comfort and dignity.[123] A prospective study of over 4000 seriously ill elderly patients who died in hospital found that more than half died with severe pain, shortness of breath, anxiety, nausea or confusion.[124] Family members reported that the patients would have preferred care that focused on comfort, even if this shortened life.

The default approach in acute hospitals should always be active treatment, but when the outlook for recovery is poor then there should be early discussion with the patient and family to consider realistic treatment goals, and palliative care is sometimes more appropriate depending on the individual situation. The clinical team may need to balance thoroughness and enthusiasm with realism and compassion. After initial treatment and assessment, goals of treatment may need to be redefined. Some patients will have an advanced directive in place that can make these decisions easier.

General principles of palliative care

All symptoms should be evaluated and a diagnosis made. Any treatments should be explained to the patient and carers. Treatment should involve correcting what can be easily corrected and prescribing to control symptoms on an individual basis. The patient should be reviewed frequently and medication stopped if ineffective or no longer required. End-of-life pathways, such as the Liverpool Care Pathway,[125] are valuable educational and audit tools, but their success in improving care depends on their application being tailored to the individual patient.

Pain management

As with all symptoms, pain should be carefully assessed as many patients suffer from more than one type of pain – each one should be evaluated. The pain may be caused by the primary diagnosis (e.g. cancer or PD), may be secondary to treatment (e.g. constipation), may be caused by immobility (e.g. pressure ulcers) or related to other associated co-morbidities (e.g. arthritis). It may be due to stimulation of nerve endings (nociceptive pain) or due to nerve dysfunction (neuropathic pain).

It is generally recommended to use the oral route whenever possible. Analgesia should be given regularly to prevent pain with additional 'as required' doses for breakthrough pain. The World Health Organization's three-step analgesic ladder should be followed to treat nociceptive pain.

1. Non-opioid analgesics (e.g. paracetamol).
2. Add weak opioid (e.g. codeine or tramadol).
3. Change weak opioid to strong opioid (e.g. morphine, diamorphine, oxycodone, fentanyl or buprenorphine).

Some situations may also benefit from the addition of adjuvant medication to any of these three steps. Examples include steroids for nerve compression or liver capsular pain; antidepressants or anticonvulsants for neuropathic pain; muscle relaxants or antispasmodics for muscular, bladder or bowel spasms; and bisphosphonates for bone pain. Additional approaches may include nerve blocks for regional pain syndromes or radiotherapy to locally invasive cancers.

Morphine is metabolised (>90%) in the liver to morphine-3-glucuronide and to smaller amounts of morphine-6-glucuronide and normorphine. All three metabolites are active and their elimination is reduced in older patients. Morphine-3-glucuronide is particularly neurotoxic and can cause delirium and seizures. For this reason, newer opiates such as oxycodone, buprenorphine and fentanyl, which have different metabolic pathways, may be preferable in the elderly.[126]

Morphine can be given subcutaneously. When converting oral morphine to subcutaneous morphine, for equivalent analgesic effect, the subcutaneous dose should be half the oral dose given over 24 hours. Fentanyl and buprenorphine can be given in the form of transdermal patches, but it is important to convert the dose carefully. A fentanyl 12 mcg/hour patch equates to around 30 to 45 mg oral morphine daily; and a buprenorphine 10 mcg/hour patch equates to around 20 mg oral morphine daily. These transdermal drugs may take 12 hours or more to get absorbed through the skin and reach their maximal effect. When titrating opioids against pain, increase the 24-hour dose by about one-third each time and the 'as required' dose should be one-sixth of the total 24-hour dose.

Neuropathic pain is often described as shooting, stabbing or burning. Recommended first-line treatment is either amitriptyline or pregabalin, and duloxetine for those with painful diabetic neuropathy.[127] In older people, small initial doses should be used (e.g. amitriptyline 10 mg) and titrated up slowly. Oral tramadol or topical lidocaine patches are possible alternatives if the first-line agents are ineffective alone or in combination.

Constipation

Constipation affects nearly everyone who is prescribed strong opioids, and laxative treatment taken regularly at an effective dose should be prescribed to all patients starting strong opioids. Constipation is also contributed to by immobility, lack of food intake and fluid depletion (*see* p. 82).

Nausea and vomiting

Nausea and vomiting are common in terminal patients. First identify the cause – for example, medication (especially opiates), hypercalcaemia or bowel obstruction. Use a regular antiemetic. Metoclopramide is suitable for gastritis and stasis, cyclizine where there is raised intracranial pressure or functional bowel obstruction and haloperidol for other causes such as hypercalcaemia.

Dyspnoea

Dyspnoea can be very distressing. Treatment depends on the cause and may include iv diuretics for heart failure or draining of a pleural effusion. The sensation of breathlessness can be at least partially relieved by small doses of opiates given regularly (e.g. morphine 2.5–5 mg 6-hourly). Lorazepam in small doses (e.g. 0.5 mg as required) may also relieve distress.

Delirium in palliative care

Delirium is common in dying patients and should be investigated and treated in the usual way (*see* p. 107). Drug causes and hypercalcaemia are particularly common. So-called 'terminal delirium' is usually due to opiate toxicity and consideration should be given to reducing the dose or changing to an alternative opiate. The mainstay of treatment of delirium in palliative care is haloperidol, which can be given in a subcutaneous infusion pump with morphine and which also acts as an antiemetic. Benzodiazepines are sedating and can worsen delirium,[128] but in the very terminal stage it may be necessary to take a pragmatic approach and use midazolam primarily for its sedative action, which can be given as a subcutaneous infusion.

Hydration and nutrition at the end of life

Artificial nutrition and hydration (i.e. that which bypasses swallowing) is a medical treatment and may be withheld. Sometimes patients who are clearly dying are labelled 'nil by mouth' in hospitals to prevent aspiration. This may cause a great deal of distress and concern to relatives. The pragmatic approach is to supply fluids, as tolerated (thickened if necessary) to patients who are in the final stages and ensure regular dental and mouth care. Sips of water are unlikely to cause problems in most patients and will provide some comfort. Parotitis, xerostomia (dry mouth), candidiasis and mouth ulcers are common treatable causes of difficulty in eating and swallowing in older frail patients. The value of artificial hydration in terminal patients is not proven,[129] but some relatives and patients may be reassured by a subcutaneous drip and this is usually well tolerated. Poor appetite and reduced nutritional intake is part of the dying process and nasogastric feeding and/or percutaneous gastrostomy feeding should only be considered if recovery is possible or if thought to be part of symptomatic care. In advanced dementia, tube feeding is generally not advocated.[130]

KEY POINTS

- At least half of older people will die in hospital and there is much that can be done to make this as dignified and symptom-free as possible.
- Acute hospital care is usually based around saving lives and reducing morbidity and mortality, but we also should provide excellent palliative care when appropriate.
- Key components of palliative care are careful assessment and treatment of symptoms, and good communication with patients and their families and carers.
- Older patients are much more sensitive to many of the drugs used routinely in palliative care and side effects are common – use smaller doses, at least initially, and be aware of potential side effects.
- There are many possible causes of pain, and each patient can have several.
- Patients should be given regular analgesia to prevent experiencing pain rather than just giving 'as required' medication when the pain occurs.
- Other common symptoms seen in the palliative phase of illnesses include constipation, vomiting, breathlessness and delirium.
- Decisions about artificial nutrition and hydration around the time of death should be informed by discussion with the patient and their family or carers. The aim should be to promote symptomatic relief.

REFERENCES

1. Jonsson R, Sixt E, Landahl S, *et al*. Prevalence of dizziness and vertigo in an urban elderly population. *J Vestib Res*. 2004; **14**(1): 47–52.
2. Maarsingh OR, Dros J, Schellevis SG, *et al*. Causes of persistent dizziness in elderly patients in primary care. *Ann Fam Med*. 2010; **8**(3): 196–205.
3. Colledge NR, Wilson JA, MacIntyre CCA, *et al*. The prevalence and characteristics of dizziness in an elderly community. *Age Ageing*. 1994; **23**(2): 117–20.
4. Lawson J, Fitzgerald J, Birchall J, *et al*. Diagnosis of geriatric patients with severe dizziness. *J Am Geriatr Soc*. 1999; **47**(1): 12–17.

5. Dros J, Maarsingh OR, van der Horst HE, *et al.* Tests used to evaluate dizziness in primary care. *CMAJ.* 2010; **182**(13): E621–31.

6. Lee H, Sohn S, Cho Y, *et al.* Cerebellar infarction presenting isolated vertigo: frequency and vascular topographical patterns. *Stroke.* 2006; **67**(7): 1178–83.

7. Kerber KA, Brown DL, Lisabeth LD, *et al.* Stroke among patients with dizziness, vertigo, and imbalance in the emergency department: a population-based study. *Stroke.* 2006; **37**(10): 2484–7.

8. Darlington CL, Smith PF. Drug treatment for vertigo and dizziness. *N Z Med J.* 1998; **111**(1073): 332–4.

9. Shin H, Yoo K, Chang HM, *et al.* Bilateral intracranial vertebral artery disease in the New England Medical Center Posterior Circulation Registry. *Arch Neurol.* 1999; **56**(11): 1353–8.

10. Caplan LR, Wityk RJ, Glass TA, *et al.* New England Medical Center Posterior Circulation Registry. *Ann Neurol.* 2004; **56**(3): 389–98.

11. Hilton D, Iman N, Burke GJ, *et al.* Absence of abdominal pain in older persons with endoscopic ulcers: a prospective study. *Am J Gastroenterol.* 2001; **96**(2): 380–4.

12. Stanley AJ, Ashley D, Dalton HR, *et al.* Outpatient management of patients with low-risk upper-gastrointestinal haemorrhage: multicentre validation and prospective evaluation. *Lancet.* 2009; **373**(9657): 42–7.

13. Yachimski PS, Friedman LS. Gastrointestinal bleeding in the elderly. *Nat Clin Pract Gastroenterol Hepatol.* 2008; **5**(2): 80–93.

14. Alkhatib AA, Elkathib FA, Abubakr SM, *et al.* Acute upper gastrointestinal bleeding in elderly people: presentations, endoscopic findings, and outcomes. *J Am Geriatr Soc.* 2010; **58**(1): 182–5.

15. Christensen S, Riis A, Norgaard M, *et al.* Short-term mortality after perforated or bleeding peptic ulcer among elderly patients: a population-based cohort study. *BMC Geriatr.* 2007; **7**: 8.

16. Chait MM. Lower gastrointestinal bleeding in the elderly. *World J Gastrointest Endosc.* 2010; **2**(5): 147–54.

17. McGuire HH Jr. Bleeding colonic diverticula: a reappraisal of natural history and management. *Ann Surg.* 1994; **220**(5): 653–6.

18. Robertson DJ, Grimm IS. Inflammatory bowel disease in the elderly. *Gastroenterol Clin North Am.* 2001; **30**(2): 409–29.

19. De Rijk MC, Tzourio C, Breteler MM, *et al.* Prevalence of Parkinsonism and Parkinson's disease in Europe: the EUROPARKINSON collaborative study. *J Neurol Neurosurg Psychiatry.* 1997; **62**(1): 10–15.

20. National Collaborating Centre for Chronic Conditions. *Parkinson's Disease: national clinical guideline for diagnosis and management in primary and secondary care.* London: Royal College of Physicians; 2006.

21. Woodford H, Walker R. Emergency hospital admissions in idiopathic Parkinson's disease. *Mov Disord.* 2005; **20**(9): 1104–8.

22. Ghosh R, Liddle BJ. Emergency presentations of Parkinson's disease: early recognition and treatment are crucial for optimum outcome. *Postgrad Med J.* 2011; **87**(1024): 125–31.

23. Woodford HJ, George J. Neurological and cognitive impairments detected in older people without a diagnosis of neurological or cognitive disease. *Postgrad Med J.* 2011; **87**(1025): 199–206.

24. Allcock LM, Ullyart K, Kenny R, *et al.* Frequency of orthostatic hypotension in a community based cohort of patients with Parkinson's disease. *J Neurol Neurosurg Psychiatry.* 2003; **75**(10): 1470–1.

25. Wood BH, Bilclough JA, Walker RN. Incidence and prediction of falls in Parkinson's disease; a prospective multidisciplinary study. *J Neurol Neurosurg Psychiatry.* 2002; **72**(6): 721–5.

26. Wenning GK, Ebersbach G, Verry M, *et al.* Progression of falls in postmortem-confirmed Parkinsonian disorders. *Mov Disord.* 1999; **14**(6): 947–50.

27. Miller N, Noble E, Jones D, *et al.* Hard to swallow: dysphagia in Parkinson's disease. *Age Ageing.* 2006; **35**(6): 614–18.

28. Miller N, Allcock L, Hildreth AJ, *et al.* Swallowing problems in Parkinson disease: frequency and clinical correlates. *J Neurol Neurosurg Psychiatry.* 2009; **80**(9): 1047–9.

29. Ghosh R, Liddle BJ. Emergency presentations of Parkinson's disease: early recognition and treatment are crucial for optimum outcome. *Postgrad Med J.* 2011; **87**(1024): 125–31.

30. Brennan KA, Genever RW. Managing Parkinson's disease during surgery. *BMJ.* 2010; **341**: 990–3.

31. Graham JM, Grunewald RA, Sagar HJ. Hallucinosis in idiopathic Parkinson's disease. *J Neurol Neurosurg Psychiatry.* 1997; **63**(4): 434–40.

32. Zahodne LB, Fernandez HH. Parkinson's psychosis. *Curr Treat Options Neurol.* 2010; **12**(3): 200–11.

33. Goetz CG, Stebbins GT. Mortality and hallucinations in nursing home patients with advanced Parkinson's disease. *Neurology.* 1995; **45**(4): 669–71.

34. National Institute for Health and Clinical Excellence. Delirium: diagnosis, prevention and management: NICE guideline 103. London: NIHCE; 2010. Available at: guidance.nice.org.uk/CG103/NICEGuidance/pdf/English (accessed 25 January 2013).

35. Quinn N. Drug treatment of Parkinson's disease. *BMJ.* 1995; **310**(6979): 575–9.

36. Serrano-Duenas M, Bleda MJ. Delirium in Parkinson's disease patients: a five-year follow-up study. *Parkinsonism Relat Disord.* 2005; **11**(6): 387–92.

37. Rabey JM, Prokhorov T, Miniovitz A, *et al.* Effect of quetiapine in psychotic Parkinson's disease patients: a double-blind labeled study of 3 months' duration. *Mov Disord.* 2007; **22**(3): 313–18.

38. Emre M, Aarsland D, Albanese A, *et al.* Rivastigmine in dementia associated with Parkinson's disease. *N Eng J Med.* 2004; **351**(24): 2509–18.

39. Keyser DL, Rodnitzky RL. Neuroleptic malignant syndrome in Parkinson's disease after withdrawal or alteration of dopaminergic therapy. *Arch Intern Med.* 1991; **151**(4): 794–6.

40. Gordon PH, Frucht SJ. Neuroleptic malignant syndrome in advanced Parkinson's disease. *Mov Disord.* 2001; **16**(5): 960–2.

41. Douglas A, Morris J. It was not just a heatwave! Neuroleptic malignant-like syndrome in a patient with Parkinson's disease. *Age Ageing.* 2006; **35**(6): 640–1.

42. Boyer EW, Shannon M. The serotonin syndrome. *N Engl J Med.* 2005; **352**(11): 1112–20.

43. Rodda J, Walker Z, Carter J. Depression in older adults. *BMJ.* 2011; **343**: 683–7.

44. Hustey FM. The use of a brief depression screen in older emergency department patients. *Acad Emerg Med.* 2005; **12**(9): 905–8.

45. Meldon SW, Emerman CL, Schubert DS, *et al.* Depression in geriatric ED patients: prevalence and recognition. *Ann Emerg Med.* 1997; **30**(2): 141–5.

46. Meldon SW, Emerman CL, Schubert DSP. Recognition of depression in geriatric ED patients by emergency physicians. *Ann Emerg Med.* 1997; **30**(4): 442–7.

47. McCusker J, Cole M, Dufouil C, *et al.* The prevalence and correlates of major and minor depression in older medical inpatients. *J Am Geriatr Soc.* 2005; **53**(8): 1344–53.

48. Royal College of Psychiatrists. *Who Cares Wins.* London: Royal College of Psychiatrists; 2005. Available at: www.rcpsych.ac.uk/PDF/WhoCaresWins.pdf (accessed 25 January 2013).

49. Goldberg SE, Whittamore KH, Harwood RH, *et al.* The prevalence of mental health problems among older adults admitted as an emergency to a general hospital. *Age Ageing*. 2012; **41**(1): 80–6.

50. Alexopoulos GS. Depression in the elderly. *Lancet*. 2005; **365**(9475): 1961–70.

51. Smyth R. Depression in physical illness. *J R Coll Physicians Edinb*. 2009; **39**(4): 337–42.

52. National Institute for Health and Clinical Excellence. Depression in Adults with a Chronic Physical Health Problem: NICE guideline 91. London: NIHCE; 2010. Available at: www. nice.org.uk/CG91 (accessed 25 January 2013).

53. World Health Organization (WHO). *The ICD-10 Classification of Mental and Behavioural Disorders: clinical descriptions and diagnostic guidelines*. Geneva: WHO; 1992.

54. Hegeman JM, Kok RM, van der Mast RC, *et al.* Phenomenology of depression in older compared with younger adults: meta-analysis. *Br J Psychiatry*. 2012; **200**(4): 275–81.

55. Farrell KR, Ganzini L. Misdiagnosing delirium as depression in medically ill elderly patients. *Arch Intern Med*. 1995; **155**(22): 2459–64.

56. Givens JL, Jones RN, Inouye SK. The overlap syndrome of depression and delirium in older hospitalized patients. *J Am Geriatr Soc*. 2009; **57**(8): 1347–53.

57. O'Connell H, Chin A, Cunningham C, *et al.* Recent developments: suicide in older people. *BMJ*. 2004; **329**(7471): 895–9.

58. Wiktorsson S, Runeson B, Skoog I, *et al.* Attempted suicide in the elderly: characteristics of suicide attempters 70 years and older and a general population comparison group. *Am J Geriatr Psychiatry*. 2010; **18**(1): 57–67.

59. National Institute for Health and Clinical Excellence. The Treatment and Management of Depression in Adults: NICE guideline 90. London: NIHCE; 2009. Available at: www.nice. org.uk/nicemedia/live/12329/45888/45888.pdf (accessed 25 January 2013).

60. Gartlehner G, Hansen RA, Morgan CL, *et al.* Comparative benefits and harms of second-generation antidepressants for treating major depressive disorder. *Ann Intern Med*. 2011; **155**(11): 772–85.

61. Coupland C, Dhiman P, Morriss R, *et al.* Antidepressant use and risk of adverse outcomes in older people: population based cohort study. *BMJ*. 2011; **343**: d4551.

62. Banerjee S, Hellier J, Dewey D, *et al.* Sertraline or mirtazapine for depression in dementia (HTA-SADD): a randomised, multicentre, double-blind, placebo-controlled trial. *Lancet*. 2011; **378**(9789): 403–11.

63. Robinson RG. Poststroke depression: prevalence, diagnosis, treatment and disease progression. *Biol Psychiatry*. 2003; **54**(3): 376–87.

64. Inzitari D, Carlucci G, Pantoni L. White matter changes: the clinical consequences in the ageing population. *J Neural Transm Suppl*. 2000; **59**: 1–8.

65. Firbank MJ, Teodorczuk A, van der Flier WM, *et al.* Relationship between progression of brain white matter changes and late-life depression: 3-year results from the LADIS study. *Br J Psychiatry*. 2012; **201**(1): 40–5.

66. Lee SJ, Eng C. Goals of glycaemic control in frail older patients with diabetes. *JAMA*. 2011; **305**(13): 1350–1.

67. Whitmer RA, Karter AJ, Yaffe K, *et al.* Hypoglycaemic episodes and risk of dementia in older patients with type 2 diabetes mellitus. *JAMA*. 2009; **301**(15): 1565–72.

68. Araki A, Ito H. Diabetes mellitus and geriatric syndromes. *Geriatr Gerontol Int*. 2009; **9**(2): 105–14.

69. Sinclair AJ, Paolisso G, Castro M, *et al.* European Diabetes Working Party for Older People 2011 clinical guidelines for type 2 diabetes mellitus. Executive summary. *Diabetes Metab*. 2011; **37**(Suppl. 3): 527–38.

70. Hermans MP, Pepersack TM, Godeaux LH, *et al.* Prevalence and determinants of impaired glucose metabolism in frail elderly patients: the Belgian Elderly Diabetes Survey (BEDS). *J Gerontol A Biol Sci Med Sci.* 2005; **60**(2): 241–7.

71. Bourdel-Marchasson I, Dugaret E, Regueme S. Disability in older people with diabetes: issues for the clinician. *Br J Diabetes Vasc Dis.* 2012; **12**(3): 135–40.

72. *National Diabetes Inpatient Audit, 2011.* London: Diabetes UK; 2011. Available at: www. diabetes.nhs.uk/document.php?o=3512 (accessed 25 January 2013).

73. George JT, Warriner D, McGrane DJ, *et al.* Lack of confidence among trainee doctors in the management of diabetes; the Trainers Own Perception of Delivery of Care (TOPDOC) Diabetes Study. *QJM.* 2011; **104**(9): 761–6.

74. English P, Williams G. Hyperglycaemic crises and lactic acidosis in diabetes mellitus. *Postgrad Med J.* 2004; **80**(943): 253–61.

75. MacIsaac RJ, Lee LY, McNeil KJ, *et al.* Influence of age on the presentation and outcome of acidotic and hyperosmolar diabetic emergencies. *Intern Med J.* 2002; **32**(8): 379–85.

76. Kitabchi AE, Umpierrez GE, Miles JM, *et al.* Hyperglycemic crisis in adult patients with diabetes: a consensus statement from the American Diabetes Association. *Diabetes Care.* 2009; **32**(7): 1335–43.

77. Joint British Diabetes Societies Inpatient Care Group. *The Management of Diabetic Ketoacidosis in Adults (Mar 2010).* London: Diabetes UK; 2010. Available at: www.diabetes. nhs.uk/document.php?o=212 (accessed 25 January 2013).

78. Savage MW, Dhatariya KK, Kilvet A, *et al.* Joint British Diabetes Society guideline for management of diabetic ketoacidosis. *Diabetic Med.* 2011; **28**(5): 508–15.

79. Matyka K, Cranston I, Evans M, *et al.* Altered hierarchy of protective responses against severe hypoglycaemia in normal ageing in healthy men. *Diabetes Care.* 1997; **20**(2): 135–41.

80. Diabetes UK. *The Hospital Management of Hypoglycaemia in Adults with Diabetes Mellitus.* London: Diabetes UK; 2010. Available at: www.diabetes.nhs.uk/document.php?o=217 (accessed 25 January 2013).

81. Pascual J, Berciano J. Experience in the diagnosis of headaches that start in elderly people. *J Neurol Neurosurg Psychiatry.* 1994; **57**(10): 1255–7.

82. Prencipe M, Casini AR, Ferretti C, *et al.* Prevalence of headache in an elderly population: attack frequency, disability, and use of medication. *J Neurol Neurosurg Psychiatry.* 2001; **70**(3): 377–81.

83. Walker RA, Wadman MC. Headache in the elderly. *Clin Geriatr Med.* 2007; **23**(2): 291–305.

84. Tonini MC, Bussone G. Headache in the elderly: primary forms. *Neurol Sci.* 2010; **31**(Suppl 1): S67–71.

85. Ramirez-Lassepas M, Espinosa CE, Cicero JJ, *et al.* Predictors of intracranial pathologic findings in patients who seek emergency care because of headache. *Arch Neurol.* 1997; **54**(12): 1506–9.

86. Nesbitt AD, Goadsby PJ. Cluster headache. *BMJ.* 2012; **344**: 37–42.

87. Suarez JI, Tarr RW, Selman WR. Aneurysmal subarachnoid haemorrhage. *N Engl J Med.* 2006; **354**(4): 387–96.

88. Nieuwkamp DJ, Rinkel GJE, Silva R, *et al.* Subarachnoid haemorrhage in patients ≥75 years: clinical course, treatment and outcome. *J Neurol Neurosurg Psychiatry.* 2006; **77**(8): 933–7.

89. Van Gijn J, Kerr RS, Rinkel GJ. Subarachnoid haemorrhage. *Lancet.* 2007; **369**(9558): 306–18.

90. Al-Shahi R, White PM, Davenport RJ, *et al.* Subarachnoid haemorrhage. *BMJ.* 2006; **333**(7561): 235–40.

91. Kowalski RG, Claassen J, Kreiter KT, *et al*. Initial misdiagnosis and outcome after subarachnoid hemorrhage. *JAMA*. 2004; **291**(7): 866–9.

92. Royal College of Physicians. *National Clinical Guideline for Stroke*. 4th ed. London: Royal College of Physicians; 2012. Available at: www.rcplondon.ac.uk/sites/default/files/national-clinical-guidelines-for-stroke-fourth-edition.pdf (accessed 25 January 2013).

93. Salvarani C, Cantini F, Hunder GG. Polymyalgia rheumatica and giant-cell arteritis. *Lancet*. 2008; **372**(9634): 234–45.

94. Nathoo N, Chahlavi A, Barnett GH, *et al*. Pathobiology of brain metastases. *J Clin Pathol*. 2005; **58**(3): 237–42.

95. Nayak L, Iwamoto FM. Primary brain tumours in the elderly. *Curr Neurol Neurosci Rep*. 2010; **10**(4): 252–8.

96. Siriwardena D, Arora AK, Fraser SG, *et al*. Misdiagnosis of acute angle closure glaucoma. *Age Ageing*. 1996; **25**(6): 421–3.

97. Winters ME, Kluetz P, Zilberstein J. Back pain emergencies. *Med Clin North Am*. 2006; **90**(3): 505–23.

98. Dionne CE, Dunn KM, Croft PR. Does back pain really decrease with increasing age? A systematic review. *Age Ageing*. 2006; **35**(3): 229–34.

99. Docking RE, Fleming J, Brayne C, *et al*. Epidemiology of back pain in older adults: prevalence and risk factors for back pain onset. *Rheumatology (Oxford)*. 2011; **50**(9): 1645–53.

100. Broder J, Snarski JT. Back pain in the elderly. *Clin Geriatr Med*. 2007; **23**(2): 271–89.

101. Ma L, Cranney A, Holroyd-Leduc J. Acute monoarthritis: what is the cause of my patient's painful swollen joint? *CMAJ*. 2009; **180**(1): 59–65.

102. Gavet F, Tournadre A, Soubrier M, *et al*. Septic arthritis in patients aged 80 and older: a comparison with younger adults. *J Am Geriatr Soc*. 2005; **53**(7): 1210–13.

103. De Leonardis F, Govoni M, Colina M, *et al*. Elderly-onset gout: a review. *Rheumatol Int*. 2007; **28**(1): 1–6.

104. Stamp LK, Jordan S. The challenges of gout management in the elderly. *Drugs Aging*. 2011; **28**(8): 591–603.

105. Quintana JM, Arostegui I, Escobar A, *et al*. Prevalence of knee and hip osteoarthritis and the appropriateness of joint replacement in an older population. *Arch Intern Med*. 2008; **168**(14): 1576–84.

106. Kerr LD. Inflammatory arthropathy: a review of rheumatoid arthritis in older patients. *Geriatrics*. 2004; **59**(10): 32–5.

107. Lopez-Hoyos M, Ruiz de Algeria C, Blanco R, *et al*. Clinical utility of anti-CCP antibodies in the differential diagnosis of elderly-onset rheumatoid arthritis and polymyalgia rheumatica. *Rheumatology (Oxford)*. 2004; **43**(5): 655–7.

108. Clarke ME, Pierson W. Management of elder abuse in the emergency department. *Emerg Clin North Am*. 1999; **17**(3): 631–44.

109. Collins KA. Elder maltreatment: a review. *Arch Pathol Lab Med*. 2006; **130**(9): 1290–6.

110. Jones J, Dougherty J, Schelble D, *et al*. Emergency department protocol for the diagnosis and evaluation of geriatric abuse. *Ann Emerg Med*. 1988; **17**(10): 1006–15.

111. Homer AC, Gilleard C. Abuse of elderly people by their carers. *BMJ*. 1990; **301**(6765): 1359–62.

112. Lachs MS, Pillemer K. Elder abuse. *Lancet*. 2004; **364**(9441): 1263–72.

113. Levine JM. Elder neglect and abuse: a primer for primary care physicians. *Geriatrics*. 2003; **58**(10): 37–40, 42–4.

114. Cooper C, Selwood A, Livingston G. The prevalence of elder abuse and neglect: a systematic review. *Age Ageing*. 2008; **37**(2): 151–60.

115. Garre-Olmo J, Planas-Pujol X, Lopez-Pousa S, *et al.* Prevalence and risk factors of suspected elder abuse subtypes in people aged 75 and older. *J Am Geriatr Soc.* 2009; **57**(5): 815–22.

116. Cohen M, Levin SH, Gagin R, *et al.* Elder abuse: disparities between older people's disclosure of abuse, evident signs of abuse, and high risk of abuse. *J Am Geriatr Soc.* 2007; **55**(8): 1224–30.

117. Action on Elder Abuse. *Hidden Voices: older people's experience of abuse.* London: Help the Aged; 2004. Available in summary form at: www.ageuk.org.uk/documents/en-gb/for-professionals/equality-and-human-rights/id3725_hidden_voices_older_people%e2%80%99s_experience_of_abuse_executive_summary_2004_pro.pdf?dtrk=true (accessed 25 January 2013).

118. Jones JS, Veenstra TR, Seamon JP, *et al.* Elder mistreatment: national survey of emergency physicians. *Ann Emerg Med.* 1997; **30**(4): 473–9.

119. Lachs MS, Williams CS, O'Brien S, *et al.* The mortality of elder mistreatment. *JAMA.* 1998; **280**(5): 428–32.

120. Wiglesworth A, Austin R, Corona M, *et al.* Bruising as a marker of physical elder abuse. *J Am Geriatr Soc.* 2009; **57**(7): 1191–6.

121. World Health Organization (WHO). *Cancer, Pain Relief and Palliative Care.* Geneva: WHO; 1990.

122. Capel M, Gazi T, Vout L, *et al.* Where do patients known to a community palliative care service die? *BMJ Support Palliat Care.* 2012; **2**(1): 43–7.

123. Dunne K, Sullivan K. Family experiences of palliative care in the acute hospital setting. *Int J Palliat Nurs.* 2000; **6**(4): 170–8.

124. Lynn J, Teno JM, Phillips RS, *et al.* Perceptions by family members of the dying experience of older and seriously ill patients. *Ann Intern Med.* 1997; **126**(2): 97–106.

125. Ellershaw J, Wilkinson S. *Care of the Dying: a pathway to excellence.* Oxford: Oxford University Press; 2003.

126. Pergolizzi J, Boger RH, Budd K, *et al.* Opioids and the management of chronic severe pain in the elderly. *Pain Pract.* 2008; **8**(4): 287–313.

127. National Institute for Health and Clinical Excellence. The Pharmacological Management of Neuropathic Pain in Adults in Non-Specialist Settings: NICE guideline 96. London: NIHCE; 2010. Available at: www.nice.org.uk/guidance/CG96 (accessed 25 January 2013).

128. Breitbart W, Marotta R, Platt MM, *et al.* A double-blind trial of haloperidol, chlorpromazine and lorazepam in the treatment of delirium in hospitalized AIDS patients. *Am J Psychiatry.* 1996; **153**(2): 231–7.

129. McCann RM, Hall WJ, Groth-Juncker A. Comfort care for terminally ill patients: the appropriate use of nutrition and hydration. *JAMA.* 1994; **272**(16): 1263–6.

130. National Institute for Health and Clinical Excellence and Social Care Institute for Excellence. Dementia: Guideline 42. Leicester: British Psychological Society; 2007. Available at: www.nice.org.uk/nicemedia/pdf/CG42Dementiafinal.pdf (accessed 25 January 2013).

CHAPTER 11

Medications

The appropriate use of medication in the frail elderly is complex but also vitally important. The clinical team have to balance potential beneficial and adverse effects. Compared with younger people there is less robust clinical evidence to base decisions on. Plus there are changes in pharmacokinetics and pharmaco-dynamics that tend to increase the risk of toxicity. Multiple co-morbidities lead to multiple medications, which increase the risk of adverse drug reactions and reduce the likelihood of accurate adherence to the regimen. Medications directly lead to around 3%–12% of admissions (*see* p. 298) and may play a minor con-tributory role to many more, through a variety of mechanisms (*see* Figure 11.1). A lot of this could be prevented by avoiding known drug–drug or drug–disease interactions, prescribing at the right dose and formulation, taking steps to improve adherence, and appropriate monitoring following any changes. All frail elderly patients should have a thorough review of their medications at the time of hospital admission.

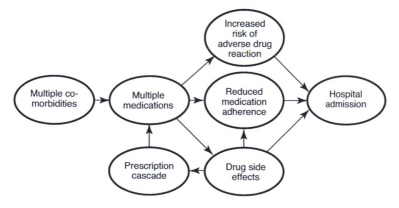

FIGURE 11.1 The complex role of medications in hospital admissions of frail elderly people

CHANGES IN PHARMACOKINETICS

Drug absorption is little affected by ageing. The main changes are seen in drug distribution, metabolism and excretion. As we age there is a change in our bodily composition (*see* p. 3), with an increased proportion of fat and less water. This causes the volume of distribution of lipophilic drugs to become increased and a reduction in that of hydrophilic ones. A larger volume of distribution tends to result in an increased half-life of the drug. An age-related increase in permeability of the blood–brain barrier can increase the risk of cognitive adverse effects of drugs. Albumin levels are not affected by normal ageing and so changes in drug protein binding are not usually significant, but low albumin states can occur in disease and precipitate toxicity of some drugs (e.g. phenytoin).

Hepatic metabolism is diminished in older age. There is a reduction in hepatic mass in the region of 20%–50% by the age of 80 years.[1] Liver blood flow and possibly enzyme activity also decline. Renal excretion is reduced. Glomerular filtration rates fall, on average, by around 10% per decade after the age of 30. The overall effect is to increase the risk of drug toxicity in the elderly.

CHANGES IN PHARMACODYNAMICS

Changes in pharmacodynamics with ageing are generally less significant than changes in pharmacokinetics, but some differences in the sensitivity of target organs to certain medications have been described. One example is the observed increased sensitivity to psychotropic medications in the frail elderly.

EVIDENCE-BASED MEDICINE

Good prescribing practices adhere to evidence-based medicine wherever possible. Unfortunately, many drug trials do not include the frail elderly. This is frequently because the researchers want a population without multiple co-morbidities or cognitive impairment (to allow accurate reporting of beneficial and adverse effects). However, the frail elderly typically have higher absolute risks of disease and so stand to gain the most from relative risk reductions.[2] Geriatricians have to make judgements on imperfect data – perhaps we could call this 'evidence-extrapolated medicine'.

POLYPHARMACY

The definition of polypharmacy can vary but is often used for patients on four or more regular medications. As older patients typically have multiple co-morbidities, they usually take multiple medications. In three studies of patients over the age of 65 (mean age, 76–79 years) presenting to the emergency department (ED) the mean number of medications used was between 3.6 and 4.2.[3–5] In a study of patients aged over 75 years presenting to an ED, 45% were on five or more medications.[6] So many come in with polypharmacy, but also patients leave hospital, on average, on more medications than when they were admitted (mean, one extra).[7] However, much of the prescribed medication may be unnecessary.[8]

PRESCRIBING FOR OLDER PEOPLE

Basic good practice in prescribing for older patients includes documentation of the indication, education of the patient, monitoring of response to treatment and for adverse effects, avoiding drugs most likely to cause side effects, and regular review (at least annually) of the ongoing need for each medication.[9] As a general rule, drugs should be given at the lowest effective dose and for the shortest possible duration of time. Care needs to be given to prescribing the optimal formulation (e.g. liquid preparations for those with impaired swallowing) and frequency of dosing (i.e. less frequent is associated with greater adherence). In those on inhaled medications it is important to consider the device and technique that they use (*see* p. 238). Judging the right amount of medications for any patient can be challenging. It involves a balance between prescribing all known beneficial treatments for their illnesses against the potential negatives of multiple drugs (i.e. difficulties with concordance, increased side effects and interactions).

When older patients present acutely to hospitals, many do not bring with them a list of medications taken, and those who do are frequently inaccurate.[10] It is vital that drug lists are checked by corroborating what the patient says they take with what their primary care team think they take. Such discrepancies are common.[11] Prescription errors (either badly written or poor choice of drug or dose) have been identified in 1.5% of inpatients, with 0.4% being judged potentially serious.[12] A study that evaluated the discharge medications of 421 patients aged over 65 (mean age, 74 years) being discharged from acute medical services, found that prescribing was suboptimal in 32% of patients.[13] Frequent problems were the prescription of inappropriate medications, inadequate monitoring, drug–drug and drug–disease interactions. Adverse events were more common in those with suboptimal prescriptions.[14]

GOALS OF THERAPY

In frail elderly patients with limited life expectancy the emphasis of importance of medications is likely to shift from disease prevention to symptom control.[15] It is appropriate to involve patients with preserved mental capacity in decisions about changes to their medications. In advanced dementia, patients lack the ability to decide about their medications and so decisions are made in their best interests. The main goal for the majority of patients with advanced dementia is palliation, yet many such patients (30%–40%) continue to receive drugs deemed inappropriate by expert consensus (e.g. statins, antiplatelets, oestrogen and cholinesterase inhibitors).[16,17]

A study of nursing home (NH) residents with advanced dementia (mean age, 85 years), of whom 55% died in an 18-month follow-up period, looked at medication use as death approached.[17] The residents took an average of 5.9 regular daily medications. The use of some medications declined (e.g. those to treat osteoporosis), but many were little changed (e.g. proton pump inhibitors, angiotensin-converting enzyme (ACE) inhibitors and lipid-lowering drugs). Antipsychotic drugs continued to be used in 20%, and cholinesterase inhibitors in 4% of patients, up to the time of death. Overall drug use tends not to decline as death approaches, but the proportion of palliative agents does increase.[18]

The time to benefit from a medication should also be considered. Some treatments take many years to show significant effects – for example, ACE inhibitors to prevent renal impairment in patients with type 2 diabetes.

ADVERSE DRUG REACTIONS

An adverse drug reaction (ADR) is a harmful or unpleasant consequence of a medicine, which necessitates the alteration of prescription or discontinuation of that agent. ADRs can be divided into different subtypes including dose-related (e.g. digoxin toxicity), non-dose-related (e.g. anaphylactic reaction to penicillin) and related to withdrawal effects (e.g. rapidly stopping long-term benzodiazepines). Elderly people are more likely to experience ADRs than younger people.[19] This is most likely due to a larger number of co-morbidities and resultant polypharmacy, which increase the risk of both drug–disease and drug–drug interactions. However, the physiological changes of ageing are also likely to be involved. As many as 32% of ADRs may to be related to impaired renal function.[20]

Around 3%–12% of hospital admissions in patients aged over 65 are because of ADRs.[3,5,21–25] This occurs more commonly in those receiving many medications. A study of frail elderly patients (mean age, 82 years; mean number of medications, 6.8) found that ADRs contributed to 14% of admissions.[20] ADRs are also associated with functional decline while in hospital, longer lengths of stay and an increased risk of death.[26,27]

More than half of drug-related hospital admissions are potentially preventable, as they are due to known drug effects (i.e. not due to idiosyncratic reactions).[3,23,28,29] Only around 50%–60% of attendances to the ED caused by ADRs are recognised as such by the attending physician.[30,31]

Many drugs are commonly blamed for precipitating ADRs (*see* Table 11.1). A recent study looking at ADRs causing older adults to be admitted to US hospitals rated 33% due to warfarin, 14% due to insulin, 13% due to antiplatelet drugs and 11% due to oral hypoglycaemics.[32] However, the ease of detecting toxicity from these drugs (e.g. high international normalised ratio, low blood sugar, digoxin level and bleeding disorders) may account for their high incidence. More subtle adverse effects, such as orthostatic hypotension from antihypertensives or delirium secondary to anticholinergics, may go unnoticed in this type of study, based on surveillance data. Other studies have found ADRs to be commonly caused by antibiotics, anticoagulants, antiplatelets, amiodarone, diuretics, calcium channel blockers, ACE inhibitors, beta-blockers, hypoglycaemics, non-steroidal anti-inflammatory drugs (NSAIDs) and digoxin.[3,5,22-24,33,34] In part, this probably reflects that these are among the most common drugs prescribed to older people. Many are still appropriate (e.g. warfarin for those with atrial fibrillation (AF)) but need more careful monitoring. However, some should be avoided (*see* p. 301).

TABLE 11.1 Drugs commonly blamed for adverse drug reactions in elderly patients[3,5,22-24,32-34]

Commonly blamed drug(s)
Warfarin
Insulin
Oral hypoglycaemics
Digoxin
Antibiotics
NSAIDs
Calcium channel blockers
Diuretics
Antiplatelets
Amiodarone
ACE inhibitors
Beta-blockers

Abbreviations: NSAID = non-steroidal anti-inflammatory drug, ACE = angiotensin-converting enzyme

Similarly, in NH populations, over 50% of ADRs are judged to be predictable and therefore preventable (commonly due to suboptimal prescribing or monitoring).[35,36] The commonest implicated agents in ADRs were antipsychotics (23%), antibiotics (typically causing rashes or *Clostridium difficile* diarrhoea) (20%), antidepressants (13%), sedatives (13%), anticoagulants (typically uncontrolled international normalised ratio values) (9%) and anti-epileptics (9%). The risk is higher in those with multiple co-morbidities and medications.[36]

Prescription cascades

Prescription cascades occur when current drug side effects are misinterpreted as new illnesses, which lead to further prescribing.[37] For example, ankle oedema secondary to a calcium channel blocker being interpreted as heart failure and a loop diuretic being commenced. This may lead to hypokalaemia and the prescription of a potassium-sparing diuretic, and so on. It is always important to consider if new symptoms could be due to a patient's medications – in which case, stopping an old agent, rather than starting a new one, is likely to be a better idea.

Drug–drug interactions

Drug–drug reactions are common among drugs with a narrow therapeutic index (e.g. digoxin, phenytoin and warfarin) or drugs affecting the cytochrome P450 isoenzymes (see Table 11.2).[38–40] Individual variation in activity exists due to genetic polymorphism. There are many other recognised interactions that potentiate drugs effects. For example, amiodarone increases digoxin levels, antiplatelets and warfarin increase bleeding risk, and ACE inhibitors and potassium-sparing diuretics can induce hyperkalaemia.

TABLE 11.2 Commonly used drugs that are either substrates, inhibitors or inducers of the P450 isoemzyme system[39,40]

Substrates	Inhibitors	Inducers
Calcium channel blockers	Cimetidine	Carbamazepine
Flecainide	Ciprofloxacin	Phenytoin
Antipsychotics	Erythromycin/clarithromycin	Rifampicin
Phenytoin	Amiodarone	Alcohol
Simvastatin	Fluconazole	Omeprazole (CYP1A2)
Theophylline	Fluoxetine/paroxetine	
Tricyclic antidepressants	Lansoprazole/omeprazole (CYP2C19)	
Warfarin	Cyclosporin	
	Grapefruit juice	

Drug–drug interactions increase in frequency according to the number of medications taken. The recent co-prescription of a medication that precipitates drug toxicity is a common cause of acute admission.[41] In a study of 1000 consecutive patients aged over 70 (mean age, 83 years) admitted to hospital with an acute illness, 89% took two or more medications (mean number of drugs was 5.1 per patient).[42] Of the 894 patients receiving two or more drugs, 538 (60%) were judged to be exposed to a potential drug–drug interaction and 130 (15%) had potentially attributable clinical presentations. Overall, 6% of admissions were judged to be directly related to a drug–drug interaction. The commonest side effects were confusion, hypotension, dehydration and electrolyte disorders. The most frequently involved drug types were cardiovascular (diuretics, ACE inhibitors, nitrates, calcium channel blockers and digoxin) and psychotropic (benzodiazepines, antipsychotics and antidepressants).

Drugs with opposing mechanisms of action

Some patients are on two or more drugs that oppose each other's actions. An example is anticholinergic and pro-cholinergic drugs (i.e. cholinesterase inhibitors). Studies have found that 11%–35% of patients on cholinesterase inhibitors concurrently receive anticholinergic medication.[43,44] This is possibly due in part to a prescription cascade – anticholinergics prescribed to treat urinary incontinence induced by cholinesterase inhibitors.[45] This combination is associated with poorer physical functioning than those on cholinesterase inhibitors alone, and may precipitate delirium.[44,46] Another example is NSAIDs (that cause fluid retention) and diuretics.

Drug–alcohol interactions

Alcohol intake may also precipitate an adverse reaction to a drug (e.g. falls with benzodiazepines). Around 20% of patients aged over 65 who are on medications that may interact with alcohol are current consumers of alcohol.[47]

Drug–disease interactions

Drug–disease interactions occur when a prescribed medication exacerbates the symptoms of a different condition. Certain diseases seem particularly susceptible, including dementia, orthostatic hypotension and constipation.[38] The prevalence of potential drug–disease interactions in a frail veteran population aged over 65 years at the time of hospital discharge was found to be 15%.[48] The commonest examples were falls and benzodiazepines or tricyclic antidepressants; peptic ulcer disease and aspirin or NSAIDs; heart failure and calcium channel blockers; diabetes and steroids; and dementia and anticholinergic drugs.

INAPPROPRIATE MEDICATIONS

Inappropriate medications are defined as those that have unacceptable side effects, are ineffective or where better alternatives are available. Their use is associated with adverse health outcomes in older adults.[49] These medications may have a role in selected situations, but in general they are unsuitable for the frail elderly.

The Beers criteria defined a list of medications that are often inappropriate in elderly patients.[50] While the list is lengthy, the key groups of medications identified are benzodiazepines, anticholinergics and NSAIDs. An alternative is the Medication Appropriateness Index, which is a numerical rating tool for individual prescribed drugs based on factors such as clear indication, evidence of efficacy and dose prescribed.[51]

Studies have found that 11%–29% of patients over the age of 65 presenting to an ED are on at least one medication judged inappropriate.[4,52,53] A number of patients then either receive an inappropriate medication in the ED or are discharged on one.[4,53–55] In addition, around 21%–32% of patients have been found to be on at least one potentially inappropriate medication at the time of hospital admission, and 10%–13% newly prescribed one or more during their stay.[27,56]

The following paragraphs in this section cover a few drugs or drug classes that are usually best avoided in the frail elderly. We recommend that patients who present to acute medical services on any of these drugs should have the ongoing need reviewed and withdrawal or change to an alternative agent considered.

Anticholinergics

Anticholinergic medications are associated with cognitive and physical dysfunction, and a higher probability of death in older adults.[57–60] They are also linked to an increased risk of delirium.[58,61] Older people seem to be more susceptible to anticholinergic side effects (*see* Table 11.3), especially when multiple drugs are used in combination. This may be because of lower levels of intracerebral acetylcholine, reduced drug elimination and/or increased permeability of the blood–brain barrier to such agents.

TABLE 11.3 The potential adverse effects of anticholinergic medications

Side effect	Possible consequence in the frail elderly
Dry mouth	Reduced swallow
	Dental decay
Pupil dilatation/loss of accommodation reflex	Blurred vision (risk of falls)
	Precipitate glaucoma (rare)
Constipation	Faecal impaction
	Pseudo-obstruction
Urinary retention	Overflow incontinence
	Catheterisation
Tachycardia	Arrhythmia
	Exacerbate heart failure or angina
Confusion	Delirium
	Reduced cognition with dementia
Orthostatic hypotension	Falls/syncope

There are a number of clinical situations where drugs with anticholinergic effects have been proposed to be beneficial, such as the treatment of overactive bladder (*see* p. 89) and Parkinson's disease (*see* p. 255). Bladder anticholinergics have been shown to have statistical benefits in reducing symptoms of urinary incontinence, but the actual size of the reduction is small, which may be of no real benefit to a patient who still has multiple episodes of incontinence and still wears pads to contain their urine, and it may not be enough to offset any side effects of treatment. It is worth asking the patient how he or she feels such drugs have affected his or her life. It may be time to try discontinuation. Drugs with a primarily anticholinergic action (e.g. orphenadrine) are not recommended for treating Parkinson's disease in the elderly.

There are also many other medications that have some degree of anticholinergic side effect (*see* Table 11.4).[61–63] In combination these drugs seem to increase the risk of harm, sometimes termed 'anticholinergic burden'. It is generally advised that medications are changed to those with the least risk of anticholinergic effect wherever possible.

Antipsychotics

Antipsychotic (also called 'neuroleptic') drugs are most commonly prescribed to the elderly to try to control agitation associated with dementia (*see* p. 119). Antipsychotics are subdivided into the older 'typical' agents (e.g. haloperidol) and the newer 'atypical' agents (e.g. risperidone, olanzapine and quetiapine). This latter group may have fewer antidopaminergic effects but more anticholinergic, serotinergic and alpha-adrenergic effects.[64] Adverse effects include drug-induced Parkinsonism (*see* p. 253), an increased risk of falls, cognitive decline, stroke and death.[65–68]

Rarely they can induce the 'neuroleptic malignant syndrome'. This is seen clinically as a combination of muscle rigidity, hyperthermia (>37.5°C), autonomic instability (e.g. tachycardia, hypertension or a fluctuating blood pressure), reduced consciousness and a raised serum creatine kinase. The mainstay of management is to stop the causative drug and ensure adequate hydration. It can potentially induce rhabdomyolysis (*see* p. 73).

Olanzapine is also associated with an increased risk of developing type 2 diabetes.[65] There is probably little overall difference in terms of safety between typical and atypical agents. Patients with dementia with Lewy bodies are particularly sensitive to antipsychotic adverse effects and should not be prescribed these drugs (*see* p. 116).

There is only limited data to suggest efficacy in agitation symptoms and this seems to be for psychosis and aggression only.[69–73] Trials typically used short time periods (around 12 weeks). These drugs have no known effect on reducing common behavioural disturbances such as wandering or shouting out. A study compared discontinuing antipsychotics with remaining on them for 165 patients (mean age, 85 years) with Alzheimer's disease who resided in care homes.[74] Behavioural scores were similar between the groups. The 12-month survival rate favoured those switched to a placebo (77% vs 70%), and after 3 years this gap had widened (59% vs 30%). It is estimated that 17%–24% of NH residents are on antipsychotic medications, but the majority (88%) are prescribed these drugs inappropriately.[75–77]

Non-steroidal anti-inflammatory drugs

NSAIDs inhibit prostaglandin synthesis. This can lead to many possible side effects, but those of particular concern in the frail elderly are:

➤ peptic ulceration (reduced gastric protection)
➤ precipitation of hypertension and/or heart failure (fluid and salt retention)
➤ renal impairment (renal vasoconstriction or interstitial nephritis) – particularly if in combination with a diuretic or ACE inhibitor/angiotensin receptor blocker.

NSAIDs are not recommended for routine pain management in the frail elderly.[78] Their use should be limited to those who are intolerant of, or whose pain is resistant to alternative means. In this situation they should be used in the lowest effective dose and for the shortest possible time period, with monitoring for adverse effects. Typically, pain should be initially managed with paracetamol and a weak opioid added (e.g. codeine or tramadol) if this is insufficient alone (*see* p. 44). Of course, opioids can cause their own side effects, including constipation, delirium and an increased risk of fractures,[79,80] but they are currently generally thought to be a safer option. Topical NSAIDs have few adverse effects and may be effective for those with osteoarthritic pain localised to a few superficial joints (e.g. hands and knees).[81]

Sedatives

Sedating drugs are associated with cognitive impairment and falls.[82,83] The use of sedative medications is associated with poorer physical and cognitive function in older adults.[57] They are also associated with increased lengths of hospital stay.[84] The most commonly prescribed sedatives are benzodiazepines, but they have few valid indications for use in the elderly. However, as many as 30% of the over-85s are on them.[82] They are sometimes prescribed to treat insomnia but have only minor beneficial effects that are frequently outweighed by harms (*see* p. 21). Chronic use appears to be associated with an increased risk of developing dementia.[85] If their use is absolutely necessary, then drugs with a shorter half-life and lower lipid solubility are probably safer (e.g. lorazepam or oxazepam).[86] A study found that around 1%–2% of elderly patients who were not previously on benzodiazepines became chronic users after discharge from hospital.[87] There are also a number of non-benzodiazepine sedating drugs available – these include zopiclone and zolpidem. It had been postulated that these drugs may be less harmful, due in part to shorter half-lives. However, a study of elderly people (mean age, 82 years) found an adjusted odds ratio of hip fracture of 1.95 (95% confidence interval, 1.09–3.51) with these medications compared with non-users, which was similar to the risk with either benzodiazepines or antipsychotics.[88]

Digoxin

The frail elderly are at an increased risk of digoxin toxicity, which can cause arrhythmias, nausea or vomiting, visual disturbances (e.g. changes in colour perception) and confusion. Factors affecting this include reduced volume of distribution, reduced renal clearance, drug interactions (e.g. amiodarone and quinine) and hypokalaemia (e.g. secondary to diuretics).[89] Digoxin does not control the rate of AF during exertion, making it an unsuitable drug for most mobile people. Nor does it control heart rate during episodes of AF in those with paroxysmal AF.[90] Its rate-limiting effect is more modest than that of most alternative agents. A randomised controlled trial that compared intravenous digoxin and placebo found that digoxin led to a small reduction in heart rate after 2 hours (105 bpm with digoxin vs 117 bpm with placebo).[91] It only has a limited role in treating AF in the frail elderly – that is, those with persisting symptomatic AF (heart rate >110 bpm), low mobility levels and unsuitable for other drugs (e.g. because of hypotension).

Digoxin has also been used in heart failure. In theory it causes an increase in intracellular calcium concentration resulting in improved cardiac muscle contraction. When compared with placebo (at a mean daily dose of 250 mcg) in patients with systolic heart failure already on standard medical therapy over a 3-year period, digoxin did not improve mortality rates, but it was associated with a significantly lower rate of hospitalisation than placebo (relative risk, 0.72; 95% confidence interval, 0.66–0.79).[92] It is unclear how relevant this benefit may be to the frail elderly, who are more prone to side effects and are unlikely to achieve such high daily doses. Its role is likely to be limited to patients with ongoing symptoms despite optimisation of other treatment options (i.e. beta-blockers and ACE inhibitors).

TABLE 11.4 Anticholinergic effects of some selected drugs commonly used in the United Kingdom – divided into those with high, medium and low risk of anticholinergic side effects

Drug type	High risk	Medium risk	Low risk
Anti-Parkinsonian	Orphenadrine Procyclidine	Amantadine	Carbidopa-levodopa Entacapone Pramipexole Selegiline
Antidepressants	Amitriptyline Imipramine	Nortriptyline	Mirtazepine Paroxetine Trazadone
Antihistamines	Chlorpheniramine Hydroxizine	Cetirizine Loratidine Cimetidine	Ranitidine
Antipsychotics	–	Olanzapine	Haloperidol Quetiapine Risperidone
Anti-emetics	–	Prochlorperazine	Metoclopramide
Bladder anticholinergics	Oxybutynin	Tolterodine	–
Others	–	Baclofen	Codeine Diazepam Digoxin Dipyridamole Furosemide Ipratropium Isosorbide Loperamide Nifedipine Prednisolone Theophylline Warfarin

Note: Data obtained from Cancelli *et al.*,[61] Rudolph *et al.*[62] and Boustani *et al.*[63]

Quinine

Nocturnal leg cramps are strong calf muscle contractions that come on at night, typically without any precipitant and lasting for a few minutes. As many as a third of people aged over 60 and half of those over 80 complain of such symptoms within the previous 2 months.[93] Although typically considered idiopathic, they can be precipitated by medications (e.g. diuretics, beta-agonists, statins and lithium) and are sometimes associated with uraemia, thyroid disease, diabetes and electrolyte disturbances (hypokalaemia, hypomagnesaemia and hypocalcaemia). First-line management strategies include looking for a reversible cause and trying stretching exercises.

The use of quinine may be considered if these measures fail in patients with frequent and severe symptoms. This drug has been found to have a modest benefit in reducing the frequency but not the severity of cramping episodes (around one less event per week than with placebo).[93] Reported side effects include potentially life-threatening thrombocytopenia and pancytopenia. In toxic levels it can cause vertigo, tinnitus, deafness, nausea/vomiting, visual disturbance and confusion. It is possible that this can occur in the frail elderly on usual therapeutic doses (200–300 mg at night). There can also be interactions with other commonly used drugs (e.g. digoxin, amiodarone, haloperidol and warfarin). For all of these reasons the role of quinine in treating leg cramps is unclear. When prescribed it is recommended that the medication be interrupted every 3 months to assess ongoing need. When patients are admitted to hospital would seem a good time to review this. It is always worth asking the patient whether he or she thinks quinine is helping the symptoms and if not, then consider withdrawal.

CONCORDANCE AND ADHERENCE

Medications are only safe and effective if taken correctly. When prescribing a medication the clinician should ensure the patient wishes and is able to take the new drug as intended. A study found that around 40% of patients discharged from the ED with at least one new medication did not adhere to their prescription.[94] The chance of taking medications consistently as prescribed reduces with increasing prescription complexity. Trials suggest that patients on once-daily medications will take those medications around 80% of the time, whereas patients on four-times-daily dosing will take only 50% of their medication as intended.[95] Other factors of relevance to the elderly include difficulty with administration (e.g. arthritis limiting the use of inhalers), cognitive impairment, depression, medications providing no symptomatic benefit (e.g. drugs for hypertension) and any side effects of the medications. Discharge from hospital on a new medication regimen can cause confusion and impair adherence. Many patients will continue to have old medicines (i.e. not currently prescribed) within their homes and these medicines may be poorly labelled.[96] Clear communication with the patient and the primary care team is essential. Discharge medications may also be provided in an unsuitable format (e.g. childproof containers).[96]

Identifying poor adherence to a medicine regimen can be challenging. A non-confrontational approach should be adopted when discussing this topic with patients, acknowledging that everyone will miss the occasional dose. Sometimes drug levels (e.g. phenytoin), physiological parameters (e.g. blood pressure) or pill counts can aid assessment. Improving concordance involves patient education on the value and rationale of their various drugs. Attempts should be made to reduce the number of medications and limit the number of times they are to be taken each day. For example, a once-daily formulation could be used in place of one taken twice daily. Medication aids may be beneficial in selected patients. These include multi-compartment and blister packs, which have individual slots for tablets to be taken in the morning, lunch, afternoon and night-time over a 1-week period. Logically, this should help adherence, but trials have not shown clear benefits.[97] Medication aids are sometimes started without adequate patient assessment and perhaps half of the patients could do as well without them.[98] Medication aids are not suitable for all drugs. Liquids or inhaled medications cannot be dispensed this way and some medications, such as bisphosphonates or levodopa, need to be taken at specific times or in specific ways. Carers can be helpful to prompt taking medications. District nurses in the community can sometimes administer drugs such as insulin.

MEDICATION REVIEW

Over time the elderly tend to accumulate multiple agents. Some of this may be due to either patient or doctor attitudes towards discontinuation.[99] However, we know that polypharmacy is associated with potential harm. The time of hospital admission is an ideal opportunity to thoroughly review a patient's medications. The supervised environment of the acute hospital allows monitoring for any adverse events due to subsequent withdrawal. Drug trials are concerned with the commencement of medications. There is little trial evidence to inform us with regard to medication discontinuation.

The clinician should work through an accurate list of the patient's current drugs and consider if each agent is still appropriate. The majority of medications can safely be withdrawn from older patients, but care is needed with certain classes (particularly some cardiovascular drugs and benzodiazepines).[100,101] The commonest adverse effects seen are exacerbations of the underlying disorder. Obvious changes that should be made are to medications that do the exact opposite of the presenting problem; for example, if dehydrated, stop diuretics; if hypotensive, stop antihypertensives; if having diarrhoea, stop laxatives; and so on. The following list is a guide to considerations when performing a medication review.

➤ Are any of the patient's medications causing or worsening the presenting problem?

➤ Are all of the medicines still required?

➤ Are there any inappropriate medications (e.g. anticholinergics, antipsychotics, NSAIDs and sedatives)?

➤ Are there any drug–drug interactions?

➤ Are there any drug–disease interactions?

➤ Do some of the medications antagonise the actions of others?

➤ Is there co-prescription of more than one drug of the same class?

➤ Is there evidence of any potential prescription cascades?

➤ Is the drug prescribed in the optimal dose, frequency and formulation?

➤ Could medication adherence be improved?

➤ Is polypharmacy a problem? Sometimes the medication burden is best limited to a small number of the most beneficial drugs.

➤ Is there inappropriate under-prescription? Are all of the co-morbidities being treated in accordance with best practice guidelines? If not are there good reasons for this, such as patient preference, unacceptable polypharmacy/side effects or life expectancy?

KEY POINTS

- All acutely unwell elderly patients should have their medications carefully reviewed.
- Changes in body composition, pharmacokinetics (mainly drug metabolism and excretion) and pharmacodynamics make the frail elderly more susceptible to adverse effects with medications.
- Multiple co-morbidities increase the risk of polypharmacy.
- Practising evidence-based medicine is often difficult in the frail elderly, as they are excluded from many drug trials.
- In patients with limited life expectancy the emphasis of medications is likely to shift from disease prevention to symptom control.
- Around 3%–12% of admissions in the elderly are related to ADRs, and this figure is probably higher for the frail.
- Look for drug–drug and drug–disease interactions among your patient's medications.
- Always consider whether your patient's symptoms could be related to an adverse effect of one of his or her medications – avoid perpetuating 'prescription cascades'.
- Anticholinergic drugs have many potential side effects in the elderly.
- There are many drugs not commonly recognised as 'anticholinergic' in mechanism of action that can increase the risk of anticholinergic-type side effects.
- It is always worth considering if your patient is taking inappropriate medications,

especially if they take any anticholinergic drugs, antipsychotics, sedatives or NSAIDs.

● Medication concordance is likely to be suboptimal in patients receiving multiple treatments. Look for ways that it could be improved – particularly education, simplification of regimens, choosing the right drug formulation and the use of devices or support from others.

REFERENCES

1. Vestal RE. Aging and pharmacology. *Cancer.* 1997; **80**(7): 1302–10.
2. Alter DA, Manuel DG, Gunraj N, *et al.* Age, risk-benefit trade-offs, and the projected effects of evidence-based therapies. *Am J Med.* 2004; **116**(8): 540–5.
3. Cunningham G, Dodd TRP, Grant DJ, *et al.* Drug-related problems in elderly patients admitted to Tayside hospitals, methods for prevention and subsequent reassessment. *Age Ageing.* 1997; **26**(5): 375–82.
4. Chin MH, Wang LC, Jin L, *et al.* Appropriateness of medication selection for older persons in an urban academic emergency department. *Acad Emerg Med.* 1999; **6**(12): 1232–42.
5. Hohl CM, Dankoff J, Colacone A, *et al.* Polypharmacy, adverse drug-related events, and potential adverse interactions in elderly patients presenting to an emergency department. *Ann Emerg Med.* 2001; **38**(6): 666–71.
6. Banerjee A, Mbamalu D, Ebrahimi S, *et al.* The prevalence of polypharmacy in elderly attenders to an emergency department: a problem with a need for an effective solution. *Int J Emerg Med.* 2011; **4**(1): 22.
7. Corsonello A, Pedone C, Corica F, *et al.* Polypharmacy in elderly patients at discharge from the acute care hospital. *Ther Clin Risk Manag.* 2007; **3**(1): 197–203.
8. Hajjar ER, Hanlon TJ, Sloane RJ, *et al.* Unnecessary drug use in frail older people at hospital discharge. *J Am Geriatr Soc.* 2005; **53**(9): 1518–23.
9. Knight EL, Avorn J. Quality indicators for appropriate medication use in vulnerable elders. *Ann Intern Med.* 2001; **135**(8 Pt. 2): 703–10.
10. Stromski C, Popavetsky G, Defranco B, *et al.* The prevalence and accuracy of medications lists in an elderly ED population. *Am J Emerg Med.* 2004; **22**(6): 497–8.
11. Frank C, Godwin M, Verma S, *et al.* What drugs are our frail elderly patients taking? *Can Fam Physician.* 2001; **47**: 1198–204.
12. Dean B, Schachter M, Vincent C, *et al.* Prescribing errors in hospital inpatients: their incidence and clinical significance. *Qual Saf Health Care.* 2002; **11**(4): 340–4.
13. Hastings SN, Sloane RJ, Goldberg KC, *et al.* The quality of pharmacotherapy in older veterans discharged from the Emergency Department or Urgent Care Clinic. *J Am Geriatr Soc.* 2007; **55**(9): 1339–48.
14. Hastings SN, Schmader KE, Sloane RJ, *et al.* Quality of pharmacotherapy and outcomes for older veterans discharged from the Emergency Department. *J Am Geriatr Soc.* 2008; **56**(5): 875–80.
15. Holmes HM. Rational prescribing for patients with a reduced life expectancy. *Clin Pharmacol Ther.* 2009; **85**(1): 103–7.
16. Holmes HM, Sachs GA, Shega JW, *et al.* Integrating palliative medicine into the care of persons with advanced dementia: identifying appropriate medication use. *J Am Geriatr Soc.* 2008; **56**(7): 1306–11.

17. Tjia J, Rothman MR, Kiely DK, *et al*. Daily medication use in nursing home residents with advanced dementia. *J Am Geriatr Soc*. 2010; **58**(5): 880–8.
18. Blass DM, Black BS, Phillips H, *et al*. Medication use in nursing home residents with advanced dementia. *Int J Geriatr Psychiatry*. 2008; **23**(5): 490–6.
19. Beyth RJ, Shorr RI. Epidemiology of adverse drug reactions in the elderly by drug class. *Drugs Aging*. 1999; **14**(3): 231–9.
20. Hellden A, Bergman U, von Euler M, *et al*. Adverse drug reactions and impaired renal function in elderly patients admitted to the emergency department: a retrospective study. *Drugs Aging*. 2009; **26**(7): 595–606.
21. Mannesse CK, Derkx FHM, de Ridder MAJ, *et al*. Contribution of adverse drug reactions to hospital admission of older patients. *Age Ageing*. 2000; **29**(1): 35–9.
22. Passarelli MCG, Jacob-Filho W, Figueras A. Adverse drug reactions in an elderly hospitalised population: inappropriate prescription is a leading cause. *Drugs Aging*. 2005; **22**(9): 767–77.
23. Franceschi M, Scarcelli C, Niro V, *et al*. Prevalence, clinical features and avoidability of adverse drug reactions as a cause of admission to a geriatric unit. *Drug Safety*. 2008; **31**(6): 545–56.
24. Cei M, Bartolomei C, Mumoli N. In-hospital mortality and morbidity of elderly medical patients can be predicted at admission by the Modified Early Warning Score: a prospective study. *Int J Clin Pract*. 2009; **63**(4): 591–5.
25. Olivier P, Bertrand L, Tubery M, *et al*. Hospitalizations because of adverse drug reactions in elderly patients admitted through the emergency department: a prospective survey. *Drugs Aging*. 2009; **26**(6): 475–82.
26. Classen DC, Pestotnik SL, Evans S, *et al*. Adverse drug events in hospitalized patients: excess length of stay, extra costs, and attributable mortality. *JAMA*. 1997; **277**(4): 301–6.
27. Corsonello A, Pedone C, Lattanzio F, *et al*. Potentially inappropriate medications and functional decline in elderly hospitalized patients. *J Am Geriatr Soc*. 2009; **57**(6): 1007–14.
28. Winterstein AG, Sauer BC, Helper CD, *et al*. Preventable drug-related hospital admissions. *Ann Pharmacother*. 2002; **36**(7–8): 1238–48.
29. Zed PJ, Abu-Laban RB, Balen RM, *et al*. Incidence, severity and preventability of medication-related visits to the emergency department: a prospective study. *CMAJ*. 2008; **178**(12): 1563–9.
30. Hohl CM, Robitaille C, Lord V, *et al*. Emergency physician recognition of adverse drug-related events in elder patients presenting to an emergency department. *Acad Emerg Med*. 2005; **12**(3): 197–205.
31. Hohl CM, Zed PJ, Brubacher JR, *et al*. Do emergency physicians attribute drug-related emergency department visits to medication-related problems? *Ann Emerg Med*. 2010; **55**(6): 493–502.
32. Budnitz DS, Lovegrove MC, Shehab N, *et al*. Emergency hospitalizations for adverse drug events in older Americans. *N Engl J Med*. 2011; **365**(21): 2002–12.
33. Wiffen P, Gill M, Edwards J, *et al*. Adverse drug reactions in hospital patients: a systematic review of the prospective and retrospective studies. *Bandolier*. 2002; June: 1–15.
34. Budnitz DS, Shehab N, Kegler SR, *et al*. Medication use leading to emergency department visits for adverse drug events in older adults. *Ann Intern Med*. 2007; **147**(11): 755–65.
35. Gurwitz JH, Field TS, Avorn J, *et al*. Incidence and preventability of adverse drug events in nursing homes. *Am J Med*. 2000; **109**(2): 87–94.
36. Field TS, Gurwitz JH, Avorn J, *et al*. Risk factors for adverse drug events among nursing home residents. *Arch Intern Med*. 2001; **161**(13): 1629–34.

37. Rochon PA, Gurwitz JH. Optimising drug treatment for elderly people: the prescribing cascade. *BMJ*. 1997; **315**(7115): 1096–9.

38. Mallet L, Spinewine A, Huang A. The challenge of managing drug interactions in elderly people. *Lancet*. 2007; **370**(9582): 185–91.

39. Goshman L, Fish J, Roller K. Clinically significant cytochrome P450 drug interactions. *J Pharm Soc Wisconsin*. 1999; May/June: 23–38.

40. Sikka R, Magauran B, Ulrich A, *et al*. Pharmacogenomics, adverse drug interactions and the cytochrome P450 system. *Acad Emerg Med*. 2005; **12**(12): 1227–35.

41. Juurlink DN, Mamdani M, Kopp A, *et al*. Drug-drug interactions among elderly patients hospitalized for drug toxicity. *JAMA*. 2003; **289**(13): 1652–8.

42. Doucet J, Chassagne P, Trivalle C, *et al*. Drug-drug interactions related to hospital admissions in older adults: a prospective study of 1000 patients. *J Am Geriatr Soc*. 1996; **44**(8): 944–8.

43. Carnahan RM, Lund BC, Perry PJ, *et al*. The concurrent use of anticholinergics and cholinesterase inhibitors: rare event or common practice? *J Am Geriatr Soc*. 2004; **52**(12): 2082–7.

44. Sink KM, Thomas J, Xu H, *et al*. Dual use of bladder anticholinergics and cholinesterase inhibitors: long-term functional and cognitive outcomes. *J Am Geriatr Soc*. 2008; **56**(5): 847–53.

45. Gill SS, Mamdani M, Naglie G, *et al*. A prescribing cascade involving cholinesterase inhibitors and anticholinergic drugs. *Arch Intern Med*. 2005; **165**(7): 808–13.

46. Edwards KR, O'Connor JT. Risk of delirium with concomitant use of tolterodine and acetylcholinesterase inhibitors. *J Am Geriatr Soc*. 2002; **50**(6): 1165–6.

47. Pringle KE, Ahern FM, Heller DA, *et al*. Potential for alcohol and prescription drug interactions in older people. *J Am Geriatr Soc*. 2005; **53**(11): 1930–6.

48. Lindblad CI, Hanlon JT, Gross CR, *et al*. Clinically important drug-disease interactions and their prevalence in older adults. *Clin Ther*. 2006; **28**(8): 1133–43.

49. Lund BC, Carnahan RM, Egge JA, *et al*. Inappropriate prescribing predicts adverse drug events in older adults. *Ann Pharmacother*. 2010; **44**(6): 957–63.

50. Fick DM, Cooper JW, Wade WE, *et al*. Updating the Beers criteria for potentially inappropriate medication use in older adults: results of a US consensus panel of experts. *Arch Intern Med*. 2003; **163**(22): 2716–24.

51. Hanlon JT, Schmader KE, Samsa GP, *et al*. A method for assessing drug therapy appropriateness. *J Clin Epidemiol*. 1992; **45**(10): 1045–51.

52. Carter MW, Gupta S. Characteristics and outcomes of injury-related ED visits among older adults. *Am J Emerg Med*. 2008; **26**(3): 296–303.

53. Nixdorff N, Hustey FM, Brady AK, *et al*. Potentially inappropriate medications and adverse drug effects in elders in the ED. *Am J Emerg Med*. 2008; **26**(6): 697–700.

54. Caterino JM, Emond JA, Camargo CA. Inappropriate medication administration to the acutely ill elderly: a nationwide emergency department study, 1992–2000. *J Am Geriatr Soc*. 2004; **52**(11): 1847–55.

55. Meurer WJ, Potti TA, Kerber KA, *et al*. Potentially inappropriate medication utilization in the emergency department visits by older adults: analysis from a nationally representative sample. *Acad Emeg Med*. 2010; **17**(3): 231–7.

56. Hustey FM, Wallis N, Miller J. Inappropraite prescribing in an older ED population. *Am J Emerg Med*. 2007; **25**(7): 804–7.

57. Hilmer SN, Mager DE, Simonsick EM, *et al*. A drug burden index to define the functional burden of medications in older people. *Arch Intern Med*. 2007; **167**(8): 781–7.

58. Campbell N, Boustani M, Limbil T, *et al*. The cognitive impact of anticholinergics: a clinical review. *Clin Interv Aging*. 2009; **4**: 225–33.

59. Carriere I, Fourrier-Reglat A, Dartigues J, *et al*. Drugs with anticholinergic properties, cognitive decline, and dementia in an elderly general population: the 3-City Study. *Arch Intern Med*. 2009; **169**(14): 1317–24.

60. Fox C, Richardson K, Maidment ID, *et al*. Anticholinergic medication use and cognitive impairment in the older population: the Medical Research Council Cognitive Function and Ageing Study. *J Am Geriatr Soc*. 2011; **59**(8): 1477–83.

61. Cancelli I, Beltrame M, Gigli GL, *et al*. Drugs with anticholinergic properties: cognitive and neuropsychiatric side-effects in elderly patients. *Neurol Sci*. 2009; **30**(2): 87–92.

62. Rudolph JL, Salow MJ, Angelini MC, *et al*. The Anticholinergic Risk Scale and anticholinergic adverse effects in older persons. *Arch Intern Med*. 2008; **168**(5): 508–13.

63. Boustani MA, Campbell NL, Munger S, *et al*. Impact of anticholinergics on the aging brain: a review and practical application. *Aging Health*. 2008; **4**(3): 311–20.

64. Neil W, Curran S, Wattis J. Antipsychotic prescribing in older people. *Age Ageing*. 2003; **32**(5): 475–83.

65. Wirshing DA. Adverse effects of atypical antipsychotics. *J Clin Psychiatry*. 2001; **62**(Suppl. 21): 7–10.

66. Hien LTT, Cummings RG, Cameron ID, *et al*. Atypical antipsychotic medications and risk of falls in residents of aged care facilities. *J Am Geriatr Soc*. 2005; **53**(8): 1290–5.

67. Schneider LS, Dagerman KS, Insel P. Risk of death with atypical antipsychotic drug treatment for dementia: meta-analysis of randomized placebo-controlled trials. *JAMA*. 2005; **294**(15): 1934–43.

68. Ellul J, Archer N, Foy CML, *et al*. The effects of commonly prescribed drugs in patients with Alzheimer's disease on the rate of deterioration. *J Neurol Neurosurg Psychiatry*. 2007; **78**(3): 233–9.

69. Schneider LS, Pollock VE, Lyness SA. A metaanalysis of controlled trials of neuroleptic treatment in dementia. *J Am Geriatr Soc*. 1990; **38**(5): 553–63.

70. Lonergan E, Luxenberg J, Colford J. Haloperidol for agitation in dementia. Cochrane Database Syst Rev. London: NICE. 2002; 2: CD002852.

71. Brodaty H, Ames D, Snowdon J, *et al*. A randomized placebo-controlled trial of risperidone for the treatment of aggression, agitation and psychosis of dementia. *J Clin Psychiatry*. 2003; **64**(2): 134–43.

72. Lee PE, Gill SS, Freedman M, *et al*. Atypical antipsychotic drugs in the treatment of behavioural and psychological symptoms of dementia: systematic review. *BMJ*. 2004; **329**(7457): 75–8.

73. Schneider LS, Tariot PN, Dagerman KS, *et al*. Effectiveness of atypical antipsychotic drugs in patients with Alzheimer's disease. *N Engl J Med*. 2006; **355**(15): 1525–38.

74. Ballard C, Hanney ML, Theodoulou M, *et al*. The dementia antipsychotic withdrawal trial (DART-AD): long-term follow-up of a randomised placebo-controlled trial. *Lancet Neurol*. 2009; **8**(2): 151–7.

75. McGrath AM, Jackson GA. Survey of neuroleptic prescribing in residents of nursing homes in Glasgow. *BMJ*. 1996; **312**(7031): 611–12.

76. Gurwitz JH, Field TS, Avorn J, *et al*. Incidence and preventability of adverse drug events in nursing homes. *Am J Med*. 2000; **109**(2): 87–94.

77. Bronskill SE, Anderson GM, Sykora K, *et al*. Neuroleptic drug therapy in older adults newly admitted to nursing homes: incidence, dose, and specialist contact. *J Am Geriatr Soc*. 2004; **52**(5): 749–55.

78. American Geriatrics Society Panel on Pharmacological Management of Persistent Pain in Older Persons. Pharmacological management of persistent pain in older persons. *J Am Geriatr Soc.* 2009; **57**(8): 1331–46.

79. Solomon DH, Rassen JA, Glynn RJ, *et al.* The comparative safety of analgesics in older adults with arthritis. *Arch Intern Med.* 2010; **170**(22): 1968–76.

80. Miller M, Sturmer T, Azrael D, *et al.* Opioid analgesics and the risk of fractures in older adults with arthritis. *J Am Geriatr Soc.* 2011; **59**(3): 430–8.

81. Barkin RL, Beckerman M, Blum SL, *et al.* Should nonsteroidal anti-inflammatory drugs (NSAIDs) be prescribed to the older adult? *Drugs Aging.* 2010; **27**(10): 775–89.

82. Vinkers DJ, Gussekloo J, van der Mast RC, *et al.* Benzodiazepine use and risk of mortality in individuals aged 85 years or older. *JAMA.* 2003; **290**(22): 2942–3.

83. Glass J, Lanctot KL, Herrmann N, *et al.* Sedative hypnotics in older people with insomnia: meta-analysis of risks and benefits. *BMJ.* 2005; **331**(7526): 1169–73.

84. Zisselman MH, Rovner BW, Yuen EJ, *et al.* Sedative-hypnotic use and increased hospital stay and costs in older people. *J Am Geriatr Soc.* 1996; **44**(11): 1371–4.

85. Billioti de Gage S, Begaud B, Bazin F, *et al.* Benzodiazepine use and the risk of dementia: population based study. *BMJ.* 2012; **345**: 14.

86. Chutka DS, Takahashi PY, Hoel RW. Inappropriate medications for elderly patients. *Mayo Clin Proc.* 2004; **79**(1): 122–39.

87. Bell CM, Fischer HD, Gill SS, *et al.* Initiation of benzodiazepines in the elderly after hospitalization. *J Gen Intern Med.* 2007; **22**(7): 1024–9.

88. Wang PS, Bohn RL, Glynn RJ, *et al.* Zolpidem use and hip fractures in older people. *J Am Geriatr Soc.* 2001; **49**(12): 1685–90.

89. Wofford JL, Ettinger WH. Risk factors and manifestations of digoxin toxicity in the elderly. *Am J Emerg Med.* 1991; **9**(2 Suppl. 1): 11–5.

90. Robles de Medina EO, Algra A. Digoxin in the treatment of paroxysmal atrial fibrillation. *Lancet.* 1999; **354**(9182): 882–3.

91. Digitalis in Acute Atrial Fibrillation (DAAF) Trial Group. Intravenous digoxin in acute atrial fibrillation: results of a randomized, placebo-controlled multicentre trial of 239 patients. *Eur Heart J.* 1997; **18**(4): 649–54.

92. Digitalis Investigation Group. The effect of digoxin on mortality and morbidity in patients with heart failure. *N Engl J Med.* 1997; **336**(8): 525–33.

93. Butler JV, Mulkerrin EC, O'Keeffe ST. Nocturnal leg cramps in older people. *Postgrad Med J.* 2002; **78**(924): 596–8.

94. Hohl CM, Abu-Laban RB, Brubacher JR, *et al.* Adherence to emergency department discharge prescriptions. *CJEM.* 2009; **11**(2): 131–8.

95. Osterberg L, Blaschkle T. Adherence to medication. *N Engl J Med.* 2005; **353**(5): 487–97.

96. Burns JMA, Sneddon I, Lovell M, *et al.* Elderly patients and their medication: a postdischarge follow-up study. *Age Ageing.* 1992; **21**(3): 178–81.

97. Huang H, Maguire MG, Miller ER, *et al.* Impact of pill organizers and blister packs on adherence to pill taking in two vitamin supplementation trials. *Am J Epidemiol.* 2000; **152**(8): 780–7.

98. Raynor DK, Nunney JM. Medicine compliance aids are a partial solution, not panacea. *BMJ.* 2002; **324**(7349): 1338.

99. Bain KT, Holmes HM, Beers MH, *et al.* Discontinuing medications: a novel approach for revising the prescribing stage of the medication-use process. *J Am Geriatr Soc.* 2008; **56**(10): 1946–52.

100. Graves T, Hanlon JT, Schmader KE, *et al.* Adverse events after discontinuing medications in elderly outpatients. *Arch Intern Med.* 1997; **157**(19): 2205–10.

101. Garfinkel D, Mangin D. Feasibility study of a systematic approach for discontinuation of multiple medications in older adults. *Arch Intern Med.* 2010; **170**(18): 1648–54.

Index

Note: page numbers in **bold** refer to tables; page numbers in *italics* refer to figures.

CPD with Radcliffe

You can now use a selection of our books to achieve CPD (Continuing Professional Development) points through directed reading.

We provide a free online form and downloadable certificate for your appraisal portfolio. Look for the CPD logo and register with us at: www.radcliffehealth.com/cpd

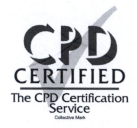